Natural Solutions for Food Allergies and Food Intolerances

Scientifically Proven Remedies for Food Sensitivities

By Case Adams, Ph.D.

Natural Solutions for Food Allergies and Food Intolerances:
    Proven Remedies for Food Sensitivities
Copyright © 2012 Case Adams
LOGICAL BOOKS
Wilmington, Delaware
http://www.logicalbooks.org
All rights reserved.
Printed in USA
Front cover image © Janice Hazeldine
Back cover image © Dianka

Publishers Cataloging in Publication Data
Adams, Case
Natural Solutions for Food Allergies and Food Intolerances:
    Scientifically Proven Remedies for Food Sensitivities
First Edition

1. Medicine. 2. Health.
Bibliography and References; Index

Library of Congress Control Number: 2010943109

ISBN-13 paperback: 978-1-936251-16-2

ISBN-13 ebook: 978-1-936251-17-9

For those who will not give up on Mother Nature

Table of Contents

Introduction: Digging Deeper

Food sensitivities are growing amongst the world's modern societies. They are increasing in prevalence, and multiple allergies and sensitivities are also increasing. What is causing this?

Knowing the cause of something is very important. We must understand what is causing food sensitivities in order to push back their increasing incidence.

While this is an important question, this is not the most important question for those currently suffering from a food sensitivity. For most people, the most important concern is or should be: *How can I get rid of my food sensitivity?*

While modern science has done a good job over the past couple of decades to study the prevalence of food sensitivities, modern medicine has not done such a good job in understanding the cause of food sensitivities, nor done a good job of figuring out how to alleviate food sensitivities. This is especially true amongst the medical and scientific community in North America.

Why? This text does not attempt to answer this question. Nor does this text assume anything regarding the motives of North American researchers and their funding sources. The only comment we can make is that research funding is a complicated and convoluted process, and research on non-patentable remedies does not typically attract investment.

The purpose of this book is to scientifically dig deeper than most of our Western conventional medical institutions, physicians and websites have been digging. To dig deeper, we use the very same tools that other researchers use to prove hypotheses. We present double-blind, placebo-controlled clinical research. We present clinical experience. We present laboratory testing. We also present the clinical application of traditional medicines upon millions of people, some for thousands of years.

And like any discovery using the scientific method, we are making logical conclusions based upon a plethora of scientific research and clinical evidence.

While the thesis may seem radical, in fact the findings of this text are supported by the piecing together of solid, corroborated scientific evidence provided by esteemed and peer-reviewed colleagues and medical institutions around the world.

The conclusions of this text might be compared to a stereogram. A stereogram presents an obvious general image at first. However, inside that obvious image is another image that is not so obvious. This second image requires a deeper look. It requires a more thoughtful and focused look at the image. We give an example of a stereogram on page 4.

The purpose of this text is not to be irresponsible. There are no broad-brush assumptions using anecdotal information. Furthermore,

1

there are no reckless panaceas being presented. This text is presenting research data and clinical documentation with meticulous analyses. None of this will replace the diagnosis and personal consultation from a health professional. But it just might offer some new information and clarity on potential strategies.

The overall purpose here is to *move along the discussion* from a very narrow bandwidth of food avoidance to one that objectively explores the evidence for scientifically sound therapies to reverse food sensitivities. This conversation is required if our medical institutions are truly dedicated to improving health: something we might loosely call *wellness*.

Consider this analogy: What if your friend was stuck in a ditch of quicksand, and you had a number of tools available to you. You had the standard tools, which included a shovel, a pitchfork and a short rope. But you also had access to several less conventional tools, such as a long bamboo stick and a couple of large stones to stand upon. What if the shovel, pitchfork and rope were all too short to reach your friend, who was quickly descending into the depths of the sand? And what if the unconventional bamboo pole was not only long enough to reach your friend, but also had a series of ridges on the outside that enabled your friend to grip onto the pole and shimmy up and out of the mud? Would you deny using the pole just because the pole was an unconventional tool? Would you worry about what your peers would say if you told them you used an unconventional tool to pull your friend out?

Medical practitioners must be armed with a tool called *knowledge* in order to help their patients. Patients too must be armed with the tool called knowledge—at least regarding their symptoms—when considering a visit with their practitioners. It is this tool of knowledge that provides responsible action from both sides.

So where does knowledge come from? Knowledge comes from scientific investigation and conclusion vetted with wisdom. Today, scientific investigation is being pursued around the world with great intensity and wisdom. Are researchers and physicians from non-western countries not as wise or scientific as Western researchers? Are these scientists not as intelligent or as educated as North American researchers? We might point out that today students of many countries around the world test ahead of North American students in math and sciences.

What would the rationale be for any arrogance on the part of Western medical institutions with regard to helping people with food allergies and intolerances given the research presented in this text?

The author has drawn from over a thousand research papers, including hundreds of controlled, randomized and double-blind clinical studies;

along with numerous case histories and historical practices of traditional medicines to compile the information presented in this text.

Furthermore, much of the research presented here has come from medical schools, prestigious universities, hospitals and/or government agencies from around the world. These present a variety of clear and proven strategies that have been successful in promoting tolerance and resolving food sensitivities.

In addition, over forty appropriate medicinal herbs and numerous botanicals are presented together with their research. This includes clinical documentation by numerous credentialed traditional doctors, naturopaths, herbalists and physicians from around the world. As the reader will find, these herbs come with medicinal benefits that produce increased tolerance and strengthen the immune system.

Unfortunately, with the amount of information being provided here, we did not have the luxury of space to add a lot of fluff and eye candy. Rather, we included, as Joe Friday from the old TV series "Dragnet" put it: *"Just the facts..."*

This does not mean that we didn't make the information easy to understand. Rather, we boiled down the data to provide a 'straight-talk' stance on each subject. This allows maximum readability and comprehension for both the health professional and the layperson—even in the face of some very technical information.

Incidentally, a couple of conventions should be noted: The use of the word "milk" without the word "breast" or otherwise before it refers to cow's milk. Similarly, "eggs" denotes hen's eggs. Furthermore, the phrase "food sensitivities" is used to describe the possibility of food allergies, food intolerances or both.

We should also note that this book may not be for those who are not comfortable with change. The information presented here is scientifically solid and substantiated, but it requires a commitment towards acquiring new information and accepting new perspectives. It requires accepting new paradigms regarding food sensitivities, and the immune system in general. It is probably not for those who are afraid of change, nor afraid to make changes.

Stereogram: Can you see the teapot inside the image?

Chapter One

Food Sensitivity Facts and Fiction

For some people, food is an absolute joy. For others, it is a nightmare. Let's consider a few nightmarish situations:

Molly

Molly is active. She is a mother of three children, two of which are under three years old. Her younger child, Raymond, is a spunky infant of two months, while Martha is two years old. The trio is rounded out by Rusty, who is five years old.

Molly stays at home to focus on the children. Her day seems to revolve around food. Her mornings are spent breastfeeding Raymond, and making breakfast for herself, her husband Tom, Rusty and Martha. She's up first in the mornings, cooking breakfast. By mid-morning, another snack is needed, and breast feedings surround each.

Raymond seems perpetually hungry, and she must feed him at least every three or four hours during the day, and at night on a rolling schedule. So Molly is a good eater. She will eat a large breakfast, a mid-morning snack, lunch, a mid-afternoon snack and then dinner. As she breast feeds and puts Raymond to sleep, she is hungry again. This is followed by fixing another meal or snack.

There is one glaring problem: Molly, and her two oldest children are all allergic to milk. This means they cannot eat butter, cheese, milk chocolate, ice cream, cottage cheese and a plethora of other foods that contain milk proteins.

This of course sets up a major challenge for Molly, especially since her husband Tom loves milk, cheese and all the other dairy foods. Tom was brought up on a farm with cows, and the entire family drank fresh whole milk from the family dairy. They also ate fresh cheese, yogurt and many other milk foods. So Tom loves to have dairy with just about every meal. He will often want cheese toppings on many of his meals, and wants a glass of milk with each meal.

This of course complicates things for Molly when it comes to making and eating meals. All milk-containing foods must be kept away from the kids and Molly, for fear of anaphylaxis.

Anaphylaxis may sound like a foreign and even technical word for some, but not in Molly and Tom's family.

Molly had her first bout with anaphylaxis 25 years ago, when she was three. She was sitting in a breakfast diner with her folks, and after they both left the table for a few minutes, Molly snuck a drink of their glass of milk. She had been told not to drink milk before, but this time, well, it just looked so good. It was so white and creamy, with a little head of foam at the top and edge of the glass. She felt compelled.

With one gulp she was rolling on the floor gasping for breath. She felt as if someone had jammed a broomstick down her throat. She couldn't breathe in or out. She felt the world closing around her and couldn't even call out for help.

She awoke hours later in the hospital, with her Mom and Dad sitting on each edge of her bed, staring inquisitively at her. They smiled as she awoke, and began to stroke her hair and thank God for her revival. Molly did not remember, of course, the emergency treatment that ensued after the diner episode. She had been taken to the hospital in an ambulance, where paramedics moved quickly to insert a breathing stoma (also called a tracheotomy) into her throat to allow her to breathe. If they hadn't, she wouldn't be around today.

While her parents had seen her get colicky and run a temperature after drinking milk, they had yet to see anything like this. They were shocked that a simple glass of milk could have taken their Molly away from them.

For the next 25 years, Molly had to be careful. She was very strict about her allergy. This meant that every label had to be carefully read, and every menu item had to be specifically questioned. This also meant that Molly didn't eat a lot of foods that many of us take for granted: Cereal with milk, toast with butter, and grilled cheese sandwiches were all sacrificed over the years.

Her milk allergy had serious effects on Molly's childhood. She was shunned by many kids in the school lunch room. She was considered a freak when her friends would go to the fast food joint for some post-football game fast food. When she went on a date it was embarrassing to ask the waitress to ask the chef for a list of the ingredients of menu items.

As a result, Molly didn't have a lot of friends in school. She tended to be a loner. Most of her classmates didn't understand, and worse, she thought, they didn't care. While she was an active youngster, she wallowed in her dairy-free foods, and became overweight in high school. This made friends even more scarce.

Molly had her music, though. She took up piano when she was eight, and could get lost in the works of the great composers. They understood her, she thought. They could relate.

Eventually, she took up the cello, and excelled in the cello. She would practice for several hours a day, and it didn't bother her that her friends were shying away from her, because she had her music.

Molly's cello playing eventually helped her earn a partial scholarship to a local university. This is where she met Tom.

"What are you eating?" said the young man disgustingly, as he sat down across from her at the long table in the main cafeteria of the university.

"Tofu," she said, embarrassingly.

"So that's what tofu looks like," blurted Tom. *"I was wondering what kind of food came in cubes like that."*

"Your food doesn't look much better," she teased. *"It looks like hog food."*

Tom wasn't taken aback at all. He had found a girl that wasn't afraid to say how she felt. Molly was just his type.

By the time both of them were university seniors they made it official. Molly's diet sure contrasted with Tom's, but they made it work. Sometimes Tom and Molly would share the same meal, but most of the time they didn't. They made accommodations. Cooking for two was really cooking for two to Molly. She became expert at having a stovetop full of pans, cooking multiple entrees.

Luckily, Tom worked during the day and Molly stayed at home. This meant that only two meals were multiplied. Molly also felt secretly lucky that both of her kids were also allergic to dairy. At this point, Tom was the only exception at the dinner table.

This also simplified shopping, and gave Molly a little better leverage when it came to deciding where to eat or what to buy at the store.

There had only been three anaphylactic events so far in Tom and Molly's house. Because Molly took courses on dealing with anaphylaxis, she handled all three situations quite easily.

The first occurred when Rusty, at age two, grabbed a milk carton out of the lower shelf of the fridge. (Not where milk is left now. Now Tom has a second fridge in the garage, which is padlocked.) Rusty shoved the neck of the carton into his mouth, and began to gulp as he had many times with a bottle of formula.

When Molly heard the choking, she immediately knew what happened. She took little Rusty to the bathroom, gave him a shot of epinephrine, stuck her finger down his throat, and made him vomit the milk contents into the toilet. Molly was relieved when Rusty belted out a loud cry, along with some gasps for air. Rusty calmed down immediately afterward.

Rusty had another event a year later, after he snuck a bit of cheese from Tom's plate. This time he began to sneeze and cough, and his eyes watered up. The cough and watery eyes lasted about an hour, and then subsided. Molly didn't force-vomit Rusty this time. She just gave him a shot of epinephrine, sat with him and gave him plenty of water to drink.

Martha's episode was a bit more traumatic. The four were at a theatre watching a Disney film, when Martha snuck a slurp of Tom's milkshake. She went into convulsions and had to be force-vomited by Molly in the ladies room. They missed the movie but were glad they also didn't ride away in an ambulance. Martha's breathing had stopped momentarily as she gasped for air in the theatre, but Molly's reaction to open her airway by arching her back and holding her neck slightly back and jaw slightly forward freed up some breathing passage for her throat. She also had a epinephrine kit in her purse, and used that.

Today Molly is careful with her kids, and Tom has slowed his love for dairy in exchange for less nervousness. Whenever he pours a glass of milk or a bowl of cereal now, the hackles go up. Molly watches the kids like a hawk, while Tom sheepishly slurps his milk.

Larry

Larry is 32 years old and married with two kids. They are now six and two. Larry works hard every day in the business of selling software, so he works from a home office most of the time, and travels to see clients.

Larry has had a skin problem for as long as he could remember. His skin breaks out in flaking, eczema-like skin rashes. He cannot figure out how to stop it either. He's tried numerous lotions, supplements, medications and alternative therapies. Nothing seems to work.

Every doctor he's visited so far has diagnosed him with psoriasis, and has given him corticosteroids to keep the inflammation down. The only problem is that the corticosteroids work for awhile, but then he has to increase the dose to get the same relief. Larry has become pretty frustrated.

Both of Larry's children have multiple food allergies. His six year old girl Wanda is allergic to tree nuts, peanuts, soy and milk. His seven year old boy, Bobby, is allergic to shellfish and peanuts, but loves dairy. Larry's wife MaryAnn has occasional asthma, which acts up after eating dairy and other animal foods.

Today Larry is walking out of an allergy specialist's office, after being given a food challenge for three foods. Last week, Larry had skin prick tests that showed high levels of sensitivity to three different foods: peanuts, soy and shellfish.

The food challenge has revealed that Larry is allergic to only one of these foods: shellfish. When the doctor challenged him with shellfish, he began to break out in hives.

This was particularly tough for Larry to hear, because he lives in Louisiana, where shellfish meals are frequent. As Larry walks back to his car from the office, he begins putting it all together. He plays back in his mind the many times that he broke out in the afternoon after a lunchtime meal of shellfish with his work buddies or clients. He also remembers breaking out on his way home from a lobster or crab dinner at one of the local restaurants.

Larry worked as a teenager on a crabbing boat during the summers. He loved going out to sea and pulling up the many traps that they had laid out the previous week. After the catch, however, Larry did not relish the evenings at the crab packing shed, as he and his shipmates brought the catch in and got it into cold storage for grading, packing and shipping out the next day.

Sometimes he would have to work in the packing shed sorting and packing the crab boxes. The smell would get to him after a few hours, especially the smell of crabs being cracked on the floor as the forklift passed by.

As Larry remembers those days, he flashes that his rashes began during the summer he graduated from high school. That summer, Larry worked sometimes seven days a week to save money for college. He also worked overtime when he could get it. It didn't matter whether it was on the boat or in the packing shed: Larry was intent on working as much as he could that summer. Sick or not, Larry always came into work.

It was late in the summer, in August, that Larry remembered suddenly breaking out in hives. He had a fever that day. He had worked a double shift in the packing house, and his clothes, hair and every part of his skin reeked with crab. His skin began to crawl during his second shift break, after eating a plate of steamed crabs. He didn't think much of it—perhaps he was just tired.

From that day on, Larry's rashes and peeling, sore skin would break out every couple of days it seemed. He would have a bad episode, and after a day or so, the redness and rash would seem to scab up and go away, replaced by dry, flaky skin. Then it seemed just as he was feeling better, he would have another attack of a fresh rash.

For 15 years, no one—none of his doctors, wife or anyone else for that matter—thought or suggested that Larry's skin issue could be related to food sensitivities. That is, until he was talking with his kids' new allergy doctor who asked Larry if he'd ever been tested for food allergies for his skin condition.

Needless to say, meals are now a bit nerve-racking for Larry, Mary-Ann and their kids. As if preparing three meals is not enough, everyone is on pins and needles while eating. Everyone is watching each other like hawks for any allergic reaction.

Going out to eat for Larry, MaryAnn and their family will now be nearly impossible. Even before Larry found out about his allergy, they had only been out to eat once in the past two years. And even that was a catastrophe. Even though everyone was careful to not order anything on the allergy list, Bobby's desert, which was not supposed to contain any dairy or nuts—had some cream mixed into the topping. That set Bobby into an anaphylactic seizure. Suddenly, they were dealing with a medical emergency right there in the restaurant. Bobby's throat seized up and had to be taken to the hospital. MaryAnn didn't bring any epinephrine. Luckily the paramedics had some on hand.

Meals at school are even more nightmarish for Bobby and Wanda. While everyone is aware of the children's allergies, the multiple allergies make eating very difficult. As a result, MaryAnn makes lunch for Bobby and Wanda every day.

Bobby and Wanda don't have many friends. Luckily they are only one year apart so they can hang out together and keep each other company during school functions. Even so, the other kids like to tease them. Some will feign choking, while others like to offer them foods they are allergic to.

The teasing doesn't bother them as much as the school nurse does. The school nurse will call each of them into her office about once a week to check on them. The appointment is announced to the whole school over the loudspeaker system. This is embarrassing to Bobby and Wanda.

Needless to say, both Bobby and Wanda want to lead normal lives. They are disgusted with the attention they get and the ignorance they face from other kids taunting them. They simply wish that more people understood food sensitivities and could possibly relate to what Bobby and Wanda go through.

It is a bit hard to ignore, however, because Bobby and Wanda both do not take their allergies seriously. While their parents are very strict and disciplined, they are not. They will frequently eat foods that are labeled as "might contain" some of their allergens. They also might eat something from the cafeteria or from a restaurant that they know might contain dairy or nuts.

As a result, sometimes they come down with allergic symptoms, and sometimes they will get anaphylaxis. Occasionally, they have had emergency room visits, because they rarely, even though often reminded by their mom, carry epinephrine with them.

Nowadays, MaryAnn is making lunches at home to help control what her kids eat at school. But this still has a short leash as the kids like to share food—especially snack food. Twice, her kids have ended up in the hospital after allergic attacks from hidden ingredients given at school.

MaryAnn's culinary life has not been so pretty either. She has a career and a full-time job on top of her home-making duties. The career has not been easy to navigate when it comes to eating either. Luncheons, company barbeques and traveling have been difficult to say the least. More like walking on eggshells. Four times in the past five years she has accidentally eaten some nuts, and succumbed to a seizure and breaking out in hives. These occasions were not pretty.

The funny thing is that MaryAnn did not remember having any allergies to tree nuts as a child. She remembers eating plenty of nuts as a child. She loved nuts in fact. Her allergies and asthma only seem to have taken hold over the past ten years.

Food is a nightmare for MaryAnn, Tom and their family. MaryAnn dreads every meal. She often worries that she'll walk away from the table for a few minutes, only to return to a table with one of her children dead.

What's Missing?

What is missing in the lives of these families? We see two families struggling with their food sensitivities. They are making considerable sacrifices, both emotionally and physically, on behalf of their conditions. Both families now carry epinephrine for emergencies. Both read labels very carefully and inquire about ingredients when they go out to eat.

Furthermore, both families have seen medical professionals and allergy specialists, and have a clear diagnosis regarding their condition and food sensitivities. They completely understand the process of avoiding certain foods and how to treat an emergency situation if one of them accidentally eats one of the foods they are allergic to. They have also read many books and websites on food sensitivities.

What is missing is any activity that might turn things around for them. There is no activity related to any change. They have all accepted their lots and they are simply living with them.

Yes, they have certainly made adjustments. They are avoiding all sorts of foods; and in order to do so, they are being creative in their recipes. They now have many tools for avoiding those foods they are sensitive to. But is this the answer to the problem?

What kind of questions will this text answer? First we will hopefully reveal to those with food allergies and food intolerances what most likely caused their conditions—from the physiological and socio-economic perspective. Secondly, we will carefully review the science on strategies that have been clinically employed around the world with success. We will also put this together with the mechanisms of how the immune system develops tolerance. In other words, we will fill in the missing elements.

First, let's cover the basics. Let's discuss the what, how, who and where of food sensitivities—which includes both food allergies and food intolerances. Let's get the facts straight.

What are Food Allergies?

Food allergies are reactions of the immune system to molecules of food—called allergens. An allergen is a portion of a food molecule that the immune system considers foreign to the body. In other words, the immune system is threatened by part of the food. Once an allergen is marked as a threat, it will be remembered as such for some time.

Once the immune system considers any molecule a threat, it stimulates a process to remove that substance from the body. Normally this is a quite docile and automatic process that happens without our perception. However, if the immune system is weakened, imbalanced and otherwise overactive, the response can be out of proportion with what would ordinarily be required to remove such a molecule from the body.

As we will discuss in more detail later, most food allergy reactions occur using a part of the immune system called immunoglobulin E, or IgE. Ordinarily, foreign molecules are removed using immunoglobulin A (IgA), which line our mucous membranes. By using IgA, the immune system can remove foreigners before they can gain access to the body's tissues.

In an IgE or other non-IgA immune response, the foreign molecules have penetrated further into the body than they would have normally. This makes them a potential threat. Once the molecules come into contact with the IgEs, the IgEs will stimulate the release of inflammatory mediators such as histamine, prostaglandins and leukotrienes. These will produce allergic reactions around the body such as rashes, wheezing, sinusitis, watery eyes and so on (see the list of symptoms on pages 24-25).

What are Food Intolerances?

Food intolerances often seem like allergies. This is because the body is also reacting to what it considers a foreign molecule. The difference is that the body simply does not know how to handle the foreigner, so it produces physiological symptoms related to its inability to handle the food.

People typically confuse food intolerances with food allergies because they consider any sort of negative physiological response to food as an allergic reaction.

An intolerance is usually the result of the body not managing or digesting a food properly. If the food is not properly managed by the body's digestive system, the food can disrupt the body in a variety of ways. This may include digestive discomfort, headaches, fever, and a host of other symptoms, which can all feel like allergic reactions. But here the food molecule is not being targeted specifically by the immune-inflammatory system. The body is simply reacting negatively to a food molecule that it cannot properly manage.

One might wonder what is the big difference. In both occurrences, the body is reacting to a foreign molecule or group of molecules. And yes, there is a lot of similarity between the two reactions sometimes. But inherent in the word "allergy" is the existence of a particular "allergen." This allergen, according to the scientific meaning, is being identified as a threat to the body. This allergen or epitope of a molecule, produces *a specific type of reaction* when it binds with immune factors. A food intolerance occurs outside of this binding system.

Also, food intolerances do not typically cause anaphylaxis. Anaphylaxis is a sometimes life-threatening reaction that requires an urgent medical response to prevent death. It is for this reason that medicine has focused more attention upon food allergies.

Because of this increased focus upon food allergies, many confuse their food intolerances with food allergies. As a result, there are far fewer food allergies than is apparent. For example, in one Italian study (Asero *et al.* 2009) of 25,601 allergy clinic patients throughout Italy, only 1,079 (8.5%) of the clinic patients were found to have IgE-mediated clinical allergic reactions.

In a food intolerance, there is a imbalance between the food's makeup and the ability of the body to process and metabolize the food. In some cases, this means that the food contains proteins, sugars or other nutrients that the digestive tract cannot properly break down. In other cases, the food may contain some constituent that the body reacts negatively to. In these cases, the food constituent may be given access to the walls of the intestine or stomach and specifically irritate those cells. Or the constituent may gain access to the bloodstream, where the liver or other metabolic process in the body may have to work to remove it.

Nearly any food can cause intolerance, but foods that often cause intolerances include dairy, soy, wheat and gluten-containing grains, nuts, seeds, particularly acidic foods such as vinegar or orange juice, and a variety of processed foods. Nightshade foods such as tomatoes, eggplants, potatoes and peppers have sometimes causing intolerances. Normally healthy glycoalkaloids such as solanine can irritate intestinal cells in an already-damaged intestinal tract (Shimoi *et al.* 2007). In a healthy person, glycoalkaloids are antioxidants that help prevent cancer (Lu, *et al.* 2010).

Again, the research has shown that people tend to self-diagnose themselves as allergic to a food when it may be a case of food intolerance. To this confusion we can add mild food poisoning cases, which can result in years of intolerance to a certain food. We can also add foods that accompanied psychological stress sometime in the past. These foods can cause years of intolerance. Sensitivity to food preservatives, processing aids and other chemical additives are also a type of food intolerance.

Credible research, including Woods *et al.* (1998) and Pereira *et al.* (2005), have suggested that actual food allergies are a quarter of the levels perceived by many in the media and population. The remainder are likely food intolerances.

Illustrating this, in a study done by researchers from France's Allergology University Hospital (Morisset *et al.* 2005), 4,737 people who consulted with allergy experts were tested for sensitivities to peanuts. The researchers found that somewhere between 1% and 2.5% of the French population has sensitivity to peanuts, while only 0.3% to 0.75% have peanut allergies. This also may be a consideration to examine for the proposed rates of peanut allergies in the U.S., U.K. and Canada.

In another example, researchers from Turkey's Karadeniz Technical University (Orhan *et al.* 2009) found in a study of 3,500 6-9-year-olds that food allergies reported by the children's parents among from urban area schoolchildren were 5.7% of the total population. However, using the (gold standard) double-blind, placebo-controlled food challenge method, only .8% of the children actually had clinical allergies.

Nearly every food can produce food intolerances, however.

Here we will be using the word *sensitivity* to cover both food intolerance and food allergies. In either case, because the body is reacting to the food, the body and/or the person has become sensitive to it.

Who Gets Food Sensitivities?

The latest analyses show that food allergies affect from 5-8% of children and 3-4% of adults within the United States, and are increasing in incidence. Food sensitivities appear to affect about 12% of the general population in developed countries. (Railey and Burks 2010, Wang 2010, Pons *et al.* 2005, Woods *et al.* 2001, Sicherer and Sampson 2010).

This rate is consistent with most other developed nations, although adult rates in the U.S. appear higher than most other countries. Research data from developed countries around the world have indicated that food allergies occur in 3-8% of children under six years of age, and about 2-3% of adults (Cingi *et al.* 2010, Moneret-Vautrin and Morisset 2005, Rodríguez-Ortiz *et al.* 2010).

Britain may be the exception, however. British researchers (Walker and Wing 2010) estimate that 25% of Britain's population suffers from one kind of food sensitivity or another.

Most of the above references concur that among undeveloped countries, allergies are much less prevalent. Furthermore, in countries such as South Africa, where there is a significant difference between those living in cities and those living in the countryside, those in the urban areas have significantly higher rates of food sensitivities (Hooper *et al.* 2008).

It appears that this is related to diet and environment. Studies in Italy (Cataldo *et al.* 2006) on rates of food allergies among immigrants from developing counties indicate that the immigrant allergy rates become similar to developed country rates following their immigration.

Confirming this, researchers from Sweden's University (Böttcher *et al.* 2006) tested 30 Estonian and 76 Swedish infants and found that the environment during the first two years of life predicated an increased risk of food sensitivities.

Among developed countries, those with more sunlight exposure appear to have less food allergies. In a large-scale international study, 17,280 adults between the ages of 20 and 44 from different countries were studied by researchers from Australia's Monash Medical School (Woods *et al.* 2001). Natives of Northern European countries such as Scandinavia or Germany, had higher levels of food sensitivities when compared with Southern European countries such as Spain and Italy. In other words, countries closer to the equator had lower food sensitivity rates.

This geographical relationship has also been seen among food sensitivities and urgent care treatments throughout the U.S. For reasons we will discuss more in depth later, those living in Southern states had lower incidence of food sensitivities and far fewer hospital room visits for food sensitivity reactions (Rudders *et al.* 2010).

French researchers (Rancé *et al.* 2003) found that a child's first allergic reaction becomes evident at about two years old. This depends, of course, on the type of food allergy. It is also recognized that atopic dermatitis allergies and food sensitivities occur more frequently among infants and younger children. Hay fever, or allergic rhinitis and allergic asthma tend to develop throughout adolescence among children.

University hospital researchers from Northern Mexico (Rodríguez-Ortiz *et al.* 2010) studied 60 patients with food allergies during 2007 and 2008. Fifty-one percent of them were under five years old.

Also, most children with food allergies tend to outgrow them. In a study by the Food Allergy Research Program of London, the food allergy rate was 5.5% in children before the age of one. This was reduced to only

2.5% of six-year-olds with food allergies. Furthermore, only 2.3% of the 11- and 15-year-olds had food allergies (Venter *et al.* 2006; Pereira *et al.* 2005).

We might also point out that more food sensitivities seem to occur among females. In the Italian study of 25,601 allergy patients mentioned earlier, 64% of the patients were women.

Food Sensitivities are Rising Worldwide

Many researchers agree that allergies are increasing globally. Others have questioned whether the increase may be related to an increase in diagnosis, or an increase of allergy awareness.

The research clearly supports increasing incidence, however; especially among developed countries.

For example, researchers from New York's Mount Sinai School of Medicine (Sicherer *et al.* 2010) exhaustively studied cases of peanut, tree nut, and sesame allergies in 2008, 2002 and 1997. They found that among 5,300 households and 13,534 subjects, 1.4% reported peanut allergy, tree nut allergy or both in 1997. In 2002, the rate was 1.2%. Peanut and tree nut allergies in children (less than 18 years old) was 2.1% in 2008, compared with 1.2% in 2002, and 0.6% in 1997. Tree nut allergy alone increased from 0.5% in 2002 and 0.2% in 1997, to 1.1% in 2008.

Many government agencies, such as the United Kingdom's Department of Health, have announced that—based on recent statistics—food sensitivities were increasing (Waring and Levy 2010).

For example, food allergy hospital admissions increased five times in the fifteen years between 1990 and 2005 in Britain (Gupta *et al.* 2006). Increased awareness could not be the only culprit for this sort of increase.

British and American researchers (Venter *et al.* 2010) studied peanut allergy prevalence among children born on the Isle of Wight, UK between 1989 and 2002. The records were reviewed at three or four years old, and a total of 4,345 subjects were studied. They found that children born in 1989 had the lowest incidence, at 1.3%. Those born between 1994 and 1996 had the greatest incidence, at 3%. Those born between 2001 and 2002 had 2% incidence. Clinical diagnosis also grew in the same way, from .5% to 1.4% to 1.2%. However, we should mention that the last group was only surveyed at the age of three years old, a full year younger than the first group and much of the second group. As other studies have shown, many peanut allergies tend to develop between three and five years of age. So it is likely that if four year olds had been included in the third group, the rates may have continued to increase linearly from the second group.

Scientists from Poland's Military Institute of Health Sciences (Bant and Kruszewski 2008) found that among the 41% of people living in towns and cities in Poland, IgE sensitivities to atopic allergens increased 52% in the 16 years from 1986 to 2002. This means that on the average, allergen sensitization increased at a rate of about 3.25% per year.

Australian researchers (Poulos *et al.* 2007) studied the prevalence of critical allergic reactions such as anaphylaxis, angioedema, and urticaria, resulting in hospitalization among developed countries. They analyzed data for three periods—1993-1994, 2004-2005 and 1997-2004. During the three periods, hospital admissions for angioedema (swelling of mucous membranes and submucosal tissues) have increased an average of 3% per year. Allergic urticaria (skin rashes) has increased an average of 5.7% per year. More significantly, hospitalizations for the sometimes-lethal anaphylaxis allergic response increased a whopping 8.8% per year. Increases in anaphylaxis hospitalization were highest among children under five years old.

A number of other studies from a variety of international agencies and universities have reported significant increases in food sensitivities around the world, particularly among Western societies and developed countries. Increases in hospital admissions and emergency room treatments have also increased among these countries (Gillman and Douglass 2010).

While studies report increasing rates of food sensitivities among industrialized countries, children and young adults are not the only victims of increasing food sensitivities. A phenomenon called *immunosenescence* occurs among the aging when the immune system must adjust to new or even repetitive environmental or dietary inputs. For this reason, as we'll discuss more later, the rates of adult food sensitivities among industrialized societies have been increasing as well.

What Foods are People Most Sensitive To?

While more than 170 foods can cause IgE-reactions, food sensitivities around the world reflect the prominent diets of those countries. Among the developed Western countries, for example, dairy consumption is quite high. As would be expected, most research illustrates that milk is the most prevalent food allergen in the United States and Britain. This is followed by eggs, peanuts and walnuts (del Giudice *et al.* 2010).

Hugh Sampson, M.D., a pediatric immunologist and researcher with nearly thirty years of experience with food allergies, points out that about 2.5% of U.S. children under the age of three have allergies to cow's milk, while 1.5% have allergies to eggs, and 0.8% have allergies to peanuts.

Other foods, he states, affect far fewer children and tend to develop later (Charles 2008).

University of Helsinki researchers (Salmi *et al.* 2010) found that cow's milk allergy (CMA) is the most common form of food allergy, affecting 2.5% of children in Finland. We should also note that Finland also enjoys the highest consumption of milk products compared to the rest of the world.

In the Mexican University hospital study mentioned earlier (Rodríguez-Ortiz *et al.* 2010), most had allergies to dairy products, eggs, seafoods, beans, soy, chili, mango, cacao and/or strawberry. Dairy, eggs and fish allergies caused the most allergies in this study.

Researchers from Turkey's Karadeniz Technical University (Orhan *et al.* 2009) found that among 3,500 6-9 year olds from urban areas, 32% were sensitive to beef, 18% to cow's milk, 18% to cocoa, 14% to eggs and 14% to kiwi (14%) were the most prevalent allergies. Other allergens reported with lower levels included soy, wheat, peanuts, fish, and hazelnuts.

In the Asero Italian study mentioned earlier, pollen-related food allergies were the highest, with 55% of all food allergies in Italy. The majority (72%) of those were from fruits and vegetables. Of those with Type I allergies, 96% lived in Southern Italy, where most of Italy's urban populations (such as Rome) are located.

Peanuts are a very popular food among developed Western countries. As a result, approximately .6% to 1.5% of the population in the United States, Britain and Canada are allergic to peanuts (Morisset *et al.* 2005, Boyce *et al.* 2010). Using the food allergy rates of 6-8% for children and 3-4% of adults, this means that peanut allergies make up somewhere in the neighborhood of 10-20% of all food allergies in these countries.

As would be expected, due to the varied diet of Western countries, there are many other foods that people are becoming increasingly allergic to.

Researchers from the McGill University Health Center in Montreal, Quebec (Ben-Shoshan *et al.* 2010) surveyed 10,596 households in 2008 and 2009—with 3,613 household responses covering 9,667 people. Of those surveyed, they found an increased prevalence of food-allergies and an increased occurrence of peanut, tree nut, fish, shellfish, and sesame allergies and anaphylaxis over the one year period. Shellfish allergies made up 1.6%; tree nut allergies were 1.2%; peanut allergies were 1%; fish allergies were 0.5%; and sesame allergies were 0.10%. This means that seafood presented the largest allergy levels, at 2.1% among Canadians. Not surprisingly, Canadians are big seafood consumers.

We should also add that people who contract food sensitivities often have multi-food sensitivities.

Fruit and vegetable allergies, for example, are typically related to pollen sensitization or latex allergy (Moneret-Vautrin and Morisset 2005). These typically occur among adults.

In a review of 934 worldwide studies by researchers from London's King's College (Rona *et al.* 2007), food sensitivity rates were reported to be anywhere from 1.2% to 17% for cow's milk; 0.2% to 7% for eggs; up to 2% for peanuts; up to 2% for fish; and up to 10% for shellfish.

In a study of specific IgE allergens among primary school children in Taipei, Taiwan, hospital researchers (Wan *et al.* 2010) found different allergens than those found among Western countries. A total of 142 primary city schools and 25,094 students 7-8 years old were screened by survey, and then tested with the IgE Pharmacia CAP system. 1,500 students (6%) had confirmed allergic sensitivities (including food). Of these 1,500, 88% had crab allergies. 23% had milk allergies, 24% had egg white allergies, and 22% had shrimp allergies. Other sensitivities among these same children were also apparent. These included various species of dust mites, including *Dermatophagoides pteronyssinus*, *D. farinae* and *Blomia tropicalis*. Allergies to dust mites ranged from 85% to 91% among the food allergenic children. Other concurrent allergies among food-allergenic children included dog dander, cat dander and cockroach allergies. Once again, the rates were higher among more industrialized areas.

Discrepencies still exist in this data, however. Danish researchers (Zuidmeer *et al.* 2008) found that among 36 studies of more than 250,000 children and adults, few used the gold standard of food challenge. Those that did showed only 0.1% to 4.3% allergies for fruits or tree nuts; only 0.1% to 1.4% for vegetables; and less than 1% for wheat, soy, and sesame. Meanwhile, IgE testing for wheat ranged as high as 3.6% and 2.9% for soy. This range of discrepancy simply indicates that food intolerance is thoroughly being mixed in with food allergy rates, and that IgE testing tends to report higher allergy rates than do food challenges.

What are the Symptoms?

Food sensitivities can cause a variety of symptoms, which can include any part of the body, including the skin, digestive system, cardiovascular system, respiratory system, nervous system and even urinary and reproductive systems. They can also cause anaphylaxis and heart conditions.

The most common allergic symptoms are hives, itching, redness, sinusitis, congestion, wheezing, inflammation and puffiness of the skin. Itchy lips or mouth is often the initial reaction in an allergy. After that, the cheeks may become swollen and red. The arms may become covered with hives and rash. The legs may become itchy and inflamed.

Skin reactions are seen as one of the highest-occurring symptoms of food sensitivities. In the Italian study mentioned earlier (Asero), nearly 50% (12,739) of the entire group had skin reactions.

Rodríguez-Ortiz et al. (2010) reported that 58% of the Mexican food allergy population had symptoms related to skin rash and hives. Digestive and respiratory symptoms followed in prominence. Coexistant conditions included urticarial angioedema (in 38%), allergic rhinitis (in 20%), atopic dermatitis (in 15%), and asthma (in 6.6%).

French researchers (Rancé et al. 2003) found that 56% of allergy patients allergic to nuts suffer from skin symptoms. A quarter had respiratory issues and 17% had digestion issues.

Respiratory symptoms will include lung congestion, breathing passage congestion, sinus congestion and in general, difficulty breathing. This may seem like asthma, a cold, hay fever or even being choked or gagged. The latter occurs when the wind pipe becomes swollen and the breathing passageways narrow. This typically occurs with anaphylaxis.

Digestive responses include irritable bowels, GERD, constipation, diarrhea, bloating, flatulence, ulcer and others. Many of these tend to be the result of food intolerances, but they can also be the result of allergies.

Allergic rhinitis is another frequent symptom of food sensitivities. Here we see watery eyes, runny nose, sneezing, stuffy nose, scratchy throat or any combination thereof. Rhinitis is frequent among peanut, shrimp and milk allergies.

The chart below summarizes a number of studies that have documented symptoms of both food types of sensitivities:

Survey of Food Sensitivity Symptoms

Symptom	Food Allergy	Intolerance
Hives	Often	Rarely
Airway constriction	Often	Rarely
Asthma	Often	Rarely
Wheezing	Often	Rarely
Itching	Often	Rarely
Drop in blood pressure	Often	Rarely
Shock	Sometimes	Rarely
Weak pulse	Sometimes	Rarely
Rapid pulse	Sometimes	Sometimes
Dizziness	Sometimes	Sometimes
Watery eyes	Often	Sometimes
Runny nose	Often	Sometimes

Skin rash	Often	Sometimes
Skin eruptions	Sometimes	Sometimes
Swollen tongue	Sometimes	Rarely
Irritable bowels	Rarely	Often
Abdominal cramping	Often	Often
Vomiting	Often	Often
Diarrhea	Often	Often
Nausea	Often	Often
Fainting	Sometimes	Rarely
Itchy mouth	Often	Rarely
Lightheadedness	Sometimes	Sometimes
Drooling	Sometimes	Rarely
Inability to swallow	Sometimes	Rarely
Change in voice quality	Sometimes	Rarely
Redness	Often	Sometimes
Fever or warmth (flushing)	Often	Sometimes
Gastritis	Rarely	Sometimes
Diarrhea	Sometimes	Often
Ulcers	Rarely	Sometimes
Bladder infections	Rarely	Sometimes
Ear infections	Sometimes	Sometimes
Joint pain	Rarely	Sometimes
Low back pain	Rarely	Sometimes
Migraine	Rarely	Sometimes
Headaches (non-migraine)	Sometimes	Sometimes
Sinusitis	Often	Often
Itchy Throat	Often	Rarely
Sore Throat	Sometimes	Often
Constipation	Rarely	Sometimes
Irritable bowels	Rarely	Often
Panic attacks	Sometimes	Sometimes
Chronic fatigue	Rarely	Sometimes
Anxiety	Sometimes	Sometimes
Depression	Rarely	Sometimes

Hives are the most frequent response to IgE-mediated food hypersensitivity according to research from Italy (del Giudice *et al.* 2010).

Rhinitis (watery eyes, sinusitis and so on) due to food allergies typically does not usually occur alone. Rather, it will likely occur with other symptoms, including eczema, asthma, urticaria, oral cavity ruptures, and various gastrointestinal problems.

What is Atopy?

Atopy is used frequently among doctors and scientists to describe food sensitivity symptoms. What is atopy anyway? Atopy is derived from the Greek word meaning *"unusual"* or *"not ordinary."* Atopic is used to describe the condition where a person is reacting to an substance in a way that is unrelated to the contact with the substance.

For example, a normal response to breathing in some dust is to sneeze. This response is normal, and will act to remove the dust. But if suddenly, rashes break out all over the body, even on the legs, then the reaction was more than a normal physiological response. It is an extraordinary response that has engaged mechanisms outside of the realm and proportion of the exposure. In the case of most allergies, the body engages antibodies such as immunoglobulin E, or IgE. This engagement with IgE produces what is called a *mediated response.* Again this response is outside of the ordinary IgA response that expels the foreigner before it penetrates the body's tissue systems. Once within the tissues, the allergen interacts with IgE, and the body will produce inflammatory mediators such as histamine, prostaglandins and leukotrienes. These stimulate a number of atopic symptoms.

If a person has atopic allergies, they will usually have hives, rashes, itchiness and respiratory issues. Atopic reactions are typically related to the mucosal membranes. These are expressed as asthma, allergic rhinitis, conjunctiva rhinitis, and even eosinophilic esophagitis. Some digestive symptoms are considered atopic, but here the response must be considered out of proportion with a typical response to a foreigner—such as indigestion, a little diarrhea or constipation or a slight stomach ache. In other words, an intense period of abdominal cramping immediately after eating might be considered atopic, while a temporary queasy feeling after eating a dinner of fried foods would be considered a normal reaction to a meal with an imbalance of fatty acids.

Eczema or dermatitis of the skin is considered atopic when the substance is not being consumed through the skin. While they can appear anywhere on the skin, atopic skin rashes will often occur at the hands, elbows or knees. These areas can feel itchy and can be very uncomfortable in an atopic condition. Over a few days of an outbreak, they can become scaly and crusted. These lesions can also worsen with by the use of chemical soaps or certain types of clothing.

On the other hand, a skin reaction to a chemical lotion we just spread onto the skin would not be considered an atopic condition. This could be considered quite normal in the case of many chemical lotions on the market today.

Diseases Related to Food Sensitivities

Food sensitivities have been associated with a number of disorders. The list can be very long, depending upon who you talk to. Some alternative practitioners associate food allergies with an extremely long list of diseases. This, however, comes with little scientific evidence.

This does not necessarily mean that sensitivities are isolated from other conditions. To the contrary, a number of conditions have been associated with food sensitivities—especially those related to the gastrointestinal system and inflammatory conditions.

For example, in a study by Polish researchers (Grzybowska-Chlebowczyk 2009), 95 children between two to 18 years old with various disease diagnoses were given IgE immunity tests for food allergies. Food allergies were found among a third of children with urticaria (skin conditions). Food allergies were also found among 21% of Crohn's disease patients.

Here is a list of common disorders that have been clinically linked to food sensitivities:

➢ Rheumatoid arthritis
➢ Colitis
➢ Irritable bowel syndrome
➢ Sinusitis
➢ Asthma
➢ Crohn's disease
➢ Migraines
➢ COPD
➢ Constipation
➢ Ulcers
➢ Urinary disorders
➢ Cardiovascular disease
➢ Mental conditions
➢ Immunosuppression

Yes, we could have extended this list quite a bit if we believed everything we heard from some of our colleagues. However, this would become speculative. Speculation in the topic of health can be misleading and even dangerous. The author chooses to remain within the realm of scientific evidence.

In some cases, the association with the conditions listed above is considered causative. In others, it may be the other way around. In fact, many of these conditions are classified as autoimmune diseases. As a matter of association then, food sensitivities might be, and often are considered autoimmune. This is supported by the fact that autoimmunity is defined as a condition where the immune system or physiology begins to attack its own cells. In the case of the food sensitivity, the body is responding to the consumption of food molecules that should otherwise provide nutrition to the body—and thus become part of the body's cells and tissues.

What is Anaphylaxis?

An anaphylactic response is considered a severe response to an allergen. Practically any symptom of a food allergy can become anaphylactic—or life-threatening. This can range from a skin response, a gastrointestinal response, a cardiovascular event, or most commonly, a respiratory event. In the latter, the throat can constrict and reduce the ability to breathe.

In the 12 years between 1993 and 2005, there were 17.3 million emergency room visits for acute allergic reactions in the United States. These represented 1.3% of all emergency room visits (Rudders *et al.* 2010). In other words, about 13 out of every 1,000 emergency room visits are for anaphylaxis.

The Food Allergy and Anaphylaxis Network (FAAN) has established through randomized phone surveys that approximately 12 million Americans—about 4% of the U.S. population—have severe allergic reactions to either peanuts, tree nuts such as cashews or pistachios, or seafood. This indicates that about two-thirds of these people are self-managing their severe allergic responses at home or without frequent urgent care responses. Many allergy sufferers or their parents carry an epinephrine injection kit, for example.

Allergy specialists report that there are generally three different types of anaphylaxis responses:

1) *Uniphasic*—a onetime rush of symptoms.
2) *Biphasic*—an initial reactive rush of symptoms, followed by another reaction later, sometimes several hours later.
3) *Protracted*—an ongoing rush of symptoms that do not abate for several hours. This is somewhat rare, but it does sometimes occur in extreme anaphylaxis.

People with food allergies and asthma have a higher risk of anaphylaxis than people who suffer from food allergies without asthma (González-Pérez *et al.* 2010). About half the deaths from anaphylaxis come from allergic responses to tree nuts or peanuts.

Researchers from California's Kaiser Permanente (Iribarren *et al.* 2010) found that the incidence of anaphylactic shock among allergic responses occurred in about 109 person-years out of 100,000 person-years, primarily when food allergies were associated with asthma. From a patient population of 526,406 cases over ten years, about one-fifth of anaphylactic shock cases (20 per 100,000 person-years) occurred in cases of asthma without food allergies. In other words, asthma sufferers with food allergies are five times more likely to experience anaphylactic shock than those with asthma alone. Other population studies have found food anaphylaxis occurs between one and 70 of every 100,000 people (Boyce *et al.* 2010).

A collaborative multicenter study from the researchers from the Massachusetts General Hospital in Boston (Clark *et al.* 2004) accumulated data on emergency room visits for food allergy complications. These visits included airway obstruction (anaphylaxis), rashes and other acute care situations. They found that 55% of the ER visits were life-threatening. Urgent care food allergy suffers had an average age of 29 years old. Emergency room visits were about 57% female. About 40% of the allergy sufferers were Caucasian.

Among the allergens that provoked the urgent care, 21% of the visits involved nut allergies, 19% were caused by eating shellfish, 12% were cause by fruit, and 10% were caused by fish.

Doctors gave 72% of the patients antihistamines. Forty-eight percent were given corticosteroids. Sixteen percent were given epinephrine. In addition, 33% were given respiratory treatments such as albuterol (inhalant). Among those with severe reactions, only 24% were given epinephrine. In all, 16% of patients were given self-injectable epinephrine to use. Twelve percent were further referred to an allergist.

It is also important to note that research has shown that anaphylaxis from food allergies has been fatal in about 1% of severe anaphylaxis cases (Moneret-Vautrin and Morisset 2005). If we consider how rare severe anaphylaxis is among the general population, we can see how rare death is. Still it does happen and those who suffer from anaphylaxis should remember this.

Most food anaphylactic deaths have co-existent asthma. Most occur among adolescents and young adults (Gillman and Douglass 2010).

Researchers have found that factors that increase the risk of severe allergic anaphylaxis include agents that tend to cause increased intestinal permeability. These include aspirin, beta-blockers, angiotensin-converting enzyme (ACE) inhibitors, and alcohol (Moneret-Vautrin and Morisset 2005). We'll discuss this topic in more depth later.

How do I Know if I Have a Food Sensitivity?

As far as allergies go, as mentioned earlier, many studies have shown that only a small percentage of those who believe they have food allergies actually have food allergies. This is especially true for parents. Many more parents believe their child has a food allergy than do. Manchester hospital researchers (Nicolaou *et al.* 2010) studied 933 children, 110 with reactions to peanuts. They found that of these 110, only 24% were found to be clinically allergic to peanuts.

Furthermore, in a study from Dutch researchers (Hospers *et al.* 2006), out of 43 children diagnosed with food allergies by a physician, only 68% were confirmed as having an allergy using double-blind challenge testing.

So what is the best way to determine whether we have a food allergy? The first thing is to consider our symptoms and their severity. See the chart earlier in this chapter. Do one or more of these rated "Often" or "Sometimes" take place within a half hour of eating? Or are the symptoms less severe and occur several hours after eating? The former, according to the research, will more likely be a food allergy, while the latter will more likely be a food intolerance.

Most of the science on diagnostic tests has focused primarily upon IgE-related food allergies, as these are most likely to cause life-threatening anaphylaxis. We should remember that there are other types of food sensitivities, such as eosinophilic gastrointestinal diseases and food protein-induced enterocolitis. Outside of these, there are a variety of sensitivities to different constituents of foods.

Regardless, we should consider getting tested to at least screen out the possibility of an IgE allergy. There are several diagnostic tests now in use:

Immunoassays

Blood may be drawn and submitted to what some refer to as a *radioallergosorbent test* (or RAST). This is more accurately called the *immunoassay for allergen-specific IgE*, however. This test will measure the content of allergen-specific immunoglobulin Es in the bloodstream.

When we say allergen-specific IgEs, know that an IgE responsive to wheat protein will not be the same as an IgE that is responsive to milk proteins. This means that the immunoassay may determine whether an food allergy exists, and if so, what the allergen might be.

A well-respected immunoassay test for accuracy is the CAP-RAST test. Because CAP-RAST immunoassay tests determine the level of an allergen-specific IgE in the blood, they are considered more accurate. Typically the test comes with a level on a 1-to-100 scale, with 100 being the highest level and one being the lowest. A score of 75 will typically produce an allergy diagnosis. On the other hand, a level that is, say, 10 or 15, might be problematic to diagnose. At this level, there may be tolerance to a food that was previously considered an allergen to the body.

Indeed, one of the problems of immunoassay testing is the fact that different people have different levels of tolerance at the same IgE levels. The immunoassay test also does little to indicate the severity or type of allergic reaction a person might have. A person, for example, might have a high immunoassay IgE number but have a strong immune system that manages the response quite well. On the other hand, an immunosuppressed person with a lower IgE level might have severe reactions to the food.

On the other hand, one of the benefits of obtaining such a clear number is that from successive tests, a person can find out whether their sensitivity is dropping or increasing with time. A higher number can indicate increasing sensitivity, while a lowering number can indicate increased tolerance. This can be truly helpful with some of the strategies we'll discuss later on.

Skin Prick Tests

In skin prick testing (often referred to as SPT), a small amount of a food that the allergist thinks we are sensitive to is inserted underneath the top layer of skin by a pricking of the skin. The skin is then monitored for response. If the skin responds with a *weal* (a small circular mark or welt), this indicates the existence of a sensitivity to that food.

There are typically three methods used to apply this skin prick test. A skin prick instrument may be soaked in the food before the skin is pricked with it. The diagnostician may also place a drop of the food onto the skin before pricking the skin underneath the drop with a needle or probe.

The diagnostician may also inject the allergen underneath the skin with a needle. This is rarely employed for food allergies.

Once the prick is done, it usually takes about 10-15 minutes for the weal to come up. It will often look like a small pimple. It is the histamine response that makes this happen. A salt water prick test is often deployed to test for skin sensitivity to the pricking alone.

Skin prick testing has proven to be one of the least accurate forms of testing, however. While a negative response (no weal) usually confirms no allergy to that food, a positive response may not indicate an actual food allergy or intolerance when the food is eaten. Research has revealed that up to 60% of positive results can be false *(false positives)*.

Food Challenges

If there is a strong suspicion of a food allergy, the allergist may invoke a food challenge by feeding the patient with first a tiny amount, and then increasingly larger doses of a food while they watch for reactions.

This can be a painstaking and extensive test. And for someone who is showing signs of allergies, this test should only be performed by or in the presence of a trained health professional prepared to react with medical care should anaphylaxis result.

There are a number of different types of food challenge tests, but the most employed method is giving the patient a capsule of the allergen (or a placebo). When a placebo is employed, it is called a *double-blind, placebo-controlled food challenge*. In other words, neither the diagnostician nor the patient will know whether the capsule contains the allergen or the placebo. This can eliminate results produced through the inclinations of either the health professional or patient.

As mentioned earlier, the double-blind, placebo-controlled food challenge is considered the gold standard among diagnostic tests for food allergies and most food sensitivities.

Enzyme-linked Immunosorbent Assays (ELISA)

This test and its relative, the ALCAT test, have been met with significant resistance and criticism from conventional Western physicians. The complaint of some physicians is that ELISA testing has not been proven to be reliable for food allergy diagnosis.

This was illustrated by researchers from India's Post Graduate Institute of Medical Education and Research (Sharnan *et al.* 2001). The scientists gave skin prick tests and ELISA tests to 64 children with food allergies previously confirmed through food challenges, along with 32 control subjects. They found that the ELISA tests had greater specificity than the skin prick tests (88% versus 64%). But while they found that ELISA provided reliability for a lack of allergy, the ELISA testing generally did not provide a reliable basis for determining an allergy was present. They concluded that ELISA provided no useful advantage over skin prick testing.

One of the issues with ELISA testing (and some say its advantage) is that it yields levels of other immunoglobulins such as IgG, IgG4 and IgA. Some research has indicated that IgG4 is indicative of a hidden food allergy (Shakib *et al.* 1986), but other research has shown that allergen-specific IgG4s can also simply indicate a recovery from a prior food allergy (Savilahti *et al.* 2010).

One of the issues that some (including the author) have with ELISA is that some of the lab results present an array of sometimes confusing and extensive sensitivity conclusions that may or may not apply to the patient. These often provide the patient with an overload of information about possible sensitivities (sometimes to hundreds of foods) that may or may not exist.

Other (Some Questionable) Diagnostic Tests

There are a variety of other diagnostic tests that health care practitioners may subscribe to. These include sublingual testing, immune-complex tests, cytotoxic tests, provocative tests, the Mediator Release Test, galvanometer skin testing and others. While some of these may have value in some instances, most have not been met with the rigor of definitive scientific study (Boyce *et al.* 2010).

Researchers from the Ospedale Civile Maggiore hospital in Varona, Italy (Senna *et al.* 2002) conducted a study of alternative food allergy tests, including the cytotoxic test, the sublingual provocation test, the subcutaneous test, the heart-ear reflex test, kinesiology, electro-acupuncture, the immunocomplex IgG test, and hair analysis. They concluded that none of these tests were reliable diagnostic tests for food sensitivities.

We might comment independently about applied kinesiology. This test is currently applied by many clinicians who subscribe to its accuracy. While not being subjected to much research, it has a relatively low cost or risk to the patient. It can also be quite immediately verified through other testing methods, which can make the test immediately verifiable to the clinician and patient.

In applied kinesiology, muscle strength is tested while the patient holds, touches or eats a suspect food. The practitioner may push against the arm of the patient before and after holding or touching the food, for example. A trained individual may also self-test, but this can be difficult.

Applied kinesiology has had a history of use among alternative practitioners, typically following special training through clinical mentorship. This is not atypical of other specialized medical treatments such as acupuncture or massage. Physicians also use mentorship. In other words, applied kinesiology should only be performed by one properly trained.

We should note that a reaction to a food is a type of kinesiological event, as nerves and muscles are typically involved in the atopic response.

Applied kinesiology is nonetheless still very controversial, as it has the potential of being highly subjective. Thus it requires a sensitive and knowledgeable practitioner, and should always be conducted using double-blind methods (where neither the patient or practitioner know what food is being held or touched).

Even with these in place, however, there is always the possibility of error. There can be a variety of environmental, muscle tension, mental or unseen influences that can skew the results. Therefore, while this test is relatively simple and inexpensive, it can also be unreliable, and results should therefore be confirmed with more established testing methods.

The Food Elimination Study

Even some of the more recognized tests discussed above are no more reliable than a simple food elimination study. Furthermore, the food elimination study can be conducted at home by oneself if the symptoms are not severe. If the symptoms are severe, the elimination program should be supervised by a health professional or observed by someone prepared for anaphylaxis if there are serious symptoms involved in the sensitivity response. This said, the only expense is time, patience, and careful record-keeping.

Here the person simply begins to eliminate suspect foods, one at a time, from the diet. If symptoms subside after the food is withdrawn, one can be fairly certain of the sensitivity. The period of elimination should be enough to confirm the test, however. A good period is seven days without a symptom, but the longer the better. The results should also probably be confirmed by returning to the inclusion diet and then eliminating the food again, assuming the symptoms are manageable and not severe or assuming there is supervision as mentioned above when the food is added back.

Elimination testing can also be conducted using foods from similar food groups to pinpoint whether there is a common protein sensitivity or otherwise. (See Chapter Three for food groups and allergen information).

To confirm the sensitivity, the food or group can also be tested with a double-blind, placebo-controlled food challenge test. Again, if symptoms are severe, this should be performed or supervised by a health professional trained in anaphylactic response.

Chapter Two

The Immune System and Food Sensitivities

To fully understand some of the research and other information presented in this text, a working knowledge of the immune system is needed. Here we will briefly survey the key elements of the immune system as updated from the latest research. Note that this is probably not all the same immune system information you might have seen in a health textbook or many websites. This is because the past decade has brought numerous breakthroughs that update our understanding of the immune system in its entirety.

Intelligent Recognition

In general, the immune system is an intelligent scanning and defense mechanism, combined with an efficient toxin removal process. There are, however, numerous systems in place to achieve these objectives.

The immune system has a number of intelligent abilities. The first is recognition, as mentioned. The immune system has the facility to memorize and then recognize threats previously memorized. The immune system focuses on the distinguishing features that identify a threatening molecule or pathogen. In the case of a pathogen, the immune system may remember proteins on the invader's cell membrane, or even the invader's excrement. Immune cells can also recognize activities of a pathogen that make it distinctive.

The immune system is set up to see, assess and memorize whether a particular molecule, cell or organism is healthy for the body. This requires a complex biochemical identification system and a process of memorization. It also means the immune system must monitor the health of the body's cells and tissue systems.

We might compare the recognition system to a criminal fingerprint search system. The computer maintains a database of fingerprints, and the program searches for matches by breaking down elements of the fingerprints into a mapping system that classifies their type and position. When enough of these elements are found, the fingerprint is declared a match.

Utilizing a database of information, the immune system also scans and checks molecular structures against its database of threat memory. If the molecular structure matches with the elements of something that threatened the body previously, the immune system begins to mobilize the appropriate mechanisms to block entry to the threat.

31

But if the threat has already entered the tissues and gained access to cells, the immune system will be forced to launch an inflammatory response to attack the foreigner and those cells the threat has invaded.

When it comes to a food molecule, the immune system scans and remembers distinctive molecular sequences or combinations—these may be polypeptides, individual peptides or a portion of a peptide. These molecular sequences are called *epitopes*. Epitopes are antigens that are often referred to more specifically as allergens, because they stimulate an allergic inflammatory response. They stimulate the inflammatory response because their epitopes are recognized by the immune system as threatening.

When the immune system first records an epitope, it also develops a special receptor for that epitope. This receptor might be compared to a lock, while the allergen epitope is a particular type of key that will only open that lock. These 'locks' are the antibodies or immunoglobulins. The lock-and-key system of immunoglobulins provides a switch for the immune system to recognize an allergen and activate the immune system to remove it.

The immune system is located throughout the body. We find immune cells on the skin, in the blood, in the lungs, in the bones and in every organ system. We also find the immune system within trillions of probiotic bacteria scattered around the body.

As we'll discuss, the body's probiotic bacteria are integral within the immune system. They also help the immune system recognize foreign entities or toxins. This information is invaluable to the rest of the immune system. Probiotic bacteria also have the ability to remember invaders and toxins. They can thus assist the body in the breakdown and ejection of foreign molecules and pathogens, and often do this before the rest of the immune system even has to get involved.

We might compare such a system to a castle from the middle ages. The castle typically has very tall walls and a moat surrounding it. It would most likely have a very large and heavy gate system. These together prevent attacking enemies from easily gaining access to the castle. But these systems would be easy to get through were it not for defending marksmen and spear-chucking warriors who stand guard in the towers and castle walls. These guards prevent enemies from climbing the walls, jumping over the moat, or setting fire to the gate. Without these living guards, the defense systems of the castle would be quite useless to any enemy with some conviction.

Our probiotics are like the castle guards. They are living within the castle. Therefore, the castle's safety is particularly important to them. Thus, they will fight to the death to defend the castle.

While this analogy is not perfect, it is close, because according to microbiologists, the probiotic immune system makes up over 70% of the body's immunity. Without probiotics, the immune system is severely weakened.

The immune system is incredible in its ability to maintain specificity and diversity. These characteristics allow the immune system to respond to literally millions, if not billions of different antigens. Moreover, each particular antigen and epitope will require a distinct type of response to get rid of it. The immune system also remembers this particular response.

This issue of recognition brings up an important question to discuss in relation to food sensitivities: How does the body distinguish between "good" food molecules and "bad" (or threatening) food molecules?

Remember that the immune system recognition process is based upon memorization. The immune system accesses a variety of databases, including the probiotic memory, the MHC memory, T-cell, B-cell and antibody memory systems. Like branches of a large but centralized database system, these memory systems interact and confirm the threat levels of particular antigens. This confirming process, of course, relies upon a balanced and strong immune system. If the system is overloaded or in emergency mode, its responses may not be balanced. We'll be discussing this in more detail later.

One of the databases the immune system utilizes comes from the body's DNA. DNA sequences code the foods that our ancestors ate, and even those foods our ancestors' bodies didn't like. This DNA coding is quite complex, but is generally an accumulated record of not just our parents, but many generations back.

For example, researchers from the Johns Hopkins Bloomberg School of Public Health (Liu *et al.* 2004) found that nucleotide polymorphisms among genes were associated with specific allergies. They found that a gene variant labeled C-1055T was associated with food or environmental allergies. They found that the variant Gln551Arg was associated with cat allergies. They found that the variant C-590T was associated with dust mite allergies.

The immune system also 'remembers' the foods our mother ate during pregnancy. Here we are sensitized to whatever nutrients managed to get through to our umbilical cord blood—which provided us with nutrition for the first nine months of our physical lives.

The next 'recognition' process takes place through our own food consumption. This also can get complicated, as this relates to our body's response to the food, how well the food was digested, how easily it accessed our bloodstream and many other factors, including even our state of mind when we began eating the food. All of these can cause the immune system to 'mark' a food in a particular way.

Once this identification takes place, the immune system will memorize the body's interaction with the food. If the body's interaction with the food was negative, the immune system may 'remember' the food as being potentially threatening to the body, and launch an immune response to rid the body of the pertinent food molecule(s).

In food sensitivities, molecules identified as foreign or harmful will initially access the body via the mouth and digestive tract, and sometimes the nose, skin and/or eyes. There are four general facilities—or strategies—the immune system's utilizes to keep foreigners out. Let's dig into each strategy a bit further:

Non-specific Immunity

The first layer of defense is called non-specific because it provides a barrier that doesn't differentiate between the bad guys This general defense utilizes a network of physical and biochemical barriers that work synergistically to block just about anything potentially threatening from getting into the body.

The barrier structures include the ability of our body to shut down its orifices. We can close our eyes, mouths, noses and ears to prevent foreigners from entering the body. Our skin is also a barrier. Within and around these lie further defenses: Nose hairs, eyelashes, tongue, tonsils, ear hair, pubic hair and hair in general are all designed to help screen out and filter invaders within and around the body's entry areas.

These barrier structures utilize the body's refined autonomic systems, which automatically respond to even the slightest indication that there may be a threat to the body. For example, if there is a little smoke in the room, the eyes will become more watery to protect the eyes from the smoke.

Nearly every one of the body's passageways is also equipped with tiny cilia, which block but also assist the body in evacuating invaders by brushing them out. These cilia move rhythmically, sweeping back and forth, working caught pathogens outward with their undulations.

The surfaces of most of the body's orifices are also covered with mucous membranes. These thin liquid membrane films contain a combination of biochemicals (also called *mucin*) and cells that prevent invaders from penetrating any further. These special biochemicals include mucoproteins, glycoproteins, glycosaminoglycans, glycolipids, and various enzymes. These are designed to stick to, alter and break down large molecules that the body is not used to consuming. These mucus films lining our passageways also contain a combination of immune cells, immunoglobulins and colonies of probiotics.

The digestive tract is equipped with another type of sophisticated defense technology. Should any foreigners get through the lips, teeth, tongue, hairs, mucous membranes and cilia, and sneak down the esophagus and through the sphincter, they must then contend with the digestive fire of the stomach. The gastrin, peptic acid and hydrochloric acid within a healthy stomach keep a pH of around two. This is typically enough acidity to kill or significantly damage or neutralize many toxins and pathogenic bacteria.

Unfortunately, many of us mistakenly weaken this protective stomach acid by taking antacids or acid-blockers. In this case, the stomach's ability to neutralize pathogens will be handicapped.

Another critical part of the body's non-specific immune system—especially as it relates to food sensitivities—is the intestinal barrier. The walls of the intestines are also lined with a special mucosal membrane chock full of the elements described above: immunoglobulins, acids, enzymes, glycoproteins, mucopolysaccharides, probiotics and more. There is also an intricate barrier system installed between the intestinal cells called the *brush barrier*. The brush barrier screens and filters larger molecules and toxins so that only certain molecules—nutrients the body can use—can gain entry into the intestinal tissues and bloodstream.

Humoral Immunity

The second layer of immune defense takes place when foreign entities (toxins, food molecules or pathogens) gain access to the body. "Humoral" originates from *"the body's humours,"* which Hippocrates and other Greek physicians used to describe the body's different physiological regions and tissue mechanisms. Allergies are most often humoral responses.

The humoral immune system involves a highly technical strategic attack that first identifies the invader's weaknesses, followed by a precise and immediate offensive attack to exploit those weaknesses.

The body can draw from more than a billion different types of antibodies, macrophages and other immune cells to execute specific attack plans. As an immune cell scans a particular invader, it may recognize a particular biomolecular or behavioral weakness within the toxin or pathogen. Upon recognizing this weakness, the immune system will devise a unique plan to exploit this weakness. It may launch a variety of possible attacks, using a combination of specialized B-cells (or *B-lymphocytes*) in conjunction with specialized antibodies—the immunoglobulins mentioned earlier.

Cruising through the blood and lymph systems, the humoral system's antibodies and/or B-cells can quickly sense and size up foreigners. Often this will mean the antibody will lock onto or bind to the foreigner to extract and confirm critical molecular information. This process will often draw upon the identity databases held within certain helper B-cells that recognize and memorize molecular vulnerabilities. In other words, the immune system will either devise or draw from a memorized strategy for breaking down and ridding the body of the invader.

As mentioned, the specific vulnerability of the foreigner is typically revealed by its molecular structures or cell membrane structures. Each pathogen will be identified by these unique structures, called antigens. The B-cell then reproduces a specific antibody designed to record and communicate that information to other B-cells through biochemical signaling. This allows for a constant tracking of the location and development of pathogenic antigens—or in the case of food allergies, allergens—allowing B-cells to manage and constantly assess the response.

Meanwhile, the B-cell's antibodies will lock on to the epitope of the antigen. This "locking on" is also called *binding*. When the antibody binds or locks on to a foreign molecule, inflammatory mediators such as histamine, prostaglandins and leukotrienes are released. This stimulates a systemic detoxification process, as we will discuss further.

Cell-Mediated Immunity

The third defense process used by the immune system is the cell-mediated immune response. This also incorporates a collection of smart white blood cells called T-cells. T-cells and their surrogates wander the body scanning the body's own cells. They are seeking cells that have become infected or otherwise have been damaged by foreigners. Infected cells are typically identified by special marker molecules (also called antigens) that typically sit atop infected cell membranes. These cell antigens have particular molecular arrangements that signal to the roving T-cells that damage has occurred within the cell, or the cell is otherwise compromised.

Once a damaged cell has been recognized by the T-cell system, the cell-mediated immune system will launch an inflammatory response against the cell and its tissue system. This response will typically utilize a variety of cytotoxic (cell-killing) cells and helper T-cells. These types of immune cells will often directly kill the damaged cell by inserting toxic chemicals into it. Alternatively, the T-cell might send signals into the damaged cell, switching on a self-destruct mechanism within the cell.

The reader may wonder why this would be important to a food sensitivity. We must remember that T-cells also carefully scan the body's intestinal cells. If the T-cells pick up that cells within the intestinal system have been compromised somehow, they will stimulate an immune response against these intestinal cells. This immune response results in an inflammatory response within the intestines. The type of inflammatory response is directly related to the T-cell helpers, also called Th-cells, as we'll discuss further.

An inflammatory response of T-cells and T-cell helpers can greatly damage the tissues of that region. In other areas, inflammation can cause arthritis, heart disease and a variety of other problems. In the intestines, this T-cell inflammatory response can compromise the barrier function that keeps certain food molecules from gaining access to the blood. It can also cause Crohn's disease, irritable bowel syndrome, polyps and a variety of other issues. As we'll discuss in greater detail, damage to the intestinal barrier function can also allow food macromolecules (typically larger peptides/proteins) into the intestinal tissues and bloodstream. When that happens, the humoral immune may also launch an allergy response.

Probiotic Immunity

The fourth and most powerful part of the immune system takes place among the body's colonies of probiotics. The human body can house more than 32 billion beneficial and harmful bacteria and fungi at any particular time. When beneficial bacteria are in the majority, they constitute up to 70-80% of the body's immune response, as mentioned earlier. This takes place both in an isolated manner and in conjunction with the rest of the body's immunity and digestive systems.

About one hundred trillion bacteria live in the body's digestive system—about 3.5 pounds worth. The digestive tract contains about 400-500 different bacteria species. About twenty species make up about 75% of the population, however. Many of these are our resident strains, which attach to our intestinal walls. Many others are transient. These transient strains will typically stay for no more than about two weeks.

The majority of our probiotics live in the colon, although billions also live in the mouth and small intestines. Other populations of bacteria and yeast can also live within joints, under the armpits, under the toenails, in the vagina; between the toes; and among the body's various other nooks and body cavities.

First, probiotics are critical to the body's recognition of foreign molecules. Remember the DNA memory system mentioned earlier? Well, probiotics also contain DNA, and this DNA also catalogs the various foods that our ancestors consumed and worked around. If a particular food is recognized by a probiotic as being typical of its historical food or working environment, there is no problem. But if the molecules are foreign, the probiotic system can signal the immune system to launch a response, as well as launch its own response to get rid of the foreigner.

In other words, probiotic colonies work alongside as well as cooperatively with the body's immune system to organize strategies to prevent toxins and pathogenic microorganisms from harming the body.

Probiotics communicate and cooperate with the immune system through complex signaling systems. Probiotics utilize complex cytokine and immunoglobulin communication processes. They will stimulate T-cells, B-cells, macrophages and NK-cells with smart messages that promote and coordinate specific immune responses. They can also activate phagocytic cells directly to mobilize an intelligent toxin-removal response.

Using this communication, probiotics can activate cell-mediated responses and humoral responses. Probiotics also organize and police the body's mucosal barrier mechanisms.

Probiotics can also quickly identify harmful bacteria or fungal overgrowths and work directly to eradicate them. This process may not directly involve the rest of the immune system. In an infection, the immune system may act in a supportive manner, by breaking up and escorting dead pathogens out of the body.

Probiotics produce chemical substances that break down some food molecules into digestible form. They also release biochemicals and nutrients that are healthy for the body.

Lactic acid produced by *Lactobacillus* and *Bifidobacteria* species sets up the ultimate pH control in the gut to repel antagonistic organisms and aid the breakdown of food.

The environment that probiotics contribute to within the mucosal membrane include a number of complex acids. These include a hydrogen peroxide complex called *lactoperoxidase*. They also include acetic acids, formic acids lipopolysaccharides, peptidoglycans, superantigens and heat shock proteins. These inhibit challengers to ultimately benefit the intestinal environment.

Probiotics also secrete a number of key nutrients crucial to their hosts' (our body) immune system and metabolism, including B vitamins pantothenic acid, pyridoxine, niacin, folic acid, cobalamin and biotin, and crucial antioxidants such as vitamin K. Research is increasingly finding that these critical nutrients are often lacking in modern society. The reason, of course, is the destruction of these important probiotic species within our intestines.

Probiotics also help the break down (or police the break down) of food molecules into useable nutrients. This is the case for the lactose in milk. Probiotics produce lactase, an enzyme that breaks down lactose into smaller, digestible sugars. The lack of this enzyme (and those probiotics) is the primary reason many people become lactose intolerant.

Probiotics also produce antimicrobial molecules called *bacteriocins*. *Lactobacillus plantarum* produces lactolin. *Lactobacillus bulgaricus* secretes bulgarican. *Lactobacillus acidophilus* can produce acidophilin, acidolin, bacterlocin and lactocidin. These and other antimicrobial substances equip probiotic species with territorial mechanisms to combat and reduce pathologies related to *Shigella, Coliform, Pseudomonas, Klebsiella, Staphylococcus, Clostridium, Escherichia* and other infective genera. Furthermore, antifungal biochemicals from the likes of *L. acidophilus, B. bifidum, E. faecium* and others also significantly reduce yeast outbreaks caused by the overgrowths of *Candida albicans* (Shahani *et al.* 2005).

Furthermore, probiotics will specifically stimulate the body's own immune system to attack pathogens. For example, scientists from Finland's University of Turku (Pessi *et al.* 2000) gave nine atopic dermatitis children *Lactobacillus rhamnosus* GG for four weeks. They found that serum cytokine IL-10 levels specific to the infection increased following probiotic consumption.

In another study (Gill *et al.* 2001), the probiotic *Bifidobacterium lactis* HN019 (or a placebo) was given to 30 healthy elderly volunteers (average age 69 years old) for nine weeks. They found that the probiotic group had significantly greater levels of helper T-cells (CD4+), activated (CD25+) T-cells, and natural killer T-cells. The probiotic strengthened their immune response in general, and stimulated the production of communication cytokines.

The research confirming the role that probiotics play with the immune system is impeccable, consistent and undeniable. We will cover some of this research in this text, but for a more complete review of the research and practical application of probiotics, see the author's book, *Probiotics: Protection Against Infection* (2009).

For now, let's discuss the other players among the body's immune system, and their interaction with food sensitivities.

The Immune Cells

The immune system is composed of a number of different cells, and most are referred to as white blood cells or leukocytes. There are at least five different types of white blood cells. Each is designed to identify and target specific types of antigens (or allergens).

Once an antigen/allergen is identified, these immune cells will initiate an attack specific to the condition of the body and the weakness of the antigen. Generally, the weaker the condition of the body's immunity, the more systemic the response. The stronger the body's immune system is relative to the threat of the antigen, the more efficient (and less systemic) the response will be. This is the reason why a high white blood cell count in a blood test will indicate that the body is fighting a big infection or toxin relative to its strength.

We might compare this to getting bit badly by red ants as we walk by an ant hill. The only reason the ants began to bite is because they felt threatened. The size of the foot was very large relative to the proximity of the ant hill. If we were walking by a few of the same ants further away from the ant hill, we probably would not get bit. They didn't feel that we threatened their ant colony and queen from that distance.

In the same way, the immune system kicks into high gear when it is most vulnerable. In the face of a less-threatening food molecule, a strong immune system would not need to launch a full scale attack. It could easily take care of the invasion by less drastic means, and with fewer white blood cells. If the attack was a lethal virus, on the other hand, then even the strong immune system will kick into high gear and launch a systemic immune response.

The main types of white blood cells are lymphocytes, neutrophils, basophils, monocytes and macrophages. Each WBC plays an important role in the antigen/allergen-identification and inflammatory process. WBCs are the body's immune response soldiers. They tackle invaders head on.

Monocytes

Monocytes are like the Neolithic ancestors of the attack soldiers. After being produced in the marrow, monocytes differentiate into either macrophages or dendrite cells. The macrophages are particularly good at engulfing and breaking apart pathogens. Dendritic cells are interactive cells that stimulate certain responses. They may, for example, isolate and present antigens to B-cells or T-cells. Dendritic cells also stimulate the production of those special communication proteins called cytokines.

Lymphocytes (T-cells and B-cells)

Lymphocytes are identification cells that code and target specific invaders. The primary lymphocytes are the T-cells (thymus cells) or B-cells (bone marrow cells). These cells and their specialized communication proteins work together to strategically attack and remove invaders. Then special memory helper cells memorize the strategy in preparation for a future invasion.

All white blood cells are initially produced by stem cells within the bone marrow. Following their release, T-cells undergo further differentiation and programming within the thymus gland. B-cells undergo a similar process of maturity before release from the spleen. Both T-cells and B-cells circulate via lymph, bloodstream and intercellular tissue fluids. Both T-cells and B-cells have a number of special types, including memory cells and helper cells to identify and memorize invaders.

As mentioned earlier, B-cells look for foreign or potentially harmful antigens moving freely. These might include allergens, toxins or microbes. Once identified, B-cells will stimulate the production of a particular type of antibody, designed to bind to and neutralize the foreigner.

Most B-cells are monoclonal, which means they will adjust to a specific type of invader. Once they set up for a particular type of invader, they can make "clones" or copies that will launch an attack and bind to the foreigners.

Most B-cells are investigative and surveillance oriented. Once activated, they launch a variety of inflammatory responses through the release of mediators such as histamine and leukotrienes. This process allows them to interrupt antigen penetration. B-cells that circulate and scan the bloodstream are often called plasma B-cells. Others—like memory B-cells—record and communicate previous invasions for future attacks.

B-cells typically work through legions of antibodies called immunoglobulins. We'll discuss immunoglobulins further in a bit. B-cells may also attach to or bind directly to antigens. In this case, their immunoglobulins are attached to their cell membrane. Once this binding takes place, the inflammatory mediators are released.

T-cells, on the other hand, are oriented toward the body's own cells, and those foreigners who get mixed up with the cells' metabolism. This means T-cells are focused upon internal cellular and tissue systems. In other words, when antigens are absorbed by or invade cells, the cell becomes damaged. T-cells look for these damaged cells. Once found, the damaged cells will be destroyed or crippled by the T-cells.

There are different types of T-cells. Each is programmed in the thymus to look for a different type of problems that may occur inside cells, such as infection or toxin contamination. This is programmed in the thymus by the major histocompatibility complex, or MHC (see the Thymus section on pages 50-51 for more on MHC programming).

Many T-cells simply respond to a pathogen that has invaded the cell by destroying the cell itself—this is the *killer* T-cell. It does this by inserting deadly (cytotoxic) chemicals into the cell or by submitting instructions into the cell to kill itself. Cell death is called *apoptosis*, and those T-cells capable of killing our cells are called cytotoxic T-cells (*cyto* refers to cells) and natural killer T-cells.

T-cells work through the communication cytokines to relay instructions and information amongst the various T-cells. Prominent cytokine communications thus take place between helper T-cells, natural killer cells and cytotoxic T-cells.

The initial screening of an infected cell by a helper T-cell utilizes an electromagnetic scanning system not unlike the scanning systems airports use to screen passengers before they get on a plane.

The T-cell's scanning system includes delta-gamma T-cells. Delta-gamma T-cells are sensitive to specific receptors on intestinal cell membranes. Thus, delta-gamma T-cells are considered key to the body's tolerance to foods, as food molecules make contact with intestinal cells.

Helper T-cells record and communicate database information on previous invaders. They also communicate previous immune responses, memorize current ones, and pass on strategic information regarding the progress of pending attack plans.

The helper T-cell scan initially surveys the cell's membrane for indications of either microbial infection or some sort of genetic mutation due to a virus or toxin. This antigen scan might reveal invasions of chemical toxins or allergens that may have intruded or deranged the cell. The scanning helper T-cell immediately communicates the information by releasing their tiny coded protein cytokines. These disseminate the information needed to coordinate macrophages, NK-cells and cytotoxic T-cells.

B-cells and T-cells often coordinate their strategies through what is called *T-cell-dependent responses*. In other words, the B-cell is activated through cytokines after a T-cell recognizes the antigen.

Most healthy cells contain tumor necrosis factor or TNF—a self-destruct switch of sorts. When signaled from the outside by a cytotoxic T-cell, TNF will initiate a self-destruct and the cell will die. These "death-switch" communications sometimes also utilize intermediary cytokines.

Under some circumstances, entire groups of cells or tissue systems may become damaged. Macrophages may be signaled to cut off the blood supply to these deranged or infected cells.

The two primary helper T-cell types are the Th1 and the Th2. The Th1 T-cell focuses on the elimination of bacteria, fungi, parasites, viruses, and similar types of invaders. The Th2 cells stimulate more B-cell activity. This focuses the immune response toward antibody and allergic responses. The Th2 cells are thus explicitly involved in the inflammatory responses of allergic reactions. The Th2 response coordinates with the B-cell-antibody system to stimulate allergic symptoms.

This is important to note on a number of levels. Research has revealed that stress, chemical toxins, poor dietary habits and a lack of sleep tend to suppress Th1 immune responses and elevate Th2 levels. With an overabundance of Th2 cells in the system compared to Th1, the body is prone to respond more strongly to allergens and toxins, causing more pronounced reactions like hay fever and food sensitivities. This is also why we sometimes see people who are under physical or emotional stress overreacting with hives, psoriasis and other allergic-type responses.

Probiotics modulate the balance between the Th1 and Th2 response. This was illustrated by Japanese researchers (Odamaki *et al.* 2007). Yogurt with *Bifidobacterium longum* BB536 or plain yogurt was given to 40 patients with allergies to Japanese cedar pollen. After 14 weeks, the peripheral blood mononuclear cell counts of the patients indicated that the probiotics reduced the body's Th2 counts and activity.

Mast Cells, Neutrophils and Basophils

Mast cells, neutrophils and basophils are granulocyte white blood cells that release inflammatory mediators. They circulate within the bloodstream and lymph, looking for abnormal behavior or toxins. Once they identify a problem or are stimulated by B-cells and immunoglobulins, they will initiate a process to clean up the area. This invokes inflammation and allergic symptoms, as they work to remove toxins.

This cleaning process is conducted by their release of inflammatory mediators such as histamines and leukotrienes. The release of these mediators in the case of an allergen is provoked by signals following the binding between immunoglobulins and allergen epitopes. Upon being signaled, the granulocyte releases mediators through its cell membrane.

Many allergy write-ups put all the histamine release upon the mast cells. Yet recent research has confirmed that both basophils and neutrophils also release histamine. Neutrophils have been associated with infective microorganisms, while basophils and mast cells have been associated with allergens. Furthermore, neutrophils have been found to release histamine within the lungs in allergic lung responses related to both allergic asthma and food allergies (Xu *et al.* 2006).

The Communicators

Cytokines are the communication systems that allow different immune cells to signal each other. Probiotics also utilize cytokines to communicate between the immune system's cells.

Cytokines come with complex names like interleukin (IL), transforming growth factor (TGF), leukemia inhibitory factor (LIF), and tumor necrosis factor (TNF). There are five basic types of cell communication: intracrine, autocrine, endocrine, juxtacrine and paracrine.

Autocrine communication takes place between two different types of cells. This message can be a biochemical exchange or an electromagnetic signal. The other cell in turn may respond automatically by producing a particular biochemical or electromagnetic message. We might compare this to leaving a voicemail on someone's message machine. Once we leave the message, the machine signals that the message has been received and will be delivered. Later the machine will replay the message. The immune system uses this type of autocrine message recording process to activate T-cells. Once the message is relayed, the T-cell will respond specifically with the instructed activity.

Paracrine communication takes place between neighboring cells of the same type, to pass on a message that comes from outside of the tissue system. Tiny protein antennas will sit on cell membranes, allowing one cell to communicate with another. This allows cells within the same tissue system to respond in a coordinated manner.

Juxtacrine communications take place via smart biomolecular structures. We might call these structures relay stations. They absorb messages and pass them on. An example of this is the passing of inflammatory messages via immune cell cytokines.

Intracrine communication takes place within the cell. First, an external message may be communicated into the cell through an antenna sitting on the cell's membrane. Once inside the cell, the message will be communicated around cell's organelles to initiate internal metabolic responses.

Endocrine communication takes place between endocrine glands and individual cells. The endocrine glands include the pineal gland, the pituitary gland, the pancreas, adrenals, thyroid, ovary and testes. These glands produce endocrine biochemicals, which relay messages directly to cells.

Endocrine communications stimulate a variety of metabolic functions within the body. These include growth, temperature, sexual behavior, sleep, glucose utilization, stress response and so many others. One of the functions of the endocrine glands relevant to food sensitivity is the production of inflammatory co-factors such as cortisol, adrenaline and norepinephrine. These coordinate and initiate instructions that help regulate inflammatory processes. Cortisol, for example, shunts or slows the inflammatory cascade, as we'll discuss more later. This is critical to the body's ability to control or balance the allergic immune response.

Cytokines Associated with Food Sensitivities

T-cell cytokines: Allergic T-cell-dependent responses utilize specific cytokines to develop and communicate response strategies. Also their cell membrane CDs (see page 50) are influenced by cytokines.

For example, University of Helsinki researchers (Savilahti *et al.* 2010) studied T-cell cytokine markers for CD4, CD25, CD127 and FoxP3 after they were stimulated by beta-lactoglobulin among milk allergy children. They also found that constant levels of these related cytokines were higher among milk-allergic children as compared with non-allergic children. These cytokines directly affected the profiles of the Th2 response.

National Institutes of Health researchers (Prussin *et al.* 2009) have found that anaphylactic food allergy and eosinophil-related GI disorders are both linked with Th2 and food-specific IgE responses, even though they have different symptoms. When they tested peanut allergy patients with allergic gastroenteritis patients together with control subjects, they found that cytokines such as interleukin-5 (IL-5) for Th2 cells were specific to the allergen. They both had IL-5 Th2 responses but with different binding. Th1s were similarly active, but dominated by the Th2 response.

Finnish medical researchers (Rautava and Isolauri 2004) found that cow's milk allergy was accompanied by increased levels of the cytokine interleukin-4 (IL-4).

University of Helsinki researchers (Westerholm-Ormio *et al.* 2010) found that particular T-regulative cells and toll-like receptors increased within the intestines of allergic subjects. These T-reg cells play a key role in the inflammation process with regard to allergies. Foxp3- and TLR4-driven cytokines were greater among food allergy patients. The Foxp3 cells stimulated primarily CD4, CTLA-4, or CD25. The researchers also found that Foxp3 mRNA cell ratios were lower among food allergy and celiac patients. Foxp3 T-cells were increased within the duodenum.

B-cell cytokines: Food allergic responses tend to utilize the CD19+CD5+ related cytokines to stimulate B-cells. Allergen-oriented B-cells tend to stimulate the further allergic response utilizing the IL-10 cytokine (Noh *et al.* 2010).

B-cells regulate immune responses with antigens in late atopic skin reactions. When eight milk allergy patients and thirteen milk-tolerant (no allergy) subjects were challenged with casein and tested for B cell subsets, researchers found that CD19+ B-cells were lower in the milk tolerant group, and apoptotic B-cells were lower in the allergy group. IL-10 producing CD19+CD5+ regulatory B-cells were also lower in the milk allergy group, compared with the no-allergy group.

The Inflammation Mediators

Our body's immune system launches inflammatory cells and factors to rid toxins, heal injury sites and prevent bleed-outs. This process is stimulated by the inflammatory factors histamines, leukotrienes and prostaglandins.

Leukotrienes

Leukotrienes are molecules that identify problems and stimulate the immune system. They pinpoint and isolate areas of the body that require repair. Once they pinpoint the site of repair, one type of leukotriene will initiate inflammation, and others will assist in maintaining the process. Once the repair process proceeds to a point of maturity, another type of leukotriene will begin slowing down the process of inflammation.

This smart signalling process takes place through the biochemical bonding formations of these molecules. Leukotrienes are paracrines and autocrines. They are paracrine in that they initiate messages that travel from one cell to another. They are autocrine in that they initiate messages that encourage an automatic and immediate response—notably among T-cells, engaging them to remove bad cells. They also help transmit messages that initiate the process of repair through the clotting of blood and the patching of damaged tissues.

Leukotrienes are produced from the conversion of essential fatty acids (EFAs) by an enzyme produced by the body called arachidonate-5-lipoxygenase (sometimes called LOX). The central fatty acids involved of this process are arachidonic acid (AA), gamma-linolenic acid (GLA), and eicosapentaenoic acid (EPA). These are obtained from the diet. Lipoxygenase enzymes produce different types of leukotrienes, depending upon the initial fatty acid.

The key considerations with regard to fatty acids and leukotrienes is that the leukotrienes produced by arachidonic acid stimulate inflammation, while the leukotrienes produced by EPA halt inflammation. The leukotrienes produced by GLA, on the other hand, block the conversion process of polyunsaturated fatty acids to arachidonic acid. This means that GLA also reduces the inflammatory (and allergic) response.

Prostaglandins

Prostaglandins are also produced through an enzyme conversion from fatty acids. Like leukotrienes and mast cells, prostaglandins are mediators that transmit inflammatory messages to immune cells. Their messaging is either paracrine or autocrine. Prostaglandins, especially PGE2, are critical parts of the allergic process. They also initiate a number of protective sequences in the body, including the transmission of irritation and pain, and some swelling from inflammation.

Prostaglandins are produced by the oxidation of fatty acids by an enzyme produced in the body called cyclooxygenase—also called prostaglandin-endoperoxide synthase (PTGS) or COX. There are three types of COX, and each converts fatty acids to different types of prostaglandins. The central fatty acid that causes inflammation is arachidonic acid. COX-1 converts AA to the PGE2 type of prostaglandin. COX-2, on the other hand, converts AA into the PGI2 type of prostaglandin.

The central messages that prostaglandins transmit depend upon the type of prostaglandin. Prostaglandin I2 (also PGI2) stimulates the widening of blood vessels and bronchial passages, and pain sensation within the nervous system. In other words, along with stimulating blood clotting, PGI2 signals a range of responses to assist the body's wound healing at the site of injury.

Prostaglandin E2, or PGE2, is altogether different from PGI2. PGE2 stimulates the secretion of mucus within the stomach, intestines, mouth and esophagus. It also decreases the production of gastric acid in the stomach. This combination of increasing mucus and lowering acid production keeps healthy stomach cells from being damaged by our gastric acids and the acidic content of our foods. This is one of the central reasons NSAID pharmaceuticals cause gastrointestinal problems: They interrupt the secretion of this protective mucus in the stomach.

This means that the COX-1 enzyme instigates the process of protecting the stomach, while the COX-2 enzyme instigates the process of inflammation and repair within the body. In the case of allergies, the COX-2 process often lies at the root of allergic wheezing.

Cyclooxygenase also converts ALA/DHA and GLA to prostaglandins. Just as lipoxygenase converts ALA/DHA and GLA to anti-inflammation leukotrienes, the conversion of ALA/DHA and GLA by cyclooxygenase produces prostaglandins that either block the inflammatory process or reverse it.

The arachidonic acid conversion process that produces prostaglandins also produces thromboxanes. Thromboxanes stimulate platelets in the blood to aggregate. They work in concert with platelet-activating factor or PAF. Together, these biomolecules drive the process of clotting the blood and restricting blood flow. This is good during injury healing, but the inflammatory process must also be slowed down as the injury heals. We'll discuss the role of fatty acids in the inflammatory process in more detail later on.

Histamine

Histamine is produced by mast cells, basophils and neutrophils as mentioned earlier. Histamine is a key mediator in the allergic response because it serves to increase the permeability of blood vessels. This in turn allows white blood cells to spread out among the various tissues of the body. As the WBCs spread, they attack any kind of foreign molecule.

As blood vessel permeability increases, the mucous membranes become fuller with fluid. This takes place concurrent with the destruction of antigens by white blood cells, producing phlegm. This also produces the watery eyes, sinus congestion and lung congestion known in allergic responses.

When histamine is released, it will bind with specific receptors located around the body. Depending upon the type of receptor, histamine will elicit a particular response.

For example, the H1 histamine receptor located within the tissues of the lungs, muscles, nerves, sinuses, and other tissues stimulates the allergic responses of congestion, watery eyes, sinusitis, skin rashes and so on. H2 receptors lie in the digestive tract and control the release of stomach acids and intestinal mucous membrane. H3 receptors stimulate the nervous system and the flow of neurotransmitters. H4 receptors involve the directional function of immune cells and intestinal cells in function.

While histamine in general might be considered a "bad guy" in the process of food sensitivity, histamine is critical for maintaining equilibrium around the body. Histamine helps establish homeostasis among cells and tissue systems. Without histamine to communicate balance and imbalance, the body would have little reference to respond to threats. When histamine is released in abundance, this will often stimulate all four receptor systems, putting the body into hyper-vigilance mode. In this mode, the body is responds on a hair-trigger.

The bottom line is that none of these inflammatory mediators are the bad guys. This type of isolation approach is what causes medications that target mediators to have so many side effects. The body is a 'smart' organism, and it operates through a series of checks and balances that intermix with information and communications. Thus, the attempt to try to shut off one process or another (such as histamines with antihistamines) with a single chemical can temporarily halt a few symptoms, but they cannot reverse or heal the basic issue of imbalance. They also come with side effects, because they can further imbalance other parts of the body's natural homeostasis.

The Immunoglobulins

Immunoglobulins are proteins that attach to the epitopes of antigens. They are either released into the blood or lymph by B-cells, or they remain on the surface of B-cells, enabling B-cells to attach to antigens. The immunoglobulins that are secreted and released into the blood and lymph are called antibodies. Those that stay attached to the B-cells are called surface immunoglobulins (sIg) or membrane immunoglobulins (mIg).

Secretory IgA (SIgA) immunoglobulins typically line the mouth, nose, ears, tears and digestive tract. Here they scan for pathogens or toxins that might harm the body. Serum IgAs look for initial tissue entry antigens. Most IgAs are SIgAs, however.

IgDs sense early microbial infections and activate macrophages. IgEs attach to early entry foreign substances (such as food molecules they do not recognize) and stimulate the release of inflammatory mediators—associated with most allergic responses. IgGs cross through membranes, responding to growing and maturing antigens within the body. IgMs are focused on earlier (but not new) intrusions into cells and body fluids that have yet to grow enough to garner the attention of IgGs.

Type	Where located	Targets
IgA	Mucus membranes, saliva, tears, breast milk (SIg), also blood/lymph (serum IgA)	Prevent initial entry of antigens or early entry into bloodstream
IgD	Blood/lymph/B-cells	Detect initial microbial infections
IgE	Blood/lymph/B-cells	Detect early toxins and allergens in blood and tissues
IgM	Blood/lymph/B-cells	Detect infections and toxins that begin to damage cells
IgG	Blood/lymph/placenta	Detect mature infections that have damaged cells and invaded tissues

Each of these general immunoglobulin categories contain numerous sub-types geared to different types of pathogens and responses. Other immunoglobulin proteins also exist. Some of these aid macrophages and lymphocytes in identifying specific pathogens.

The status of the body's immunoglobulins indicates the immune system's strength and health. An immune system with a large number of IgAs (SIgAs and serum IgAs) and healthy mucosal membranes will typically be more tolerant of all foods, toxins and pathogens, because antigens will typically be taken out before they can access the body's bloodstream and tissue systems. On the other hand, high IgE counts indicate a hypersensitivity mode for allergens and/or other toxins. Likewise, high IgM and

IgG levels indicate a past infection or toxicity that is being increasingly managed or tolerated.

For example, a Swiss allergy study (Bell and Potter 1988) found that following the consumption of milk and whey, children allergic to milk produced more milk-specific IgE antibodies.

An element of immunoglobulins is the CD glycogen-protein complex. CD stands for *cluster of differentiation*. CDs are molecules that sit on top of immune cells to navigate and steer their behavior. They will sit atop T-cells, B-cells, NK-cells, granulocytes and monocytes, identifying threats and infected cells. They will also sometimes negotiate with and bind directly to pathogens. This allows the lymphocytes to proceed to strategically attack the threat.

Clusters of differentiation are identified by their bindable molecular structure: This is also referred to as a ligand. The specific molecular arrangement (or CD number) will also match a specific type of receptor at the membrane of the cell or pathogen. Each CD number maintains a bonding relationship with a certain receptor structure on the cell to allow the accompanying immunoglobulin or lymphocyte to have interactivity with the pathogen. This gives the immunoglobulin or lymphocyte an access point from which to attack the perceived threat, and a coding vehicle to remember the invader later on.

Immunoglobulins and CDs are also tools probiotics utilize to define or influence appropriate responses for the immune system. Probiotics stimulate IgAs through CDs, for example, when they discover a pathogen has invaded the body's mucous membranes.

CDs are also utilized by probiotics to alert the immune system to intestinal cells and tissues that have been damaged by toxins, bacteria, or viruses. Probiotics signal back and forth with the immune system to maintain a check and balance system among the intestines. This signaling process can stimulate particular immune responses as needed.

The Thymus

One of the most important players in the immune system is the thymus gland. The thymus gland is located in the center of the chest, behind the sternum. The thymus is one of the more critical organs of the lymphatic system. Some have compared the thymus gland of the lymphatic system to the heart of the bloodstream.

The thymus gland is not a pump, however. The thymus activates T-cells and various hormones that modulate and stimulate the immune and autoimmune processes. The thymus converts lymphocytes called thymocytes into T-cells. These activated T-cells are released into the lymph and bloodstream ready to protect and serve. Within the thymus, the T-cells are infused with CD surface markers—which identify particular types of problematic cells or invading organisms. Their CD markers define the mission of the T-cells.

In other words, the thymus codes the T-cells with receptors that will bind to and damage particular cells or toxins. The types of cells or toxins they bind to or identify are determined by the *major histocompatibility complex*, or MHC determinant. During the process of converting thymocytes to T-cells, their CD receptors are programmed with MHC combinations. This allows them to tolerate particular frailties within the body while attacking what the body considers to be true invaders (Kazansky 2008).

Therefore, it is the MHC that gives the T-cell the ability to identify the difference between the "self" and "non-self" parts of the body. A non-self identification will produce an immunogen—a factor that stimulates an immune response. Once the immunogen is processed, it stimulates the inflammatory cascade.

The thymus gland develops and enlarges from birth. It is most productive and at its largest during puberty. From that point on, depending upon our diet, stress and lifestyle, our thymus gland will shrink over the years. By forty, an immunosuppressed person will often have a tiny thymus gland. In elderly persons, the thymus gland is often barely recognizable. For many people today, the thymus is practically non-functional.

Throughout its productive life, the thymus gland processes T-cells with the appropriate MHC programming. If the thymus gland is functioning, it will continue to produce T-cells with MHC programming that reflects the body's current status. Its constantly updated programming will accommodate the various genetic changes that can happen to different cells around the body as we age and adapt to our changing environment. With a shrunken and non-functioning thymus, however, its ability to reprogram T-cells with a new MHC—enabling them to identify the body's cells that have adapted—is damaged. The T-cells will have to keep working from the old MHC programming. This means the T-cells will not be able to properly identify "self" versus "non-self" within the body's cells.

With this progression of thymus weakness and the resulting lack of updated MHC determinants, T-cells begin attacking the body's own tissues instead of becoming tolerant to their new conditions.

The Liver

The liver is the key organ involved in detoxification and the production of a variety of enzymes and biochemicals. The liver produces over a thousand biochemicals the body requires for healthy functioning. The liver maintains blood sugar balance by monitoring glucose levels and pro-ducing glucose metabolites. It manufactures albumin to maintain plasma pressure. It produces cholesterol, urea, inflammatory biochemicals, blood-clotting molecules, and many others.

These functions are major reasons for the liver's involvement in food sensitivities.

The liver sits just below the lungs on the right side under the dia-phragm. Partially protected by the ribs, it attaches to the abdominal wall with the falciform ligament. The *ligamentum teres* within the falciform is the remnant of the umbilical cord that once brought us blood from mama's placenta. As the body develops, the liver continues to filter, purify and enrich our blood. Should the liver shut down, the body can die within hours.

Interspersed within the liver are functional fat factories called stellates. These cells store and process lipids, fat-soluble vitamins such as vitamin A, and secrete structural biomolecules like collagen, laminin and glycans. These are used to build some of the body's toughest tissue systems.

Into the liver drains nutrition-rich venous blood through the hepatic portal vein, together with some oxygenated blood through the hepatic artery. A healthy liver will process almost a half-gallon of blood per min-ute. The blood is commingled within cavities called sinusoids, where blood is staged through stacked sheets of the liver's primary cells—called hepatocytes. Here blood is also met by interspersed immune cells called kupffers. These kupffer cells attack and break apart bacteria and toxins. Nutrients coming in from the digestive tract are filtered and converted to molecules the body's cells can utilize. The liver also converts old red blood cells to bilirubin to be shipped out of the body. Filtered and purified blood is jettisoned through hepatic veins out the inferior vena cava and back into circulation.

The liver's filtration/purification mechanisms protect our body from various infectious diseases and chemical toxins. After hepatocytes and kuppfer cells break down toxins, the waste is disposed through the gall bladder and kidneys. The gall bladder channels bile from the liver to the intestines. Recycled bile acids combine with bilirubin, phospholipids, cal-cium and cholesterol to make bile. Bile is concentrated and pumped through the bile duct to the intestines. Here bile acids help digest fats, and broken-down toxins are (hopefully) excreted through our feces. This is assuming that we have healthy intestines containing healthy mucous membranes, barrier mechanisms and probiotic colonies.

The liver's filtration and breakdown process is critical to food sensi-tivities. If an allergen gets through the intestinal IgA process of removal, the liver gets a crack at removing it. If the liver is not able to metabolize and neutralize the molecule, the body must rely upon the inflammatory immune response to rid the body of the molecule. Often this process is concurrent, but a strong liver will reduce the body's dependence upon the inflammatory processes for removing macromolecules. If the hepatocytes and kuppfer cells are abundant and resilient, they can remove many toxins. Should those cells be damaged or overwhelmed by too many toxins at once, their ability to break down and remove problematic macromolecules becomes diminished.

Research and a wealth of clinical evidence tells us that the liver is damaged by chemical and food-based toxins. This is the very reason that alcohol (ethanol) causes liver disease: ethanol damages the liver's hepatocytes and kuppfers.

Today our diets, water and air are full of many other chemicals that produce the same result. These include plasticizers, formaldehyde, heavy metals, hydrocarbons, DDT, dioxin, VOCs, asbestos, preservatives, artificial flavors, food dyes, propellants, synthetic fragrances and more. With every additional chemical comes a requirement for the liver to work harder to break down these synthesized chemicals.

Frankly, most modern livers—especially those in urban areas of industrialized countries—are now overloaded and beyond their natural capacity. What happens then? Generally, two things. First, the hepatocytes collapse from toxicity, causing an overactive immune system due to the additional burdens placed upon it. Second, liver exhaustion leads to increased susceptibility to infectious diseases such as viral hepatitis. The combined result is a downward spiraling of hypersensitivity.

Liver disease—where one or more lobes begin to malfunction due to the death or dysfunction of hepatocytes—can result in a life-threatening emergency. Cirrhosis is a common diagnosis for liver disease, often caused by years of drinking alcohol or taking prescription medications combined with other toxin exposure. During this progression towards cirrhosis the sub-functioning liver can also produce symptoms such as jaundice, high cholesterol, gallstones, encephalopathy, kidney disease, clotting problems, heart conditions, hormone imbalances and many others. As cirrhosis proceeds, it results in the massive die-off of liver cells, and the subsequent scarring of remaining tissues, causing the liver to begin to shutdown.

While most of us have heard about the damage alcohol can have on the liver, many do not realize that pharmaceuticals and so many other synthetic chemicals can also be extremely toxic to the liver. The liver must find a way to break down these foreign chemicals. The liver's various purification processes can become overwhelmed by these synthetic molecules.

As liver cells weaken and die, their enzymes leak into the bloodstream. Blood tests for AST and ALT enzymes reveal this weakening of the liver.

We must therefore closely monitor the quantity and types of chemicals we put into our body. Eliminating preservatives, food dyes and pesticides in our foods can be done easily by eating whole organic foods. We can eliminate exposures to many environmental toxins mentioned above by simply replacing them with natural alternatives.

A number of herbs help strengthen liver function. These include goldenseal, dandelion, milk thistle and others.

Probiotics also play a large role in liver disease. When pathogenic bacteria get out of control in the intestines, they can overload the liver with endotoxins—their waste products. This bombardment of endotoxins onto the liver produces a result similar to alcohol or pharmaceuticals: During the putrefaction of pathogenic bacteria such as *Clostridium* spp., for example, one of the endotoxins is ammonia. Like ethanol, ammonia is toxic to the liver (Shawcross *et al.* 2007). Ammonia from pathogenic bacteria in the gut damages the liver, in other words.

Because probiotics reduce pathogenic bacteria, probiotics prevent these metabolites and endotoxins from affecting the liver. For example, researchers from the G.B. Pant Hospital in New Delhi (Sharma *et al.* 2008) gave 190 cirrhosis patients a combination of probiotics or placebo for one month. The probiotic group experienced a 52% improvement in cirrhosis symptoms and significantly lower blood ammonia levels.

Intestinal Immunity

The intestines utilize non-specific, humoral, cell-mediated and probiotic immunity to protect intestinal tissues from larger peptides, toxins and invading microorganisms. This is all packaged nicely into the mucosal membrane that lines the intestines—also referred to as the intestinal brush barrier.

The intestinal brush barrier is a complex mucosal layer of mucin, enzymes, probiotics and ionic fluid. It forms a protective surface medium over the intestinal epithelium. It also provides an active nutrient transport mechanism. This mucosal layer is stabilized by the grooves of the intestinal microvilli. It contains glycoproteins, mucopolysaccharides and other ionic transporters, which attach to amino acids, minerals, vitamins, glucose and fatty acids—carrying them across intestinal membranes. Meanwhile the transport medium requires a delicately pH-balanced mix of ionic chemistry able to facilitate this transport of useable nutrient. The mucosal layer is policed by billions of probiotic colonies, which help process incoming food molecules, excrete various nutrients, and control pathogens.

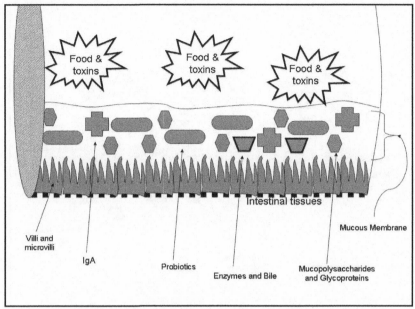

The Healthy Intestinal Wall

The brush barrier is a triple-filter that screens for molecule size, ionic nature and nutrition quality. Much of this is performed via four mechanisms existing between the intestinal microvilli: tight junctions, adherens junctions, desmosomes, and colonies of probiotics. The tight functions form a bilayer interface between cells, controlling permeability. Desmosomes are points of interface between the tight junctions, and adherens junctions keep the cell membranes adhesive enough to stabilize the junctions. These junction mechanisms together regulate permeability at the intestinal wall.

This mucosal brush barrier creates the boundary between intestinal contents and our bloodstream. Should the mucosal layer chemistry become altered, its protective and ionic transport mechanisms become weakened, allowing toxic or larger molecules to be presented to the microvilli junctions. This contact can irritate the microvilli, causing a subsequent inflammatory response. This is now considered a contributing cause of IBS.

The breakdown of the mucosal membrane causes it to thin. This depletes the protection rendered by the mucopolysaccharides and glycoproteins, probiotics, immune IgA cells, enzymes and bile. This thinning allows toxins and macromolecules that would have been screened out by the mucosal membrane to be presented to the intestinal cells.

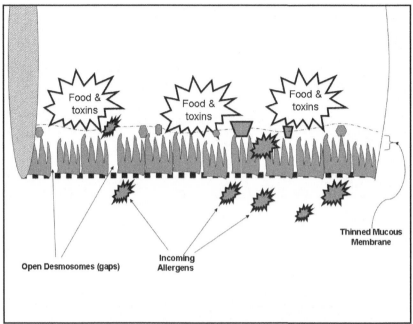

The Unhealthy Intestinal Wall

This mucous membrane thinning, intestinal cell irritation and inflammatory immune response cause desmosomes and tight junctions to open. These gaps allow food macromolecules to enter the tissues.

The Inflammatory Process

Most people think of inflammation as bad. Especially when they hear that allergies involve inflammation.

Inflammation simply coordinates the various immune players into a frenzy of healing response. This is a good thing. Imagine for a moment cutting your finger pretty badly. First you would feel pain—letting you know the body is hurt. Second, you will probably notice that the area has become swollen and red. Blood starts to clot around the area. Soon the cut stops bleeding. The blood dries and a scab forms. It remains red, maybe a little hot, and hurts for a while. After the healing proceeds, soon the cut is closed up and there is a scab left with a little redness around it. The pain soon stops. The scab falls off and the finger returns to normal—almost like new and ready for action.

Without this inflammatory process, we might not even know we cut our finger in the first place. We might keep working, only to find out that we had bled out a quart of blood on the floor. Without clotting, it would be hard to stop the bleeding. And without some continuing pain, we would be more likely to keep injuring the same spot, preventing it from healing.

Were it not for our immune system and inflammatory process slowing blood flow, clotting the blood, scabbing and cleaning up the site, our bodies would simply be full of holes and wounds. Our bodies simply could not survive injury.

The probiotic system and immunoglobulin immune system work together to deter and kill particular invaders—hopefully before they gain access to the body's tissues. Should these defenses fail, they can stimulate the humoral immune system in a strategic attack that includes identifying antigens and recognizing their weaknesses. B-cells and probiotics coordinate through the stimulation of immunoglobulins and CDs.

This progression also stimulates an activation of neutrophils, phagocytes, immunoglobulins, leukotrienes and prostaglandins. Should cells become infected, they will signal the immune system from paracrines located on their cell membranes. Once the intrusion and strategy is determined, B-cells will surround the pathogens while T-cells attack any infected cells. Natural killer T-cells may secrete chemicals into infected cells, initiating the death of the cell.

Leukotrienes immediately gather in the region of injury or infection, and signal to T-cells to coordinate efforts in the process of repair. Prostaglandins initiate the widening of blood vessels to bring more T-cells and other repair factors (such as plasminogen and fibrin) to the infected or injured site. Histamine opens the blood vessel walls to allow all these healing agents access to the injury site to clean it up.

Prostaglandins also stimulate substance P within the nerve cells, initiating the sensation of pain. At the same time, thromboxanes, along with fibrin, drive the process of clotting and coagulation in the blood, while constricting certain blood vessels to decrease the risk of bleeding.

In the case where the pathogen is an allergen, the inflammation response will also accompany an H1-histamine response. As mentioned earlier, histamine is primarily produced by the mast cells, basophils and neutrophils after being stimulated by IgE antibodies. This opens blood vessels to tissues, which stimulates the processes of sneezing, watering of the eyes and coughing. These measures, though sometimes considered irritating, are all stimulated in an effort to remove the toxin and prevent its re-entry into the body. As histamine binds with receptors, one of the resulting physiological responses is alertness (also why antihistamines cause drowsiness). These are natural responses to help the body and mind remain vigilant in order to avoid further toxin intake.

At the height of the repair process, swelling, redness and pain are at their peak. The T-cells, macrophages, neutrophils, fibrin and plasmin all work together to purge the allergen from the body and repair the damage.

As macrophages continue the clean up, the other immune cells begin to retreat. Antioxidants like glutathione will attach to and transport the byproducts—broken down toxins and cell parts—out of the body. As this proceeds, prostaglandins, histamines and leukotrienes begin to signal a reversal of the inflammation and pain process.

One of the central features of the normalization process is the production of bradykinin. Bradykinin slows clotting and opens blood vessels, allowing the cleanup process to accelerate. A key signalling factor is the production of nitric oxide (NO). NO slows inflammation by promoting the detachment of lymphocytes to the site of infection or toxification, and reduces tissue swelling. NO also accelerates the clearing out of debris with its interaction with the superoxide anion. NO was originally described as endothelium-derived relaxing factor (or EDRF)—because of its role in relaxing blood vessel walls.

The body produces more nitric oxide in the presence of good nutrition and lower stress. Probiotics also play a big role in nitric oxide production in a healthy body. Lactobacilli such as *L. plantarum* have in fact been shown to remove the harmful nitrate molecule and use it to produce nitric oxide (Bengmark *et al.* 1998). This is beneficial to not only reducing inflammation: NO production also creates a balanced environment for increased tolerance.

Low nitric oxide levels also happen to be associated with a plethora of diseases, including diabetes, heart failure, high cholesterol, ulcerative colitis, premature aging, cancers and many others. Low or abnormal NO production is also seen among lifestyle habits such as smoking, obesity, and living around air pollution.

There is more to the food sensitivity process than simply an allergen being met by immunoglobulins and releasing histamine (as simplified by many health writers). The intestinal cells are often damaged first by other toxins, resulting in an inflammatory cascade. Once the intestine's cells are damaged, macromolecules/allergens can enter the system through the damaged intestinal wall.

Thus a food sensitivity is usually the result of two events: The first being an inflammatory process responding to an injury to the cells of the intestinal wall. These cells can be damaged by an assortment of toxins, poor dietary choices, microorganism pathogens, stress, smoking, alcohol, pharmaceuticals and toxins. Food macromolecules or allergens can also produce this damage to the cells of the intestinal walls.

Once the cells of the intestinal wall are damaged, the immune system will launch an inflammatory injury response through the T-cell system as described earlier. The T-cells will "repair" the problem by killing off these intestinal cells. This is often described as an autoimmune issue, but in reality, the T-cells are responding to real damage of toxins to these cells. They are not confusing "self" with "non-self."

While this damage and response is active, the intestinal cell wall barrier is altered. This alteration creates a problem called *increased intestinal permeability*. In an increased permeable condition, large food molecules (macromolecules) and/or allergens may enter the tissues and bloodstream, stimulating the IgE-histamine allergic immune response and/or other physiological and immune responses that produce food sensitivity symptoms.

The Hypersensitivity Response

There are four kinds of hypersensitivity responses within the body once an intruder gains access to the body: Type I, Type II, Type III and Type IV. These might sound very similar but they are actually quite different. Let's review these:

Type I: Immediate Hypersensitivity

This response occurs when IgE antibodies bind to food antigens. Food antigens include proteins, fatty acids, and polysaccharides among others. They may also be combined subparts of any food. When this binding between an antigen and IgE takes place, the bound IgE will typically set off the release of inflammatory mediators from mast/basophil/neutrophil white blood cells. These mediators include histamine, prostaglandins and leukotrienes. Depending upon the location and type of mast/basophil/ neutrophil cells, these mediators will spark an allergic response within the airways, sinuses, skin, joints and other locations. This kind of response will typically be immediate, within about two hours of ingestion of the offending food.

Type II: Cytotoxic Response

In this type of immune response, food antigens have penetrated the tissues, and the body responds to kill these cells. This typically takes place through an antigen binding to IgG or IgM immunoglobulins in a delayed immune response. This response can happen concurrently to other allergic responses; though it is still most often a delayed response.

Should the red blood cells be involved in the antigen absorption, hemolysis (the destruction of red blood cells) and anemia (a lack of red blood cells) may result.

Type III: Immune-Complex Response

Here the allergen-bound antibody complex actually penetrates cell tissues and injures them. This can occur within the intestinal cells, liver, or virtually anywhere around the body. In some instances these immune complexes can increase vascular permeability or intestinal permeability, as we've discussed.

This type of response is also often a delayed response, occurring hours or even a day or two after eating the offending food.

Sometimes the immune complexes will stimulate mast/basophil/neutrophil cell degranulation of histamine, prostaglandins and leukotrienes, and stimulate inflammation within the tissue system. This can result in a variety of conditions, which are sometimes attributed to autoimmunity.

Type IV: T-Cell Responses

This type of response is independent of other types of sensitivity. For example, the Type III may generate a T-cell response once the cell and tissue damage begins. But this Type IV occurs without the binding of an antigen by an antibody. In this response, a cell is directly affected by the allergen or food constituent. Conditions of colitis are typical of this type of response, because the antigen directly stimulates toxicity within the intestinal cells. Once the intestinal cells are damaged, T-cells launch an immune response to clear out the invaded cells. As mentioned, this response is also often attributed to autoimmunity. Rather it is an immune response to cellular toxicity.

This type of response will typically take from two to four days from exposure to response.

Other Responses

There are a variety of other types of immune responses to food that result in food sensitivity. A food may spark an inflammatory response by stimulating any number of inflammatory mediators, including prostaglandins, serotonin, platelet-aggregating factor, kinins and others. In these instances, any number of conditions may result.

To this we can add that some foods actually contain histamine, as we'll discuss later. These can sometimes stimulate an inflammatory response, especially among immunosuppressed people with hair-trigger immune systems.

While most of these different types of responses might relate to the body's immune system, most of them are not often referred to as a food allergy by physicians and researchers. Many refer only to the IgE form of allergen-antibody response (Type I) as a pure food allergy. The others sometimes are present in food allergies, but some are often simply food intolerances that have involved the immune system.

Furthermore, the **Type I** allergic response can be broken down into two stages: sensitization and elicitation.

Sensitization

The food molecule sensitization process takes place when a potential protein antigen happens to come into contact with a type of immune cell called a progenitor B-cell. As part of their immune system responsibilities, these B-cells will break apart the protein into smaller peptides. These will be attached to hystocompatibility complex class II complex molecules.

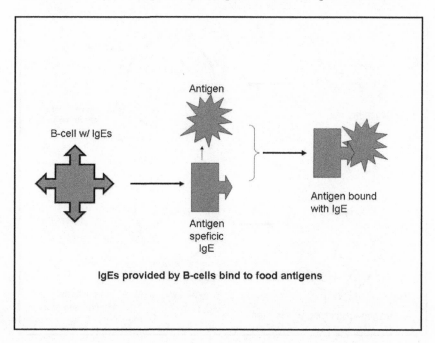

IgEs provided by B-cells bind to food antigens

The T-cell hystocompatibility complex is transferred onto the surface of the B-cell, which binds to a particular allergen. Once upon the B-cell surface, T-helper cells take notice of this foreign particle stuck to the B-cell. The T-helper cell cytokine CD4 receptors trigger a response, and this stimulates the production of the IgE immunoglobulins. These particular IgE immunoglobulins are now sensitized to the particular epitope of the antigen in the future.

Elicitation

Once sensitized, the IgE associates with the specific IgE receptors that lie on the surface of the neutrophil, basophil or mast cells. Within these cells are packages called granules.

The granules are stock full of a variety of inflammatory mediators. The most notorious of these in food allergies is histamine as we've been discussing. As the allergen-specific IgEs connect with the IgE receptors on these immune cells, the immune cells will release the inflammatory mediators such as histamine and leukotrienes into the bloodstream and lymph. This is what drives much of the symptoms of an allergic attack, including but not limited to hives, asthma, uritica, sinusitis and others.

The below diagram illustrates elicitation:

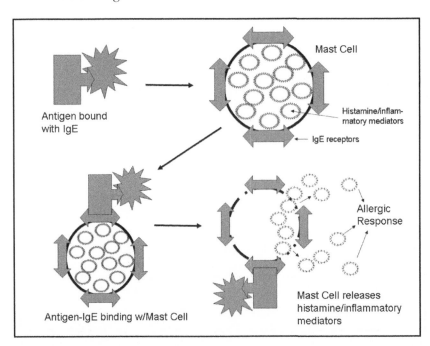

The Role of Probiotics in Immune Response

Probiotics play a critical role in many of the processes of the immune system described in this chapter. They also temper and balance the immune response so that the body responds in less allergic fashion. Let's discuss some of the science that illustrates the important role probiotics play in the immune system:

Probiotics tend to increase IgA responses within the intestines and reduce the IgE allergic response. Finnish scientists (Ouwehand *et al.* 2009) gave healthy elderly volunteers *Lactobacillus acidophilus* or a placebo. Immune factors were tested, and the probiotics had modulated their IgA and PGE2 levels. They also observed improved spermidine levels—an enzyme involved in DNA synthesis. The researchers concluded that these improvements suggested increased mucosal and intestinal immunity among the probiotic group.

Researchers from the Teikyo University School of Medicine in Japan (Araki *et al.* 1999) gave *Bifidobacterium breve* YIT4064 or placebo to 19 infants for 28 days. IgA levels significantly increased among the probiotic group.

In a study of 105 pregnant women, University of Western Australia scientists (Prescott *et al.* 2008) found that *Lactobacillus rhamnosus* and *Bifidobacterium lactis* stimulated higher levels of cytokine IFN-gamma, higher levels of TGF-beta1, and higher levels of breast milk IgA. Plasma of their babies had lower CD14 levels, and greater CB IFN-gamma levels. These indicated that the probiotics strengthened immunity and moderated hypersensitivity.

Researchers from the Turku University Central Hospital in Finland (Rinne *et al.* 2005) gave 96 mothers either a placebo or *Lactobacillus rhamnosus* GG before delivery and continued the supplementation in their infants after delivery. At three months of age, immunoglobulin IgG-secreting cells among breastfed infants supplemented with probiotics were significantly higher than the breastfed infants who received the placebo. In addition, the non-hypersensitivity IgM-, IgA-, and IgG-secreting cell counts at 12 months were significantly higher among the breastfed infants who supplemented with probiotics, compared to the breastfed infants receiving the placebo.

Probiotics help modulate the inflammatory processes. In research from Poland's Pomeranian Academy of Medicine (Naruszewicz *et al.* 2002), scientists found that giving *Lactobacillus plantarum* 299v to 36 volunteers resulted in a 37% decrease in inflammatory F2-isoprostanes. Isoprostanes are similar to prostaglandins, formed outside of the COX process.

Probiotics also stimulate a healthy thymus gland. Illustrating this, medical researchers from the University of Bari (Indrio *et al.* 2007) gave a placebo or a probiotic combination of *Bifidobacterium breve* C50 and *Strepto-*

coccus thermophilus 065 to 60 newborns. The thymus glands of the probiotic group was significantly larger compared to babies that consumed the standard (placebo) formula.

Scientists from the Nagoya University Graduate School of Medicine (Sugawara *et al.* 2006) found in a study of 101 patients that supplementation with probiotics increased NK activity and lymphocyte counts. Proinflammatory IL-6 cytokines also decreased significantly among the probiotic group. Serum IL-6, white blood cell counts, and C-reactive protein also significantly decreased among the probiotic group.

Furthermore, probiotics have the ability to *uniquely* modify cytokines depending upon the condition and disease of the person. Illustrating this, a probiotic drink with either placebo or a probiotic combination of *Lactobacillus paracasei* Lpc-37, *Lactobacillus acidophilus* 74-2 and *Bifidobacterium animalis* subsp. *lactis* DGCC 420 (*B. lactis* 420) was given to 15 healthy adults and 15 adults with atopic dermatitis. After eight weeks, CD57(+) cytokines levels increased significantly among the healthy group taking probiotics, while CD4(+)CD54(+) cytokines decreased significantly among the atopic patients who were taking the probiotics, compared with the placebo group and compared to the levels at the beginning of the trial (Roessler *et al.* 2008).

In another study, researchers from Poland's Pomeranian Academy of Medicine (Naruszewicz *et al.* 2002) gave *Lactobacillus plantarum* 299v or placebo to 36 healthy volunteers for six weeks. Monocytes isolated from probiotic subjects had significantly reduced adhesion to endothelial cells, and the probiotic group had a 42% reduction in pro-inflammatory cytokine interleukin-6. No changes were observed among the placebo group.

Probiotics are often involved in the production of intermediary fatty acids used for LOX and COX enzyme conversions, producing anti-inflammatory effects. To illustrate this, scientists from the University of Helsinki (Kekkonen *et al.* 2008) measured lipids and inflammation markers before and after giving probiotic *Lactobacillus rhamnosus* GG to 26 healthy adults. After three weeks of probiotic supplementation, the subjects had decreased levels of intermediary inflammatory fatty acids such as lysophosphatidylcholines, sphingomyelins, and several glycerophosphatidylcholines. Probiotics also reduced hyper-inflammatory markers TNF-alpha and CRP in this study.

The bottom line is that our body's probiotics and our immune system are interconnected. They are inseparable. At least 70% of the immune system *is* probiotic. Consider this carefully: If the intestine's probiotics were decimated by either a lethal bacteria infection or a course of antibiotics, *we would lose nearly three quarters of our gut's immune system.*

Chapter Three

Specific Food Sensitivities

Food sensitivities are highly variable. They can start as a sensitivity to one food, and another sensitivity may develop later. Many children develop a food allergy as an infant and outgrow it within a few years. Or a person can be sensitized to a food as a child and—given no later immune modulation—that allergy may follow them for much of their lives. Or an adult may develop a food sensitivity without warning.

Food sensitivities are variable because our immune systems are variable. Our immune system may be have provided us with a strong defense for most of our lives, and then suddenly break down and become vulnerable for a host of reasons. Or we may be born with or develop a weakened immune system for any number of reasons, as we'll discuss further in the next chapter.

Research discussed in the first chapter indicates that the type of allergy we get is likely to reflect the typical diet of our family or shared cultural diet of the society in which we live. Among Western diets, allergies tend to be to milk, eggs, fish, shellfish, and peanuts. Seafood allergies are more prevalent in societies that eat more fish and shellfish. In societies that drink more milk (such as Northern Europe), dairy allergies dominate. In Southern European countries that tend to consume more fruits and vegetables, there are more allergies to these foods—although their food allergy rates are significantly lower than Northern European countries.

Let's review some of the different foods that people become sensitive to. This is not a compendium on each type of sensitivity, but this information can give an allergy sufferer some insight into some of the who's, what's and when's. In some cases, the research presents causative issues. We will discuss causes of food sensitivities with more detail in the next chapter. For now, let's get to know some of the facts that food sensitivity research has unveiled.

Milk

Milk contains three principle parts: whey, butterfat and milk solids. The whey is the major protein component, while the butterfat contains a variety of different fatty acids, including butyric acid, palmitic acid, myristic acid, stearic acid, caproic acid, oleic acid, conjugated linolenic acid and linoleic acid (Månsson 2008). Milk solids will also contain proteins, together with various sugars such as lactose.

As we'll discuss in detail, the proteins casein and beta-lactoglobulin are the primarily allergens in milk. Meanwhile, lactose is the primary cause for milk intolerance.

About 2.5% of young infants among industrialized countries have allergies to cow's milk. This number also is closely reflected in the United States (Schouten *et al.* 2010). University of Helsinki researchers (Salmi *et al.* 2010) found that cow's milk allergy is the most common form of food allergy in Finland.

Cow's milk allergy and intolerance is often short-lived. In a study by researchers from the Pediatric Allergy Clinic at the Coimbra Pediatric Hospital (Santos *et al.* 2007), 139 children who were either intolerant to milk or IgE-allergic to milk were studied. Case reporting revealed that 34% of the children became tolerant by two years of age. Fifty-five percent were tolerant by age five. Sixty-eight percent were tolerant of milk by the age of ten. Among children with IgE-mediated milk allergies, the tolerance was 0% at two years, 22% at five years and 43% at ten years old.

Medical researchers from Rome's University La Sapienza (Cantani and Micera 2004) studied 115 infants with milk allergies. The researchers followed food-allergic children after an average age of six months, for up to eight years. They found that the average age for becoming tolerant to cow's milk was seven years and 11 months. However, during those years, many of the children, whether they became tolerant or not, developed other, sometimes multiple allergies. Of the total, 57% achieved tolerance of food allergens in the end. Disturbingly, asthma later occurred in 54% of the early-allergic children—many by then tolerant of milk.

Note also that the researchers also determined that most children are not born with milk allergies. Rather, milk allergies usually appear within the first few months after birth, and sometimes even later.

Spanish researchers (Sanz Ortega *et al.* 2001) followed 1,663 breast-fed newborns for a year after birth. They confirmed that 0.36% had milk allergies. The first reaction typically occurred within a week after milk formula was introduced. They also determined that among infants of allergic mothers, the risk of developing an allergy to milk rose over ten times, from .36% to 3.8%.

The body begins to set up its tolerance to some milk proteins from birth. Finnish researchers (Kuitunen and Savilahti 1995) measured IgA antibodies for cow's milk in the saliva, feces and blood of 20 term and 20 preterm infants for eight months after birth. All the infants had IgA for cow's milk in their saliva within the first week after birth. The IgA levels peaked at one month, and decreased until three months, and stabilized after that. Normal term infants had more IgA than preterm infants. There was no difference in IgA between infants who were breastfed from cow's milk-fed infants, however.

Research from Finland's National Institute for Health and Welfare (Metsälä *et al.* 2010) found that of all children born between 1996 and 2004 in Finland, 16,237 children were diagnosed with milk allergies by 2006. Cesarean section increased the risk of cow's milk allergies by 18%. Mothers being over 35 increased the risk by 23%. On the other hand, low socioeconomic status, several previous children and multiple pregnancies significantly decreased the risk of the child having milk allergies.

Researchers from Portugal's Coimbra Pediatric Hospital (Santos *et al.* 2010) studied milk-allergic children in under-two-year-olds at their Pediatric Allergy Clinic between 1997 and 2006. Among the 139 children tested, 74% suffered from more than one symptom. Fifty-one percent had multiple organs involved in the allergy. Eighty-one percent had skin rashes or other skin irritations. Fifty-five percent had gastrointestinal issues. Sixteen percent had respiratory symptoms. Three percent had anaphylaxis reactions. Over time, 32% developed asthma, 20% developed eczema and 20% developed rhinoconjunctivitis. Nineteen percent of the children developed other food allergies over time.

While wheezing and skin rashes are prevalent, other symptoms of milk allergy are often overlooked. Acid reflux is one example. Researchers from Denmark's University of Southern Denmark (Nielsen *et al.* 2004) studied 42 patients with cow's milk allergies. Eighteen of the 42 had severe acid reflux (GERD).

Helsinki University Central Hospital researchers (Suomalainen and Isolauri 1994) found that IFN-gamma levels were low in active milk allergy but higher among those who were recovering from milk allergies. After over a year on a milk elimination diet, IgA response to milk had increased among those who became tolerant to milk.

A variety of research has confirmed that casein and beta-lactoglobulin (beta-LG) are the major allergens related to cow's milk allergies.

Japanese researchers (Nakano *et al.* 2010) found that casein and beta-lactoglobulin were the main allergens in cow's milk. They also found that 97% of 115 milk allergy children had casein-specific IgE antibodies, while 47% had IgE antibodies against beta-lactoglobulin (beta-LG).

Oslo researchers (Sletten *et al.* 2006) determined that beta-LG is resistant to enzymatic breakdown. This makes it available for non-immunoglobulin-mediated gastrointestinal symptoms should it be presented to intestinal tissues and bloodstream. Patients tested for serum levels of beta-LG IgG and IgE levels were found to also have delayed gastrointestinal food sensitivity symptoms.

The LG-immunoglobulins in the study above were about 40 times lower in milk-tolerant people when compared to allergic patients. This was accompanied by a 90-fold increase in IgA-dominated immune responses in tolerant persons as compared with active allergy patients. This of course means that those who are tolerant of milk still respond to the beta-LG molecule. They simply respond differently (without a hypersensitivity response) than those with active allergies. Milk-tolerant people respond with more mucosal membrane-IgA response initially—keeping beta-LG from invading the body.

This, by the way, is the normal way to respond to molecules that are not considered nutritious to the body. There are innumerable molecules like this in every meal. Our bodies respond quite normally, by simply preventing their inclusion into our tissues.

Italian researchers (Paganelli *et al.* 1985) found beta-lactoglobulin-specific antibodies within the blood of patients with ulcerative colitis and Crohn's disease. The IgG and IgM antibodies to beta-LG were found to be significantly higher as compared with non-allergic individuals. This indicated a prior immune system issue with beta-LG.

Researchers from the University of Helsinki (Salmi *et al.* 2010) studied the urinary concentrations of 37 organic acids in 35 infants under one years of age who had atopic eczema. Sixteen of the infants also had diagnosed milk allergies. The milk allergy infants had different urinary levels of hydroxybutyrate, adipate, isocitrate, homovanillate, suberate, tartarate, 3-indoleacetate and 5-hydroxyindoleacetate. This of course indicates that milk-allergic children metabolize milk components substantially differently. This points to differences within the intestinal probiotic content, the health of the intestinal wall, and the health of the liver.

Eggs

Egg allergies are the second-most prevalent allergy in most Western countries. They occur primarily among children, but also occur among adults. Egg allergies typically involve the OVO proteins ovomucoid, ovotransferrin, ovomucoid, or apovitillin, vosvetin, livetin, and/or ovalbumin.

Australian researchers (Palmer *et al.* 2005) found that when lactating mothers ate cooked eggs, OVO concentrations within their breast milk increased substantially. The researchers concluded that this was the primary pathway for egg allergy development among infants who contract egg allergies prior to eating any eggs.

Furthermore, it is difficult to differentiate between egg protein allergens and chicken protein allergens. This is not surprising, since eggs are essentially the fetuses of unhatched chickens. This is confirmed by testing with the DNA-based PCR method of protein analysis, which cannot distinguish egg protein from chicken meat protein (Lee and Kim 2010).

In addition, researchers (Swiderska-Kiełbik *et al.* 2010) have found that people regularly exposed to birds—which include zoo keepers, pet shop workers, food industry employees and even pet bird keepers—have an increased risk of allergies to feathers, egg proteins, latex and disinfectant allergies.

Contrary to what many believe, egg whites also contain egg allergens. Researchers from South Korea's Chung-Ang University's College of Pharmacy (Lee and Kim 2010) tested various products for egg allergens, and found the same allergens among egg whites, egg yolks, ovomucoid, alpha-livetin, ovalbumin, votransferrin, and lysozyme portions of eggs.

Asthma symptoms are prevalent among egg allergies. Researchers from Malaysia's Kebangsaan University (Yusoff *et al.* 2004) found that the removal of eggs and milk significantly improved wheezing symptoms and lung function of 22 asthmatic children.

Wheat and Grains

Despite its reference, gluten is not a single protein. It is better described as a category of proteins. Rather, the proteins in wheat are primarily either gliadins or glutenins. Within these two types are many different specific proteins. Furthermore, the types of glutinous proteins in wheat are not like the glutinous proteins in most other grains. In fact, between these two types, gliadins are considered the most prevalent allergen—common in both baker's asthma and wheat allergies (Ueno *et al.* 2010).

There also many other possible wheat allergens. They include alpha-amylase inhibitor, peroxidase, thaumatin-like protein (TLP) and lipid transfer protein 2G (LTP2G) and low-molecular-weight glutenins. These allergens are heat resistant and do not readily cross-react with grass pollen allergens (Pastorello *et al.* 2007).

Noting this, it appears the reason why people react to proteins in wheat and other grains is through cross-reactivity among similar strings of amino acids, called peptides. While the full proteins (complex strings of hundreds of amino acids will be different between wheat, barley and oats, for example, they will share similar peptide strings. These are also sometimes referred to as protein fractions.

French researchers (Bodinier *et al.* 2007) found that hydrolyzed omega5-gliadin fractions and lipid transfer proteins were detected within the epithelial layers after wheat consumption. We've discussed the repercussions of macromolecule intestinal wall contact in the previous chapter, and we'll dig into this topic further later.

These common protein fractions may be present in wheat, rye and barley. They may also be (depending upon the sensitivity) present in oats, corn and rice. However, these latter three grains have significantly-different protein fractions, so it is less likely that a wheat sensitivity will cross over to oats, rice and corn.

However, a full carryover of gliadin or glutenin sensitivity may leave one sensitive to foods that use wheat proteins such as blue cheese, bouillon cubes, chocolate, curry, food colorings, starches, grain alcohols (including beer, ale, rye, scotch, bourbon or grain vodka), gum base, hydrolyzed vegetable protein, malts, marshmallows, modified food starches, monosodium glutamates, non-dairy creamers, processed meats, pudding, wheat/soy sauce, and even distilled vinegars.

This of course significantly changes the perspective that most people have as they consider "gluten sensitivities." In fact, gluten-free is somewhat of a misnomer, because nearly every grain elevator and trucking company transports or holds a variety of grains, which include those fractions considered "glutens." In these facilities, there is a strong likelihood of cross-contamination between grain proteins because the same bins and trucks will shift variably from one type of grain to another.

This doesn't mean that there aren't facilities dedicated to non-gluten-type protein grains. These may not mix bins and may carefully wash trucks. However, the risk of cross-contamination is still there, because grains can also cross-pollinate via the wind.

Thus practically any grain can have some level of a crossover protein fraction. Some grains will certainly have less, albeit. But it is a very hard road to hoe, as it were.

For example, in a study published in the *Journal of the American Dietetic Association* (Thompson *et al.* 2010), 22 grains, seeds, and flours that were supposedly inherently gluten-free (but not labeled gluten-free)—including flours from sorghum, buckwheat and millet—were analyzed for gluten-type protein fraction content in a laboratory in June of 2009. The lab found that nine of the 22, or 41% of the supposedly gluten-free samples contained more than the limit considered as quantification for gluten-free, of five ppm (parts per million). In addition, seven of the 22 samples, or 32%, contained gluten levels that averaged more than 20 ppm. Under the FDA's proposed rule for gluten-free labels, these would not qualify to be labeled as "gluten-free."

The Food Allergen Labeling and Consumer Protection Act (FALCPA) took effect in January 1, 2006. This act, passed in 2004, says that food labels from products that contain one or more of the major food allergens must state the allergen either on the ingredient panel or elsewhere on the label in plain English. The major allergens in the law include milk, eggs, fish, shellfish, peanuts, tree nuts, wheat and soy.

Certainly other foods can be allergenic outside of these. It is therefore assumed that ingredients are clearly stated on the ingredient panel. This is not always the case, however. Many ingredients will contain known allergens without the allergen being listed. This of course presents a very complex situation for food processors, because the list of food allergens has been growing significantly over the past few years.

The Food Allergen and Consumer Protection Act is also being updated for gluten-free products. Within the language of the currently proposed rule, many foods are considered gluten-free. Millet is a good example. However, a millet label cannot, under the rule, be labeled as "gluten free" without stating that all millet foods are inherently gluten-free. For example: "all millet is gluten free." In addition, the limit for being able to describe the product as gluten-free under the new ruling is 20 parts per million.

Liquid chromatography-mass spectrometry (LC-MS) based assays, and the enzyme-linked immunosorbent assays (ELISAs) are the best methods of analyzing grain foods for their gluten or allergen content.

Spanish researchers (Palacin *et al.* 2010) found that wheat allergies are rising. They also found that the wheat flour lipid transfer protein (LTP) Tri a14 appears to be the key allergen responsible for baker's asthma and wheat sensitivities among their test population. And because cross-reactivity is common among the LTPs, there is often a transference between asthmatic bakers so that they become allergic to eating bread at some point. This has been termed *LTP syndrome*. The researchers confirmed this effect among eight adults who suffered from anaphylaxis after eating wheat foods.

Many children with wheat allergies become tolerant as they get older. In the Cantani and Micera study mentioned earlier, the average age for becoming tolerant to wheat was seven years and two months.

Celiac Disease

Celiac disease occurs among both infants and adults, and often among Caucasians. It is characterized by scarred lesions (sprue) and inflammation within the small intestines, which produce a variety of symptoms.

While many pathology texts estimate that celiac appears in about one in about 5,000 people, real incidence is higher. Researchers from the University of Maryland School of Medicine (Fasano *et al.* 2003) found in a blood screening of celiac antibodies of 13,145 people that one in 113 people in the U.S. may suffer from celiac disease.

Furthermore, recent ELISA testing has offered the possibility that about one of 100 are now celiac (Leffler and Schuppan 2010).

Another recent study (Rubio-Tapia *et al.* 2009) illustrated that celiac disease has increased by four to five times over the past fifty years.

It is important to note the variance with celiac disease around the world. Among Europeans, the high portion of the range occurs in Western Ireland. However, celiac disease occurs rarely among African and Asian countries (Laghi *et al.* 2003).

Why is this? Is this only genetics?

Celiac disease is considered an autoimmune disorder, although many also consider it hereditary. Genetic predisposition aggravated by epigenetic variables including diet and local environment are more likely. (See the genetic section in the next chapter.) This is because celiac mechanisms are comparable to the inflammatory intestinal response that takes place in other food sensitivities. This response is seen in lesions along the villi and walls of the small intestines. These of course, derange nutrient absorption and produce a variety of metabolic symptoms around the body caused by macromolecules entering the bloodstream and tissues.

Celiac sprue are the inflamed and damaged epithelial cells inside the intestines. They are often worse in the jejunum. The cells become flattened, and this will deform the villi. The intestinal wall will also often become thickened, and be teeming with a variety of immune cells, cytokines and plasma cells.

This is also consistent with the fact that the symptoms of celiac disease are extremely variable. They can range from weight loss, fatigue, diarrhea, flatulence, irritable bowels, malabsorption issues (nutrient deficiencies) and so many others. Upon examination, celiac patients may have high cholesterol, anemia, hypocalcaemia, high albumin levels, blood clotting issues and elevated liver enzymes. Gluten ataxia may also result. This can cause disorientation, headaches, fevers and other issues.

The genetic link in some celiac sufferers has been seen in the HLA class II D-region of chromosome 6 in the DNA. However, it has been estimated that about 90-95% of sufferers have genetic markers for celiac disease haplotypes (Heap and van Heel 2009). Yet we know from epigenetics that those genes will still have to be switched on. How might this happen? Through choices related to consumption, environment and lifestyle, as we'll discuss further.

Adults can contract celiac disease at any age. The middle ages are most prevalent. This poses the question of why the late onset if the disease is hereditary? Celiac disease also occurs among children during the first three years of life, but typically after the first year. The symptoms will often include ongoing diarrhea, slow growth and a large belly. These symptoms might go away during the teenage years. Adults might suffer severe weight loss and nutrient absorption problems, which can in result in bone loss, rickets, osteoporosis, eye problems, hormone disruption, seizures, ataxia and infertility. Worse, celiac disease increases the risk of stomach cancer, intestinal cancer or lymphoma by forty to one hundred times. Celiac children also have an increased risk of Down's syndrome. Nutrient deficiencies and their symptoms are common among celiac patients, and depression is also prevalent.

ELISA-derived tests for gliadin-specific IgA, IgG and antigliadin antibodies (AGAs) are often signs for celiac disease. AGAs will not be present during a gluten elimination diet, however.

Peanuts

Peanuts are not nuts. Really. Peanuts are actually legumes. They are closer relatives to beans and roots than they are to nuts, which typically grow on trees.

Peanut allergies are primarily a concern among developed countries of the Western world. Major studies have shown that developing countries exhibit far less prevalence of peanut allergies among these populations (Yang 2010).

Researchers from France's Allergology University Hospital (Morisset *et al.* 2005) calculated that peanut allergies are one of the most prevalent food allergies among Western countries, and third or fourth in prevalence in the U.S., the U.K. and Canada. In these countries, peanut allergy rates range from about 0.8% to 1.5% of the population. This calculates to nearly 20% of all food allergies in these countries.

This research also found that the peanut allergy rate in France was between 1% and 2.5% of the French population—the highest rate globally.

Furthermore, peanut allergy rates have been rising dramatically. In a study mentioned earlier, researchers working with the David Hide Asthma and Allergy Research Centre and St. Mary's Hospital on the Isle of Wight (Venter *et al.* 2010) studied the incidence of peanut allergies between 1994 and 2004 in thousands of children. The first group, born in 1989, were reviewed at four years old. The second group, born between 1994 and 1996 were reviewed between three and four years old. The third group, born between 2001 and 2002, were studied at three years old. Peanut sensitization levels increased from 1.3% in the first group to 3.3% in the second group. In the third group, sensitization to peanuts reduced to 2.0%. Peanut allergies were 0.5%, 1.4% and 1.2% respectively among the three groups. It should be noted that peanut allergies often occur between three and four years old, so the third group would still represent significant growth from the second group, as the second group included four year olds while the third group did not.

Peanuts are one of the most severe allergies. Researchers from the Alfred I. duPont Hospital for Children in Wilmington, Delaware (Simpson AB *et al.* 2010) studied children with peanut allergies older than three years old. They found that children with peanut allergies had more than double the chance of hospitalization than other children, and 1.6-times the risk of being prescribed systemic steroids. They also found that peanut allergies are often a predictive factor for having asthma and even dying from asthma.

Other researchers have estimated that severe reactions to peanut allergies affect about 1% of Americans, and comprise the majority of severe food reactions (Nielsen and Lindsey 2010).

At the same time, research has illustrated that about 20% of young people with peanut allergies outgrow them. On the other hand, about 8% of those who outgrow a peanut allergy experience a recurrence. This is more significant among those who completely abstain from eating peanuts or only rarely eat them. Several studies have shown that a recurrence is less likely among those who consistently eat at least small amounts of peanuts periodically (Byrne *et al.* 2010).

The proteins in peanuts most known to cause allergies are the Ara protein epitopes. Specific IgE and IgG antibody levels (PN-IgE and PN-IgG) are prominent in most peanut allergies. Researchers from the University Medical Center in Utrecht, The Netherlands (Flinterman *et al.* 2007) tested 20 peanut allergy children between the ages three and fifteen years old. IgE reactions were to the peanut proteins Ara h1, Ara h2, Ara h3 and Ara h6. Sixteen of the children had IgE reactions to Ara h2 and Ara h6 proteins, and 10 children had IgE reactions to Ara h1 and Ara h3.

The Ara h8 protein was the main peanut allergen in research from Zurich's University Hospital (Mittag *et al.* 2004). Ara h8-specific IgE antibodies were found in 85% of 17 peanut allergy patients.

However, UK researchers (Lewis *et al.* 2005) found that in studies of 40 peanut allergy sufferers that IgE binding and subsequent allergic response can also occur with multiple peanut proteins.

More importantly, they also found that the Ara h8 protein becomes unstable in roasting and during gastric digestion. In some patients, however, Ara h8 histamine release is mitigated by the birch allergen protein, Bet v1.

Research shows that the large increase in peanut allergies coincided with the mass distribution of roasted peanuts in the 80s and 90s. We will discuss peanut roasting in more detail in the next chapter.

This may also be one of the reasons some of the research on peanuts is confusing. A review of research by the British Nutrition Foundation (Thompson *et al.* 2010) evaluated the effects of exposure to peanuts and eventual peanut allergy during the maternal years and beyond. While the research was sometimes confounding, it suggested that lower peanut consumption during childhood can lead to peanut sensitivity while higher consumption can lead to tolerance.

As with eggs, many children have peanut allergies though they have not eaten any peanuts yet. Others have peanut allergies when they just begin to eat peanuts. How do these children contract their allergies if they have yet to be exposed to them?

Researchers from Montreal's Immunology-Allergy Department at Sainte-Justine's Hospital (DesRoches *et al.* 2010) tested 403 infants with peanut allergies under the age of 18 months, together with their mothers. Their focus was on exposure: How did the child gain exposure? Was it from the home? Or possibly from the mother or her breast milk?

They found that infants with mothers who consumed more peanuts during breastfeeding were over four times more likely to have peanut allergies than infants with mothers who did not eat peanuts during breast-feeding. They also found that mothers of infants with peanut allergies were over twice as likely to eat more peanuts during pregnancy as mothers of non-allergic children. Outside of this exposure from their mother, the peanut-allergic children were no more exposed to peanuts in their environments than were the non-allergic children.

Contrary to the fear of incidental peanut exposures, allergic responses from casual inhalation of peanut fumes or skin is quite rare. Illustrating this, researchers at New York's Mount Sinai School of Medicine (Simonte *et al.* 2003) tested 30 children with peanut allergies with peanut skin contact and inhalation of peanut butter fumes to gauge their responses. None of the children experienced a systemic reaction or a respiratory reaction to either tests. In the skin contact tests, three children had slight skin redness and five children had slight itch without redness, and two of the children had minor weal reactions. The researchers concluded that, *"90% of highly sensitive children with peanut allergy would not experience a systemic-respiratory reaction from casual exposure to peanut butter."* They also said: *"Casual exposure to peanut butter is unlikely to elicit significant allergic reactions."*

French researchers (Rimbaud *et al.* 2010) developed a model of calculating the risk of incidental allergen food reactions as a result of contami-

nation during food processing. Using second-order Monte Carlo simula-
tions, they determined that peanut allergens occur in about 36% of
chocolates. The amount of allergen renders an average exposure of 0.2
mg of peanut proteins per average chocolate eating session. This concluded a risk of reaction of about 0.57% per chocolate eating occasion
(or one in 175), among peanut-allergic adults.

Lupin and other legume sensitivities are often seen in those with peanut allergies—including peanut (Hieta *et al.* 2010).

Tree Nuts

While real nuts all grow on trees, most people refer to nuts as tree
nuts to avoid any confusion with peanuts. That said, nut sensitivities typically appear later than most other sensitivities. Nut allergies also tend to
have a high risk of anaphylaxis. A good number of nut allergy sufferers
will also be allergic to more than one nut. Crossover allergies between
nuts and peanuts are less likely, but they do happen. Still, many allergy
specialists will say that having a peanut allergy increases the risk of nut
allergies; yet this is confounded by the fact that having any food allergy
increases the risk of having multiple food allergies.

Walnuts

The two allergens thought to cause most walnut allergies are 2S albumin and vicilin-like protein.

However, Italian researchers (Pastorello *et al.* 2004) studied 46 people
with walnut sensitivities, and found that the allergens that caused sensitization were 9-kd lipid transfer protein—which affected 37 patients—and
two vicilin proteins. Interestingly, the IgE response to walnut LTP was
halted by LTP from peaches.

Cashews

Among cashew nut allergy sufferers, French researchers (Rancé *et al.*
2003) found that the average age of diagnosis was 2.7 years old. Out of
these only one in five, or 12% were exposed to nuts prior to their diagnosis. They also found that 56% suffered from skin symptoms. A quarter
had respiratory issues and 17% had digestion issues. Many also had food
allergies for other nuts, eggs, mustard, shrimp and milk.

Pistachios

The same researchers found that nearly one-third of those children
allergic to cashews are also allergic to pistachios—which belong to the
same botanical family as cashews.

Manganese Superoxide Dismutase (MnSOD) may be the allergen most responsible for allergic responses to pistachios, however. Iranian researchers (Noorbakhsh *et al.* 2010) found that MnSOD had the greatest potential for cross-reactivity as well.

Hazelnuts

Hazelnut's allergens include homologues to Bet v1 and Bet v2 proteins, a sucrose-binding protein, a legumin, a 2S albumin, and a lipid transfer protein.

Research has confirmed that those allergic to hazelnuts are most sensitive to lipid transfer proteins rCor a1.04, rCor a2, rCor a8 and rCor a11. Spanish researchers (Hansen *et al.* 2009) also found that where a person lived often determined which type of LTP the person was allergic to. In other words, Italians and Spaniards were allergic to different LTPs than most of the Swiss or Danish allergic subjects.

Furthermore, some sufferers of hazelnut allergies are not allergic to roasted hazelnuts. Researchers from Denmark's National University Hospital (Hansen *et al.* 2003) found that roasting hazelnuts reduced their allergenicity for majority of cases. They tested 17 confirmed hazelnut food allergy sufferers with roasted hazelnuts, and found that twelve were not sensitive to roasted hazelnuts. However, five of the 17 tested sensitive to the roasted nuts. That is still significant enough to be concerned.

Seeds

Seed allergies are quite rare. Sesame seed allergies are probably the most known, but are still rare. Sensitivities to other seeds such as flax and rapeseed, are even more rare, but do occur.

Sesame Seeds

Sesame seed sensitivities seem to be growing, however. The average age of occurrence is at one years old. As in many allergies, skin rashes, digestive issues and respiratory difficulties are seen the most in sesame seed allergy sufferers. Many sesame allergies will also continue long after childhood (Cohen *et al.* 2007).

Researchers from the Ambroise Paré Hospital (Agne *et al.* 2004) studied 14 children with sesame seed allergies from three allergy centers in France. They found that the average age of allergy contraction was five years old, with 16 years being the oldest. Inflammation occurred among 48%, skin eruption among 27% and vomiting, rhinitis, conjunctivitis, asthma and/or anaphylactic shock also occurred among some. Only three of the 14 patients outgrew their sesame allergies.

Research from the Children's Hospital in Boston (Stutius *et al.* 2010) has shown that children with peanut and tree nut allergies have an increased risk of sesame seed sensitivities.

Flax

Flax sensitivity is fairly rare, but it is growing. Recent French research from the Biologie Moléculaire Laboratory in Nancy, France (Fremont *et al.* 2010) has indicated that among allergy sufferers, flax allergy exists in about 6%. In testing 1,317 people, they found some cross-reactivity of flax sensitivity with peanut, soybeans, rapeseeds, lupine and wheat. They surmised that cross-reactivity with these other seeds was possible.

As we'll discuss more later, these researchers also found that flax sensitivity seems to be growing with the increased distribution of milled and extruded flax.

Soy

The Gly m4 protein is considered soy's central allergen. However, the content of the soy allergen Gly m4 in soy foods depends on the amount and type of processing, and whether it has been fermented. Fermenting reduces Gly m4 levels. This means that someone allergic to soy flour or raw soybeans may not be very sensitive to tempeh or tofu.

This said, soy and a number of other beans also contain a particularly difficult saccharide called raffinose. Many people who are intolerant of soy cannot digest this saccharide well. Raffinose requires a special enzyme termed by some as raffinase, but its more technical name is alpha-galactosidase. Alpha-galactosidase is not produced by the human body.

However, alpha-galactosidase *is* produced by probiotic bacteria. For this reason, a person with healthy colonies of probiotic bacteria in their intestines should have no problem breaking down raffinose into sucrose and galactose. We should also note that other foods, such as broccoli, beans, cabbage and Brussels sprouts also contain raffinose.

Another complex saccharide in soybeans is stachyose. Stachyose contains similar properties as raffinose. Broccoli, Brussels sprouts, cabbage and other plant foods contain stachyose as well.

Alternatively, the probiotics used to produce fermented soy foods will also break down much of the raffinose and stachyose. See the section on fermented foods in the last chapter.

The incomplete breakdown of raffinose from beans into sucrose and galactose also has an interesting byproduct: flatulence. Many choose to add alpha-galactosidase with over-the-counter supplement solutions. Supplementing with probiotics is another possible strategy.

Back to soy allergies. Swiss researchers (Ballmer-Weber *et al.* 2007) have found that only 10 mg to 50 grams of soy will produce symptoms recognized by the allergic person. They also showed that it would take from 454 mg to 50 grams of soy to produce "objective symptoms" (symptoms recognizable by health professionals). This number decreases dramatically when soy isolates are considered.

Researchers from Johns Hopkins University School of Medicine (Savage *et al.* 2010) studied soy allergies among 133 soy-allergic patients. Of the 133, 64% had asthma, 71% had allergic rhinitis and 85% had atopic dermatitis. A full 88% also had peanut allergies. The average age of occurrence was one year old and ranged from two months to 17 years old. The average follow-up period was five years, but ranged from one to 19 years. The researchers calculated resolution of soy allergies at 25% of the children by four years old, 45% by six years old, and 69% resolution by age ten years old. Their model calculated that by the age of seven, about half of soy-allergy children will have outgrown their soy allergies.

It also should be noted that IgE sensitization to soy is rare, and particularly rare during early infancy. It is more frequently seen following pollen sensitization contracted during school-age childhood. Birch pollen allergies have been known to cross-react with soybean allergies.

Pollen-related Food Sensitivities

Plants use pollens to stimulate the sexual activity that results in seeds being produced. Without seeds, plants cannot procreate. Therefore, pollens are all around us. Most plants pollinate periodically, and many do at the same time each year—during the springtime.

When an immunosuppressed person (notably a person with weakened mucosal membrane immunity) breathes in pollen, should the pollen escape the mucosal membrane shield within the sinuses and respiratory tract, the pollen may penetrate the epithelial layer and reach the body's tissues and bloodstream. When this happens, especially among the immunosuppressed, the immune system can overreact with hypersensitivity. The immune system will also remember the pollen protein as an invader for the next time it is consumed.

Later, when foods are eaten that contain elements of those pollen proteins, the immune system may again respond in the same way it overreacted to the pollen, resulting in a pollen-related food sensitivity.

Note that hypersensitivity to pollens is limited to plants that carry their pollen through the air by wind. Those plants that pollinate strictly through insect pollination, such as dandelion, goldenrod and similar flowering plants do not typically cause pollen allergies.

Researchers from the Institute of Internal Medicine at Italy's University of Ferrara (Boccafogli *et al.* 1994) studied 169 allergic patients who were sensitized to grass pollen. They compared them to a 50-patient control group who were sensitized to dust mites. The grass pollen allergy sufferers reported more adverse food reactions than the dust mite group.

The pollen-sensitive group reported sensitivities to peanut, garlic, tomato, onion; and some fruits. They also reported sensitivities to egg whites and pork. The researchers concluded a cross reactivity between pollen and food allergens.

Researchers from Japan's Yokohama City University Hospital (Maeda *et al.* 2010) studied food allergies and pollen allergies among adults. After studying IgE antibodies for five pollens among 622 allergy sufferers with an average age of 37 years old, they found twice as many of those allergic to pollens had food allergies than existed in the general population.

However, when considering the rare types of allergies of the subjects—apples, peaches and melons—the increase in rates was significantly higher. Cedar, ragweed, orchard grass, mugwort, and alder pollen were the most common pollen allergies. Apple allergies correlated more with alder pollen allergies. Peach allergies correlated with alder and orchard grass sensitivity. Mellon allergy correlated with alder, orchard grass and ragweed sensitivity. The researchers commented that allergies relating to trees in the Betulaceae family (alder, birch, hazel, hornbeam and some tree nuts) are implicated with similar tree pollen allergies.

Pollen allergies affect different people differently, however. In the Italian study mentioned in the first chapter (Asero *et al.* 2009) of 25,601 allergy clinic patients throughout Italy, pollen-related food allergies were the highest, at 55% of all allergies. Of those pollen-related allergies, 45% had Type I allergies, and the majority (72%) of those had allergies to fruits and vegetables.

Of the pollen-allergy group, 96% of those with Type I food allergies lived in Southern Italy and most of these were related to lipid transfer protein sensitization. The researchers indicated a link between diet and pollen exposure because of this geographical trend. Most Italians understand that the diet of Northern Italy is significantly different from the diet of Southern Italy. South Italy also has significantly more urban dwellers.

Here are a few pollen-allergy foods and some of the research evidence linking several of these associations:

Peaches

Spanish researchers (Fernández-Rivas *et al.* 2003) studied peach and related Rosaceae fruit allergies. They found that cross-reactivity of IgE antibodies to lipid transfer proteins (LTPs) were prevalent among the subjects.

The scientists studied 98 people with peach sensitivities. IgE allergies were found among 77% of the patients. They also found that 76% of the peach allergy subjects had allergies to pollens. Furthermore, all of the 22 nonallergic patients also had pollen allergies.

The proteins most sensitized to were Pru p3, rBet v1, and rBet v2. IgE responses to rBet v2 were greatest among pollen allergy sufferers. They concluded that Pru p3 is the major protein allergen in peach.

Peach allergy sufferers in the north of Spain are sensitive to different allergens than sufferers from the South of Spain (Gamboa *et al.* 2007). Those from the north have more systemic responses, with the protein Pru p3 being the key allergen mixed with a profilin-Bet v1 protein sensitivity. This is often referred to as an LTP-profilin-Bet v1 sensitization—also common in Northern and Central Europe.

Apples

Apple sensitivity is quite common in some parts of Europe due to cross-reactivity. Research has established that about 2% of people who live in Northern and Central Europe are sensitive to apples.

Danish researchers (Hansen *et al.* 2004) found that among 74 patients allergic to birch pollen, 69% were also allergic to apples.

Denmark National University Hospital researchers (Skamstrup *et al.* 2001) tested the seasonal occurrence of apple sensitivity among 27 patients allergic to birch pollen. They were tested for reactions to apples before and during the 1998 birch pollen season. The results of their oral challenge testing concluded that sensitivity to apples significantly increases during birch pollen allergy season, and decreases or disappears after the season is over.

However, while birch pollen can cross-react and cause apple and other fruit allergies, it can also significantly reduce allergies among certain fruits, including some varieties of apples (Bolhaar *et al.* 2004).

In other words, not every apple variety has the same allergic potential. Some apples produce more sensitivity than others. For example researchers at Groningen University Medical Centre found that among three different apple cultivars—Santana, Golden Delicious, and Topaz—a majority (53%) of the allergic patients were not sensitive to the Santana apple variety. Those who were sensitive were far less sensitive to the Santana apple than to the other two. After the study, 73% of the participants said that they would eat Santana apples in the future.

Cherries

While cherry allergies occur throughout Europe, they occur with more severity and more systemic reactions in Southern Europe. Cherry allergy sufferers among the Central and Northern European countries have primarily oral responses. This appears related to the sensitization to LTP, which occurs more in the Northern countries, and sensitivity to cherry proteins, such as Pru av3, which occurs primarily in Southern locations such as Spain and Italy (Reuter *et al.* 2006).

Figs

Fig allergies can occur among those also allergic to both rubber latex and birch pollens.

In an Austrian study (Hemmer *et al.* 2010) of 85 patients with birch pollen allergies, 78% of them were also sensitized to fresh figs and (interestingly) only 10% were sensitized to dried figs. In addition, 91% were sensitive to mulberries, 91% to jackfruit, 77% to Rosaceae fruits (which include almonds, apples, apricots, cherries, peaches, pears, plums, raspberries, strawberries as well as ornamentals such as firethorns, hawthorns, meadowsweets, photinias and roses).

The researchers concluded that other fruits of the Moraceae family should also be cross-reactionary with fig allergies. These include breadfruits and many other trees.

Spanish researchers (Cuesta-Herranz *et al.* 2010) found in a study of 806 patients from eight hospitals that people suffering from both pollen and pollen-related food allergies have significantly more respiratory symptoms than pollen-only allergies.

Kiwifruit

Kiwis may be an exception to pollen allergies in some cases. In a study of 33 people with kiwi allergy symptoms, food challenge was positive in 23 patients. Twenty-one percent were not allergic to pollen, however. Twenty-eight percent of the kiwifruit allergy sufferers had sensitivities to latex (Alemán *et al.* 2004).

Kiwifruit's main allergens are Act d1, Act d2, Act d4, and Act d5, Bet v1, Act d8 and profilin rAct d9 (Bublin *et al.* 2010). Italian researchers (Fiocchi *et al.* 2004) found that children allergic to fresh kiwifruit were by and large not allergic to steam-cooked (100 degrees C for five minutes) and homogenized kiwifruit. Twenty kiwi-allergic children were tested. Only one child reacted to the cooked kiwi food challenge.

Melon

Spanish researchers (Rodriguez *et al.* 2000) found in testing 53 patients complaining of melon allergies that only 42% had IgE allergy and 42% were positive using the skin prick test. Eighteen of these confirmed melon-allergy patients were also allergic to up to 15 other foods. The most prevalent included banana (39%), kiwi (33%), watermelon (33%), and peach (28%).

Melon allergies first occurred among the patients at an average age of 20, with a range of six years old to 45 years old. In addition, 88% had seasonal rhinitis (sinus issues, watery eyes and so on) and/or asthma symptoms.

The chart below summarizes the foods that relate to specific types of pollens:

Pollen-Food Allergy Associations

Pollen Type	Food Allergy Associations
Birch	almonds, apples, apricots, avocados, bananas, carrots, celery, cherries, chicory, coriander, fennel, figs, hazelnuts, kiwifruit, nectarines, parsley, parsnips, peaches, pears, peppers, plums, potatoes, prunes, soy, strawberries, wheat, walnuts
Ragweed	banana, cantaloupe, cucumber, honeydew, watermelon, zucchini, echinacea, artichoke, dandelions, hibiscus, chamomile
Alder	almonds, apples, celery, cherries, hazel nuts, peaches, pears, parsley, strawberry, raspberry
Grass	figs, melons, tomatoes, oranges
Mugwort	carrots, celery, coriander, fennel, parsley, peppers, sunflower

(Adapted from Zarkadas *et al.* 1999)

Lipid Transfer Protein Foods

While many LTPs relate to pollen, we've separated a section on LTP to dig deeper. The reader might have noticed that many of the foods listed above included LTP as an allergen. This includes apples, peaches, kiwifruit, melon, cherries and many other fruits and vegetables. As we'll see, LTPs are even more pervasive among allergies than this indicates.

Italian researchers (Asero *et al.* 2002) selected 20 patients who were lipid transfer protein allergic out of 600 Rosaceae (apples and related fruits) allergic patients. They found that all the patients also had allergic reactions to a large number of other plant foods, including nuts, peanuts, legumes, celery, rice, corn and others. The researchers concluded that LPT was a *"pan-allergen."*

Spanish researchers (Palacin *et al.* 2010) found that the rise in wheat allergies may relate to the rise in sensitivity to LTP. They found that the wheat flour lipid transfer protein Tri a14 appears to be the key allergen responsible for baker's asthma and wheat food allergy. And because cross-reactivity is common among the LTPs, there is often a transference between asthmatic bakers so that they become allergic to eating bread at some point. This has been termed *LTP syndrome.* The researchers confirmed this effect among eight adults with anaphylaxis after eating wheat foods.

Researchers (Hartz *et al.* 2010) have discovered that allergies to hazelnuts and cherries are mediated by non-specific lipid transfer proteins and often stem from an initial sensitization to the Pru p3 protein from peaches. They found that sensitization occurred with nsLTPs in 88% of peach allergies, 85% of hazelnut allergies and 77% of cherry allergies.

Corn allergies with anaphylaxis have been found to be mostly in response to the IgE reaction to alpha-amylase inhibitor and a 9-kDa LTP. The 9-kd lipid-transfer protein (LTP) is the major allergen of corn. The binding capacity to IgE was tested among different corn hybrids, and all showed about the same sensitization rates. Furthermore, cooking did not seem to affect this LTP allergen content in corn (Pastorello *et al.* 2003, Pastorello *et al.* 2009).

The major allergen of green beans (*Phaseolus vulgaris*) is the non-specific lipid transfer protein called Pha v3. This was confirmed in tests of 10 Spanish allergic patients (Zoccatelli *et al.* 2010).

About 1.1% of children with food allergies have allergies to mustard (Morisset *et al.* 2003). Researchers have found that nsLTP and profilin are the allergens in mustard seeds (Sirvent *et al.* 2009).

The bottom line is the LTP is now being considered by a growing legion of researchers as the allergen most responsible for a majority of food sensitivities, especially those with multiple cross-reactive food allergies.

Yeast

Yeast (*Saccharomyces cerevisiae*) is a type of fungus that is a considered healthy and even probiotic among most people. It is commonly used to prepare a variety of foods, including many breads. It is also found within the colons of healthy people, and is thus considered as a probiotic microorganism.

Like any microorganism, however, there must exist a balance between the species and strains within the gut in order the maintain health. Persons without that balance, or who have become infected with overgrowths of other not-so-probiotic yeast colonies such as *Candida spp.*, may become sensitive to foods containing yeast. Yeast sensitivities may also yield or be a symptom of other intestinal problems.

Australian researchers from Ninewells Hospital and Medical School (McKenzie *et al.* 1990) studied IgG antibodies in 15 Crohn's disease patients, 15 patients with ulcerative colitis, and 15 healthy subjects. They exposed the subjects to 12 strains of yeast (*Saccharomyces cerevisiae*). The Crohn's patients had heightened IgG antibodies to 11 of the 12 *S cerevisiae* strains.

Meat

Despite the lack of attention, meat allergies do exist. Researchers (Theler *et al.* 2009) from Zürich's University Hospital found people with IgE allergies to pork, beef and chicken. Those with meat allergies complained of skin rashes, nausea, diarrhea, vomiting and/or abdominal pain.

Other research has confirmed that beef allergies can have symptoms of skin rash, respiratory difficulty, artery inflammation, digestive difficulties and anaphylaxis. Basophil testing can expose immunoglobulin E-mediated allergies for beef protein (Kim *et al.* 2010).

Albumin is often the central allergen. This protein is contained in most animal foods. Albumin-specific IgE antibodies are frequently found. Bovine serum albumin (or BSA) is often the culprit (Fiocchi *et al.* 1995).

Seafood

Researchers from Canada's McGill University (Ben-Shoshan *et al.* 2010) surveyed nearly 10,000 people in 2008 and 2009, and found that seafood allergies were greater than any other food allergy, with a 2.1% total between fish (.5%) and shellfish (1.6%).

Parvalbumin is the central protein allergen among fish seafood. Cod seems to be one of the more allergic fish, as it contains significant parvalbumins. Often cod brings on the initial sensitivity, and other fish such as carp, salmon, tuna, halibut, flounder and others become cross-reactive as they are consumed. Once sensitive, even inhaling cooked fish vapors can set off a significant reaction (de Martino *et al.* 1993; O'Neil *et al.* 1993).

Fish allergies often come with severe reactions, which include severe skin rashes and anaphylaxis. This means that bronchospasm, wheezing, and choking can arrive almost immediately after eating seafood or breathing fish cooking fumes.

Mollusk allergies include squid and other cephalopods. The protein seen as most allergic is the 36 kDa protein from squid tropomyosin (muscle). The heat-sensitive protein is 50 kDa. This can cause increased sensitivity when squid is eaten raw (Yadzir *et al.* 2010).

Tropomyosin is also suspected as the major source of crab allergies (Liu *et al.* 2010). It is resistant to stomach pepsin, but trypsin and chymotrypsin enzymes can break it down if available (Ueno *et al.* 2010).

How Much Does it Take?

As we will discuss at length, tolerance to specific foods is highly unique to each food-sensitive person. That said, research has indicated that most IgE-mediated food allergies require a specific range of dosage before allergy sufferers will react. Foods will require anywhere from five to 5,000 milligrams to produce a clinical response. For oils including peanut, sesame, sunflower, and soy oil, up to 30 milliliters can cause a response. Here is a chart based on the research:

Food	Respiratory Symptoms	Reaction at 65mg/.8mL	Lowest Reactive Dose
Eggs	12%	16%	2 mg
Peanuts	20%	18%	5 mg
Milk	10%	5%	0.1 mL
Sesame	42%	8%	30 mg

(Morisset *et al.* 2003)

Multiple Sensitivities: Primary vs. Secondary

While many people who are allergic appear to be sensitive to only one food or food type, multiple food sensitivities increasing occur. Food intolerances are similar, but not enough research has been done to confirm whether most food intolerances are multiple. From the author's clinical experience, and a growing opinion among other clinicians, the majority of food sensitivity sufferers have sensitivities to multiple foods.

When children present with multiple allergies, doctors attempt to find which allergy was primary to the others. The primary allergy is typically the one that the child became sensitized to first. The primary allergen likely also produced the cross-reactivity that caused the second sensitivity. In other words, often once there is an initial allergy, subsequent allergies follow that are related to the first in the antigen structure.

To explain this relationship more, researchers from Germany's Charité University Medical Center (Matricardi *et al.* 2008) followed 1,314 children for up to thirteen years from birth. They found that sensitization to milk and eggs decreased over years, from levels of 4% at two years old to less than one percent at ten years old. On the other hand, allergies to soy and wheat increased as the children got older: From about 2% at two years old to about 7% at 13 years old for soy; and from 2% to 9% for wheat allergies.

When the children were ten years old, confirmed allergies to grass pollen were from 97% to 98% of those children who were also allergic to soy and wheat. In addition, allergies to birch pollen among the soy and wheat allergy children occurred in 86% and 82%, respectively.

The researchers concluded that the pollens were the primary allergens in most cases. They found that soy or wheat allergies were primary to grass or birch pollen in only 4% and 8% of participants sensitized to soy and wheat, respectively.

University of Chicago researchers (Sahin-Yilmaz et al. 2010) found that when peanut, shrimp, and milk allergies are compared, peanut is associated with multiple allergies and milk is more associated with later asthmatic symptoms. In 283 allergic adults, they found that peanut and shrimp are most commonly seen with allergic rhinitis.

A peanut allergy is often a predictor for other IgE allergies (Sahin-Yilmaz et al. 2010). About a third of peanut-allergy sufferers may also be allergic to or at least sensitive to lupin (Shaw et al. 2008)

Legume (peanuts, beans and so on) allergies can also carryover to fenugreek, a legume often used as a key part of the spice blend that makes up curry. Researchers (Faeste et al. 2010) have found that fenugreek contains protein homologies similar to peanut allergens.

Histamine Foods

Foods like cheese, sausage, sauerkraut, tuna, tomatoes, and alcohol can contain up to 500 mg/kg of histamine. Eating foods that contain high levels of histamine may sometimes cause allergic symptoms, even in adults with no current allergies.

To test this, researchers from the Floridsdorf Allergy Center in Vienna, Austria (Wöhrl et al. 2004) gave 75 mg of liquid histamine dissolved in tea or the tea alone to ten healthy non-allergic females between the ages of 22-36 years old. After testing with a standardized symptom protocol over 24 hours, they found that five of the ten subjects experienced reactions to the histamine. These included tachycardia, mild hypotension, sneezing, runny nose and itchy nose, most within the first hour. Four of the five also had diarrhea, flatulence, headaches and other delayed symptoms that began after three hours of consuming the histamine.

French INSERM researchers (Kanny et al. 1996) also studied histamine levels in food and intestinal permeability. They had previously demonstrated that ingested histamine could promote or stimulate chronic urticaria (hives). The researchers fed seven urticaria patients with 120 mg of histamine. They found that histamine stimulated diarrhea, urticaria, headaches, increased heart rate and a drop in blood pressure among five of the seven within an hour of the histamine exposure. The researchers performed intestinal biopsies on the urticaria patients before and after the histamine. They found that the histamine also caused inflammation within the intestinal intercellular regions.

These studies gave pure liquid histamine to their subjects. The question of course is whether eating otherwise healthy foods high in histamine, such as tomatoes and sauerkraut, will necessarily produce this kind of reaction. The answer is that healthy foods also contain a variety of nutrients (tomatoes contain over 10,000 healthy constituents, for example) that are anti-inflammatory. These buffer histamine reactions and balance out the role of histamine within the tissues.

However, an unhealthy source of histamine, such as sausage or alcohol, may be another matter altogether, because these sources contain other elements (nitrites, ethanol and so on) that can stimulate inflammation in considerable amounts. These foods have been associated with damaged livers and an increased risk of cancer.

Salicylate Food Sensitivity

A large number of foods also contain salicylates. Foods particularly high in salicylates include peppers, broad beans, radishes, tomatoes, zucchini, chicory, endive, fava bean, spinach, watercress, broccoli, artichoke, eggplant and squash. These of course are also very nutritious foods, and in fact salicylates are abundant in the plant kingdom. Nearly every plant contains some salicylates. Furthermore, salicylate levels will significantly decrease as the fruit or vegetable ripens.

Salicylate sensitivity has been known to cause bronchial congestion, wheezing, hives, GI pain, upset stomach, indigestion and other symptoms.

At the same time, salicylates are extremely healthy constituents in plants. They balance the immune system and slow inflammation. They have also been shown to reduce cardiovascular disease and even reduce some cancers (Din et al. 2010). Many of these properties stem from the fact that salicylate constituents are produced to help plants themselves defend against disease.

Often salicylate sensitivity begins from the overuse of aspirin and other salicylate-containing medications such as aspirin. Over time, the isolated salicylates in aspirin can damage the mucosal membrane in the stomach and intestines, producing sensitivity (Goldstein et al. 2008).

Salicylate-containing herbs such as peppermint, meadowsweet and willow, in contrast, contain a number of natural constituents that buffer and balance the effects of their salicins (Schmid *et al.* 2001).

At the end of the day, when it comes to histamine and salicylate food sensitivity, a lot depends upon the health of the mucosal membrane, intestinal tract and immune system. For a person whose mucosal membrane is thinned, intestinal walls have been damaged, and/or the immune system has been compromised and burdened with toxins and other foreigners (immunosuppressed, in other words), histamine and salicylate foods—along with any number of other food components—can certainly trigger a hypersensitivity response, as we will discuss further in the next chapter.

Chapter Four

What Causes Food Sensitivities?

This is a critical chapter for not only understanding what causes food allergies, but how to resolve them. According to conventional Western medicine, there are several causes for food sensitivities. They include genetic factors, diet and environmental impacts (Hamelmann *et al.* 2008).

General enough for you? This is what most doctors will tell us; and what most informational websites will tell us. Some of the texts on food allergies may delve a bit deeper into histamine and IgE responses—as we included in the second chapter. But IgE responses, histamine mediators and so on are not the *causes*. These are the *mechanisms*.

This chapter will focus upon the causes of food allergies and sensitivities with the practical issues in mind: Is it genetic or was some dietary, lifestyle or environment factor involved? Here the facts are laid out that illustrate not just the science, but the mechanisms that produce the cause-effect relationship. The purpose here will be to understand what, if any, changes to our diet, environment or other lifestyle choice can turn things around.

How Important are Genetic Factors?

A number of large scale studies have confirmed that a person's risk of food sensitivities rises dramatically if ones parents are allergic to foods, allergic otherwise (pollen, mites, mold), or asthmatic. This risk rises if both parents are allergic. Does this mean that our genes cause food sensitivities? The simple (heretical yet more scientific) answer is no.

Can we back up this statement with research? Let's review some of the research directly regarding allergies and genetics.

Researchers from the Department of Pediatrics of Brazil's State University of Campinas (López *et al.* 1999) studied allergies among 114 newborns (including three twin pairs) starting at birth through one years old. They measured IgE levels of the umbilical cord blood, and again after three months, six months and at 12 months. They also correlated the relative influences of race, sex, family income, birth month, family allergy history, breast-feeding, parents' smoking, and symptoms. At one year, they found no association between IgE (allergy) levels and a family history of allergies. They concluded that, *"immune response for atopy was in a large degree influenced by environmental factors and serum IgE at 12 months was a good marker for identifying infants with risk of atopic disease in early life."*

Researchers from Germany's Philipps University of Marburg (Pfefferle *et al.* 2008) found that 24% of newborns had allergen-specific IgE antibodies when they tested blood samples from 922 infants and mothers. The only allergen-specific IgEs found to be common between mother and infant were for milk, eggs, and soybeans IgE. Note also that these three types of allergies are often outgrown during the first few years of childhood.

Our understanding of genetics is still in its infancy. This is indicated by the progress of our genome research. Over the last two decades, geneticists have focused on assembling the combined gene combinations that together would make up the genome of particular organisms. Genome research has expanded into a worldwide focus on establishing the genome of humans and other species. The assumption in the beginning of this research project—which has involved hundreds of scientists from different specialties over two decades—was that we would find within the genome the answers to all the mysteries of nature. In other words, we'd find out the cause for every disease and why people die when they do.

The hypothesis that the genome would provide this was erroneous. The first invalid assumption was that the combination of genes in humans would uniquely indicate the occurrence of disease pathologies. And preliminary research seemed to connect certain gene combinations to particular diseases. It was assumed that every disease came with a particular genetic sequence. This worked out pretty well in the beginning until researchers began discovering that many people with gene sequences associated with a particular disease never contracted that disease. And sometimes two or three diseases were associated with the same genetic trait. For example, Angelman syndrome and Prader-willy syndrome both occur with the same chromosome 15 deletion.

These and other problems revealed that perhaps our understanding of genes and disease etiology was not as advanced as we'd like to think.

Consider obesity. It was assumed by geneticists that obesity was a genetic disorder that could be switched off by switching off a particular gene sequence. However, researchers from the Massachusetts General Hospital (Ashrafi *et al.* 2003) went through 16,757 worm genes (most of which are common with humans), and found that 303 genes switched on reduced fat and 112 genes switched on increased fat storage. This means that at least 415 genes are involved in obesity.

The other mystery for geneticists is that monozygotic twins—which share the same DNA at conception—do not necessarily develop the same diseases later in life. In other words, identical twins often have very different pathological outcomes.

This is supported by the research. Many twins have dramatically unique and individual disease pathologies from each other.

For example, in a study of genetically identical twins and lung capacity from Pennsylvania State University (Whitfield *et al.* 2004), lung expiration capacity was only 14% attributable to genetic factors. About 30% was found to be due to shared environments and 56% was due to non-shared environmental effects. These and other studies confirm that our environment (including what we eat) has a much greater affect upon our health than do genetic factors.

Among autoimmune diseases, genetic associations among twins and families exist, but the stronger factor is also related to environmental issues. For example, a study from the University of Western Ontario's Clinical Neurological Science Department (Ebers *et al.* 1996) reviewed the research on twins and autoimmune complexes such as multiple sclerosis. They also conducted a genome search of 100 sibling pairs, looking for MS gene markers. Their research on multiple sclerosis concluded that while monozygotic twins showed higher concordance levels (matching pathologies) than dizygotic twins and siblings (25-30% versus 4%), they found that *"environmental factors strongly influenced observed geographical differences."* They also concluded, *"Studies of candidate genes have been largely unrewarding."*

This of course is because twins make different choices and have different behavior; and behavior directly relates to changes in environment.

But don't twins also maintain similar environmental conditions? Certainly they do. Especially during childhood. They also share the same mother and the same breast milk. They also share the same birthing canal, where they receive similar doses of immunoglobulins and probiotics— just as they receive in breast milk.

However, depending upon how much time they spend together, they will typically make distinctly different choices in life. In general, they display significantly unique and often diverse behavior. Hur and Rushton (2007) studied 514 pairs of two to nine year old South Korean monozygotic (identical) and dizygotic (non-identical) twins. Their results indicated that 55% of the children's pro-social behavior related to genetic factors and 45% was attributed to non-shared environmental factors. It should also be noted that shared environmental factors could not be eliminated from the 55%.

The environmental versus genetic association could well be higher if the twin's early shared environments had been removed. In another recent study (Forget-Dubois *et al.* 2007), an analysis of 292 mothers demonstrated that maternal behavior only accounted for a 29% genetic influence at 18 months, and 25% at 30 months.

In a study done at the Virginia Commonwealth University's Institute for Psychiatric and Behavioral Genetics (Maes *et al.* 2007), a large sampling revealed that individual behavior was only about 38-40% attributable to genetics, while shared environment was 18-23% attributable and un-shared environmental influences were attributable in 39-42%.

Studies of arthritis have revealed a range of only 12-15% concordance between monozygotic twins for rheumatoid arthritis (RA). This indicates an even weaker connection between genetics and RA exists—contradicting a decades-old assumption that RA was generally a genetic disease. If RA were significantly genetic, then we would see that among twins with the RA genetic traits, both twins would contract the disease at least more than 50% of the time, instead of 12-15% of the time (Silman *et al.* 1993, Jones *et al.* 1996; Aho *et al.* 1986).

To further close the door on the genetic-arthritis association, the *British Medical Journal* (Swendsen *et al.* 2002) published a nationwide study from Denmark on RA among monozygotic twins and dizygotic twins. This concluded no significant difference between monozygotic twins and dizygotic twins with regard to 1) onset of RA; 2) presence of RA factor; or 3) any other RA association. In other words, RA occurrence was no more shared between genetically identical twins than non-genetic identical twins—the opposite of what should happen if RA was genetic.

At the same time, this does not mean that genetic disposition has nothing to do with the contraction of allergies and many other diseases. A genetic disposition can increase the likelihood of contracting the disease *given susceptibility genes are switched on.*

We might compare this to automobile ownership. Say two people purchase the exact same make, model and year automobile at the same time. Comparing the two cars in the future will reveal the cars had vastly different engine lives and mileages. They each had different types of breakdowns, and different problems. This is because each car was driven differently. One was likely driven harder than the other was. One was likely better taken care of than the other was. They may have been the same make and model, but each had different owners with different driving and maintenance habits. While the model might have a particular weakness in its design, this weakness may only affect performance if the car is pushed and not maintained.

Because twins have the same genetics—just as the cars shared the same make, model and manufacturer—their unique disease factors stem from the fact that each body is operated differently by a different individual under different conditions.

This distinction between inherited genes and continued environmental inputs is a realm that scientists are just beginning to explore. Realizing that even the same genes or the same genetic abnormalities will not render the same pathologies, researchers want to better understand the full matrix of causation in differentiated gene expression. Even twins who shared the same diet and environment will still have vastly different disease pathologies. This means there are missing elements that future research must take into consideration.

These missing elements have forced a re-calibration of the genetic theory, and the rise of the concept of *epigenetics*. In general, epigenetics is the acceptance of environmental or dietary factors that *switch off and on* the expression of genes. In other words, it has been hypothesized—and confirmed by the research—that ones DNA is not as important as how gene expressions—or *phenotypes*—are switched on or off. If the genes are expressed, particular metabolism consequences result. If they are not expressed, there are different consequences. Furthermore, even if the susceptibility gene is not present, certain activities can *create* the epigenetic sequences that switch a particular disease event on (and often produce the susceptibility for future generations).

The original concept of epigenetics was penned by geneticist Conrad Waddington in the early 1940s to explain in general how environmental circumstances could affect ones genetic instructions. The concept, however, got lost until the 1990s and early 2000s, as scientists have discovered the many gaps in the genetic assumptions.

The biochemical relationships of gene expression have focused upon the action of DNA histone regulation. These biochemical messengers have been observed switching gene alleles on or off. For example, mice experiments at McGill University's Douglas Hospital Research Center (Szyf *et al.* 2008) found that phenotype switching could be turned on and off with increased nurturing from the mother. Those baby mice receiving affectionate nurturing from mama would switch on genes differently than those mice that received less nurturing.

Biochemical mechanisms like phosphorylation, sumoylation, acetylation, methylation, and ubiquitylation appear to be further mechanics responsible for phenotype expression—which connect gene expression to the availability of nutrients like oxygen, water, vitamin B, Co-Q-10 and so on. This of course confirms the link between genes and diet.

As stated clearly by esteemed nutrition researcher Dr. T. Colin Campbell:

> *"Genes do not determine disease on their own. Genes function only by being activated or expressed, and nutrition plays a critical role in determining which genes, good and bad, are expressed."*
> (Campbell and Campbell 2006)

As we review food sensitivity research, it becomes evident that even if a parent has had food sensitivities, the child's environmental factors play a stronger role. It is these environmental factors that switch on, or express a particular genetic trait.

For example, a component that is often missed in the genetic discussion is the common diet and common living environment between parents and their children. With rare exception, children consume the foods and recipes chosen by their parents. Dinners and cooking methods, for the most part, are passed down from generation to generation. As a result, the diet the children have may be practically identical, with the exception of brand names and packaging, to the diet the parents, grandparents and great-grandparents ate.

In the case of mothers who provide the womb, the birthing canal and breast milk, the health of their own bodies becomes part of the baby's environment.

The mother and the infant share the same food and blood for nine months. This means that whatever the mother eats directly affects the child via the umbilical cord. It also means that whatever food sensitivities the mother has will also impact the baby. This has been supported by the research, as we've discussed.

Furthermore, the house and those environmental toxins present in its furniture and building materials are presented equally to the parents and the children. The outside environment—automobile pollution, pesticides and so on—is also mutually presented to parents and children. And because they are developing, children are more sensitive to environmental conditions. Children are also more vulnerable to the influences of their parents' diets and lifestyles.

Even if the child does not assume the lifestyle choices of the parent as an adult, the environmental exposure has already been accomplished. In other words, we can prevent further exposures to our bodies and to the next generation's. But we still will have to deal with our own childhood exposures.

This "passing" of lifestyle habits is undoubtedly more important than the genes parents pass on to their children. Why? Because even if the children received the genes predisposing some weakness towards a particular issue such as allergies—those genes still have to be switched on in order for the sensitivity to be expressed. And how do we switch on the genes? By our environment and lifestyle choices—including diet, air, water consumption and exercise.

As we'll discuss further, food-borne and environmental chemical toxins can become potent free radicals once inside the body. They can damage the mucosal membrane and expose intestinal epithelia to the toxins.

Here they can damage the intestinal cell membranes and brush barriers, allowing larger molecules into the intestinal wall and bloodstream.

In such exposures, the immune system must launch into high gear, using whatever available resources it has to try to correct the damage. Sometimes this means launching a high-scale alert against the intruder (maybe a simple food protein) and then maybe even quarantining that part of the intestinal tissue and launching an all-out cleanse of the damaged cells (autoimmunity) as dictated by genetic disposition.

This interaction between genes and environment was concluded in a report from University of North Carolina's Department of Rheumatology and Immunology (Dooley and Hogan 2003):

> *"Rather than disease-specific genes for individual autoimmune disorders, there may be "autoimmunity genes" that increase the risk for development of autoimmune disorders in families. Autoimmune disorders may result from multiple interactions of genes and environmental factors."*

In other words, for those of us who may have had parents with allergies, we may have inherited certain gene sequences that establish how the immune system will respond when it is in a compromised state.

This epigenetic conclusion was confirmed by researchers from China's Sun Yat-Sen University (Fu *et al.* 2010) who studied late embryo maturation among peanut allergy children. They found that an epigenetic change took place during the developmental stages related to the environment. Their nucleosomes on the assigned match for the Ara h3 peanut protein were depleted. Histone H3 levels were significantly reduced. Because these factors changed during development, they were determined not to be genetic. They were epigenetic. Gene developmental changes that evolve during embryo maturation are responses to environmental changes. This relates to the diet of the mother and the mother's environment.

Another important element to consider is the genome of our probiotic colonies. A thriving population of more than three trillion organisms renders the conclusion that our bodies have ten times more bacteria than cells. This resounding fact has led scientists to the concept of the *microbiome*—an extended genome of the genetics of our resident microorganisms. Recent research indicates that our probiotics' genes better reflect our body's predispositions and pathologies than does our own cellular DNA (Kinross, *et al.* 2006).

Margaret McFall Ngai, Ph.D., microbiome researcher and professor of microbiology and immunology at University of Wisconsin's School of Medicine has said:

"Understanding the human microbiome may be as or more important to understanding human health than mapping and understanding the human genome."

Increased Intestinal Permeability

The consensus of the research is that the gastrointestinal tract, from the mouth to the anus, is the primary defense mechanism against antigens as they enter the body. The mucous membrane integrity, the probiotic system, digestive enzymes, and the various immune cells and their mediators work together to orchestrate a "total defense" structure within the mucosal membrane. However, should this barrier be weakened or become imbalanced, hypersensitivity can result. The weaknesses in the barrier can be influenced by a number of factors, including toxins, diet, genetics, and environmental factors (Chahine and Bahna 2010).

In other words, poor dietary choices, toxin exposures and environmental forces related to lifestyle and living conditions can wear down and thin this mucosal membrane. Once the membrane is damaged, the intestinal cells become exposed to the foods and toxins we consume.

The intestines also have a microscopic barrier function. The tiny spaces between the intestinal epithelial cells—composed of villi and microvilli—are sealed from the general intestinal contents with what are called tight junctions. As we discussed earlier, should the tight junctions open up, this barrier or seal will be broken.

This results in increased intestinal permeability, as we've mentioned before.

When tight junctions are open—as they are normally in the bladder or the colon—the wrong molecules can cross the epithelium through a transcellular pathway. Researchers have found more than 50-odd protein species among the tight junction. Should any of these proteins fail due to exposure to toxins, the barrier can break down, giving access to what are called macromolecules—molecules that are larger than nutrients that the intestinal cells, liver and bloodstream are accustomed to. Once these macromolecules access the intestinal tissues, they can stimulate an immune response: an inflammatory reaction.

The epithelial mucosal immune system has two anti-inflammatory strategies: The first is to block invaders using antibodies, probiotics and acids. This controls microorganism colonies and inhibits new invasions. The body's immune response counteracts local and peripheral hypersensitivity by attempting to remove them before a full inflammation attack is launched. This is referred to as oral tolerance when it is stimulated in the intestines.

The biochemical constituents of the mucosal membrane (glycoproteins, mucopolysaccharides and so on) also attach and escort nutrients across the intestinal barrier, while resisting the penetration of unrecognized and potentially harmful agents. Intestinal permeability allows molecules that are normally not able to cross the intestines' epithelial barrier access to the bloodstream.

When the intricate balance between the intestinal epithelial layer is destroyed by exposure and inflammation, abnormal protein antigens gain access to the intestinal subepithelial compartment. Here they stimulate the release of immune cells and degranulation (Yu 2009).

Let's examine the research supporting these conclusions:

Medical researchers at Norway's University of Bergen (Lillestøl *et al.* 2010) found that self-reported food hypersensitivity was highly associated with irritable bowel syndrome and intestinal permeability. Of the 71 adult subjects, 93% had irritable bowel syndrome and increased intestinal permeability, while 61% had atopic disease—primarily rhinoconjunctivitis. All the atopic sufferers had respiratory allergies, and 41% had food allergens.

Louisiana State University researchers (Chahine and Bahna 2010) found that the intestinal wall uses specific immunologic factors to defend the body against antigens. They showed that integrity of the mucous membrane lining of the intestine is critical. A defective lining, on the other hand, leads to allergic responses and hypersensitivity reactions, according to their research. They named the cause of these *"defects in the gut barrier."*

Medical researchers (Jackson *et al.* 1982) gave polyethylene glycol to eight eczema patients with food allergies and 10 patients with supposed non-allergic eczema in order to investigate intestinal permeability. Both groups absorbed macromolecules in excess of the normal subjects. They concluded that eczema with and without food allergy was associated with *"intestinal mucosal defects"* (increased intestinal permeability).

Hungarian researchers (Kovács *et al.* 1996) tested intestinal permeability among 35 food allergic patients and 20 healthy controls. Intestinal permeability was determined using EDTA. Of the 35, increased intestinal permeability was determined in 29 of the food allergy patients. Of these 29, 21 volunteers were tested for intestinal permeability five years later. IgA antibody titers were increased, among wheat, soy and oat antigens. Significant correlations between intestinal permeability and IgA antibody titers was found, especially against soy and oat proteins.

French researchers (Bodinier *et al.* 2007) studied wheat proteins with patients with intestinal permeability syndrome. They compared the translocation of native wheat proteins with those in a pepsin-hydrolyzed state.

They found that the native wheat proteins were crossing the intestinal cell layer, and were able to associate this with their allergic responses.

Hospital Saint Vincent de Paul researchers (Dupont *et al.* 1991) pointed out in their research that the extent of intestinal permeability depends upon the molecule size and the state of the intestinal mucosa. Some intestinal *"porosity,"* as the researchers put it, is normal. However, when macromolecules that were normally not allowed to enter the bloodstream gained entry—primarily protein macromolecules—this stimulated the immune system, according to their research.

The Intestinal Permeability Index

So how do scientists and physicians test for increased intestinal permeability? Intestinal permeability is typically measured by giving the patient molecules that do not break down in the intestines. For example, alcohol-sugar combinations such as lactulose and mannitol are often used. These indicate intestinal permeability because of their different molecular sizes. After ingestion, the patient's urine is tested to measure the quantities that these two molecules were absorbed through the intestinal walls.

Because lactulose is a larger molecule than mannitol, it will thus be more present in the urine compared to mannitol when there is greater permeability of the intestinal wall. Intestines with normal permeability will have little lactulose absorption. This creates a ratio between lactulose and mannitol, which scientists call the L/M ratio. This L/M ratio is used to quantify intestinal permeability. When the lactulose-to-mannitol ratio is higher, more permeability exists. When it is lower, less (and normal) intestinal permeability exists. Higher levels are graduated using what many researchers call the *Intestinal Permeability Index.*

Other large molecule markers are also sometimes used to detect intestinal permeability using the same protocol of measuring recovery in the urine over a period of time (typically 5-6 hours). Substances used include polyethylene glycols of various molecular weights, horseradish peroxidase, EDTA (ethylenediaminetetraacetic acid), rhamnose, lactulose and cellobiose. Because these substances are not readily metabolized in the intestine or blood, and they also happen to have large molecular sizes, they can also give accurate readings on the level of intestinal permeability. Let's see how researchers have used the Intestinal Permeability Index to discover how food sensitivities are related to intestinal permeability:

Researchers from Italy's University of Bari Medical School (Ventura *et al.* 2006) studied intestinal permeability among 21 patients with food allergies, and 20 patients with food intolerances who were on an allergen-free diet. They measured intestinal permeability using the L/M ratio from urinary excretion. Their results found a progressive state of intestinal permeability among all the allergy and food sensitive subjects. They also found that clinical symptoms were increased among those with higher scores on the Intestinal Permeability Index. In other words, intestinal permeability was greater among those with IgE food allergies with worse symptoms. This was also the case to a lesser degree among those with food intolerances.

Researchers from the Charité University Medical School in Berlin (Buhner *et al.* 2004) studied 55 patients with non-IgE allergic (food intolerant) chronic urticaria (hives). The researchers used a triple-sugar-test to determine duodenal permeability, and the lactulose/mannitol ratio to measure intestinal permeability. Gastroduodenal and intestinal permeability levels were both significantly higher among urticaria patients as compared to controls. After the 55 patients were given an allergen-free diet, 29 of the patients displayed reduced or eliminated skin eruptions. These 29 "responders" had significantly greater levels of intestinal permeability than those who did not respond to the diet.

Researchers from the Department of Pediatrics of the Cochin St Vincent de Paul Hospital in Paris (Kalach *et al.* 2001) studied intestinal permeability and cow's milk allergy among children as they aged. The research included 200 children who exhibited symptoms of cow's milk allergies. Of this 200, 95 were determined as allergic using challenge testing. This left 105 children as control subjects. The researchers measured intestinal permeability using the L/M ratio. They found that the L/M ratio was significantly greater among the milk-allergic children. Abnormal intestinal permeability levels were present among 80% of the milk-allergic children who had digestive symptoms, and 40% of children who exhibited anaphylactic symptoms. Furthermore, L/M ratios improved among older children who became more tolerant to milk.

Researchers from the French national research institute, INSERM (Andre *et al.* 1987) compared intestinal permeability between 90 healthy persons and 60 food allergy patients using the mannitol-lactulose test. In healthy subjects, the average urinary excretion of mannitol was 14.11% and of lactulose 0.26%. The food allergy patients had levels of 11.57% and 1.04% after eating a meal that included the allergen—a considerable difference from the healthy controls.

Researchers (Fälth-Magnusson *et al.* 1984) utilized sodium cromoglycate (a similar test to L/M) to determine intestinal permeability among 22 children between eight and ten years of age. Half of the children were previously diagnosed as allergic using history and laboratory tests. Half of the children were healthy. The sodium cromoglycate test revealed that the allergic children had significantly greater levels of intestinal permeability.

Researchers (Ukabam *et al.* 1984) used the lactulose-mannitol ratio to test 11 allergic eczema patients plus control subjects. Lactulose absorption was significantly greater among eczema patients, and their excretion ratios were significantly higher than control subjects. The researchers concluded that small intestinal permeability was greater among the patients with atopic eczema.

Medical researchers from Kuwait University (Hijazi *et al.* 2004) studied 32 asthmatic children together with 32 matched controls. The lactulose/mannitol test was performed to determine intestinal permeability. The asthmatic children had significantly higher levels of intestinal permeability.

Medical researchers from Italy's University of Naples (Troncone *et al.* 1994) tested intestinal permeability among 32 children aged from three months old to 84 months old. They utilized a ratio related to L/M called the cellobiose/mannitol (C/M) ratio. Of those who had allergy symptoms after a challenge with milk, 90% had significantly increased C/M ratios, indicating increased intestinal permeability.

INSERM scientists from the Lyon-Sud Center Hospital in France (Andre *et al.* 1991) compared 15 healthy volunteers with 20 food allergy patients using the L/M ratio. When both groups were fasting, there was little difference between their L/M indices. However, when the allergic group ingested food containing their allergen, the absorption of lactulose doubled among this group.

Researchers (Fälth-Magnusson *et al.* 1986) gave 16 children with milk allergies different-sized polyethyleneglycolsy molecules (approx. 400 and 1000 Daltons—the same principle as the L/M ratio), and then measured their urinary recovery over six hours. The children with the most severe allergic symptoms also had the greatest levels of permeability. The molecule and milk challenge among healthy children produced only minor permeability symptoms. In other words, the allergic subjects had significantly greater changes in the absorption of large molecules.

Researchers from France's St. Vincent de Paul Hospital (Dupont *et al.* 1989) measured intestinal permeability using mannitol and lactulose among 12 children with milk allergy, 28 children with atopic dermatitis and 39 healthy children. They found that while the allergy sufferers' L/M ratio was similar to the healthy group while fasting, intestinal permeability was three times higher than the healthy group when the allergic group drank milk.

Researchers (Pike *et al.* 1986) tested permeability among 26 children with food-sensitive atopic eczema together with 29 non-allergic children. This time they used urinary excretion rates of di- and monosaccharides lactulose and rhamnose after eating. The average absorption ratio was significantly higher among the 26 allergic children as compared with the control group of 29 children. The researchers concluded that: *"This increased permeability may be a primary abnormality of the gut or may reflect intestinal mucosal damage caused by local hypersensitivity reactions to food antigens."*

The Link Between Intestinal Permeability and GI Issues

French researchers (Heyman and Desjeux 2000) found that not only can intestinal permeability cause various disorders, disorders can worsen intestinal permeability. They pointed out that as undigested food antigens are transported through the intestinal wall, the immune system launches an inflammatory response. Intact proteins and large peptides, they pointed out, stimulate inflammation among the mucosa of the intestinal wall. IFN gamma and TNF alpha are cytokines that are often part of this inflammatory response. These two—IFN gamma and TNF alpha—also so happen to increase the further opening of the tight junctions.

Researchers from Ohio State University's Medical School Zhou *et al.* 2009) studied 54 patients with irritable bowel syndrome along with 22 controls. They found that those patients with higher pain intensity and higher levels of diarrhea also had greater levels of increased intestinal permeability.

Researchers from Brazil's Federal Fluminense Medical School (Soares *et al.* 2004) studied the associations between IBS and food intolerance. The researchers used 43 volunteers divided into three groups: an IBS group, a dyspepsia group, and a group without gastrointestinal difficulties. All test subjects were given skin prick tests for nine food allergens. The IBS group presented the highest level of positive allergen responses. The researchers concluded that, *"The higher reactivity to food antigens in group I compared to groups II and III suggests that intestinal permeability may be increased in patients with IBS."*

Researchers (Forget *et al.* 1985) tested intestinal permeability using EDTA in ten normal adults, eleven healthy children, seven children with acute gastroenteritis, and eight infants with eczema. They found significantly greater intestinal permeability among those with either gastroenteritis or eczema.

Researchers from Paris' Cochin-St Vincent de Paul Hospital (Kalach *et al.* 2001) studied 64 children with cow's milk allergy symptoms, and found that higher intestinal permeability levels were also associated with anemia.

Researchers from London's Middlesex Medical School tested intestinal permeability among eight patients with food-intolerance using EDTA testing. While fasting levels were normal, after they ate the sensitive foods, permeability levels changed some, but not that significantly.

Researchers from Paris' Saint-Vincent de Paul Hospital (Barau and Dupont 1990) tested intestinal permeability using the lactulose and mannitol test with 17 children with irritable bowel syndrome (IBS). Of the 17, nine tested positive to IgE food allergies. Among these, permeability levels increased when the children were given foods they were sensitive to, illustrating the link between IBS, food allergies and intestinal permeability among many IBS sufferers.

Russian researchers (Sazanova et al. 1992) studied 122 children, four months old to six years old with food intolerances. Symptoms included atopic dermatitis among 52 children, and chronic diarrhea among 70 children. They found antibodies to food antigens among all the children. They also found chronic gastroduodenitis (duodenum and stomach inflammation) among every child with atopic dermatitis and among 95% of those with chronic diarrhea. They observed that lactase deficiencies and microorganism growth in the duodenum increased the levels of intestinal permeability and subsequent allergy response.

Increased Intestinal Permeability Immune Mechanisms

Once permeability is increased in the intestinal tract, there is no telling what the immune system will begin responding to. At this point it is likely that the immune system is greatly burdened by the many strange and different molecular structures now gaining entry into internal tissues and the bloodstream. What is known is that once permeability is increased, a self-perpetuating cycle of increased permeability and immune response produces more intestinal dysfunction and more immune response (Heyman 2005).

Researchers from Ontario's McMaster University (Berin et al. 1999) studied the role of cytokines in intestinal permeability. They found that interleukin-4 (IL-4) increased intestinal permeability and increased horseradish peroxidase (HRP) transport through intestinal walls. They found that IL-4 was inhibited by the soy nutrient genistein, and anti-IL-4 antibodies also reduced the HRP transport. The researchers concluded that:

"We speculate that enhanced production of IL-4 in allergic conditions may be a predisposing factor to inflammation by allowing uptake of luminal antigens that gain access to the mucosal immune system."

Research has indicated that CD23 encourages the transport of intestinal IgE and allergens across intestinal epithelium. This opens a gateway for antigen-bound IgE to move across (transcytose) the intestinal cells. This sets up the immune response of histamine and atopic environmental conditions (Yu 2009).

Researchers from the University of Cincinnati College of Medicine (Groschwitz *et al.* 2009) determined that mast cells are critical to the regulation of the intestinal barrier function. The type and condition of the mast cells seems to affect the epithelial migration through intestinal cells.

Researchers from the Cincinnati Children's Hospital Medical Center (Forbes *et al.* 2008) found that interleukin-9 appears to help stimulate, along with mast cells, increased intestinal permeability. The researchers found that this *"IL-9- and mast cell-mediated intestinal permeability"* activated conditions for food allergen sensitization.

What Causes Increased Intestinal Permeability?

The causative forces of increased permeability are a bit complicated. Infections, toxins, pharmaceuticals, probiotic deficiencies, breast milk deficiencies, metabolic stress and others have been identified as potential causes of increased intestinal permeability.

Accordingly, French INSERM researchers (Desjeux and Heyman 1994) concluded that increased protein permeability in milk allergies follows what they called *abnormal immunological response.* This abnormal immune response, they observed, leads to mucosal inflammation and a dysfunction of intestinal cellular endocytic processes (endocytosis is the process the cells undertake when they engulf or absorb amino acids and polypeptides). The researchers based this conclusion on the observation that the milk protein beta-lactoglobulin stimulated lymphocytes that released increased levels of cytokines tumor necrosis factor-alpha (TNF alpha) and gamma interferon. The cytokines stimulated an inflammatory response that in turn disturbed the intestinal cell wall barrier.

In other words, first an irritating toxin, abnormal macromolecule or other stressor disrupts the intestinal mucous membrane. This produces inflammation, which in turn opens gaps in the intestinal barrier.

On a biochemical level, electrogenic chloride secretion is involved in an ion transport chain that stimulates the inflammatory prostaglandin E2 (PGE2) response within the intestinal mucosa. This secretion is balanced by the chloride channel blocker diphenylamine-2-carboxylate in healthy persons. In unhealthy persons, inflammatory cytokines alter the balance among intestinal barrier cells, with the effect of increasing permeability.

Medical researchers from the University Hospital in Groningen, The Netherlands (van Elburg *et al.* 1992) point out that the intestinal immunity mechanisms, which include IgA immunoglobulin and cell-mediated immune factors—and the brush barrier in general—do not completely mature until after about two years of age. Until this time, the barrier is sensitive to toxins and feeding problems.

Researchers from the Medical University of South Carolina (Walle and Walle 1999) found that mutagens formed when frying meat may be implicated in opening the transport process in intestinal permeability. These mutagens, such as phenylimidazo-pyridine, were studied for their possible transport across human Caco-2 intestinal cells. The absorption was characterized as *"extensive and linear."* Equilibrium exchange tests showed that the mutagens form substrates with intestinal transporters. This indicates that these fried meat byproducts directly increase intestinal permeability.

A biochemistry researcher from Germany's Otto-von-Guericke University (Schönfeld 2004) discovered that dietary phytanic acid increases intestinal permeability through a function of ionic exchange and disruption of mitochondrial energy production. Damage to mitochondria may also explain the production of the inflammatory cytokine IL-4 within intestinal cells.

Researchers from the Department of Pediatrics at Italy's University of Federico II (Raimondi *et al.* 2008) found that bilirubin modifies the intestinal barrier. They also found among infants that cow's milk protein intolerance had higher levels of bilirubin and higher stool excretion. Those infants that had higher levels of bilirubin in the first year also had a greater risk of contracting cow's milk allergy.

To this, the French INSERM researchers added that stomach and upper intestinal infections with microorganisms such as *Helicobacter pylori* also increase intestinal permeability. Their observations led them to conclude that this was caused by an increased burden upon the immune system, and the resulting increase in inflammatory cytokines.

Medical researchers from Finland's University of Helsinki (Kuitunen *et al.* 1994) studied permeability using beta-lactoglobulin from cow's milk with 20 infants through eight months old or until they began weaning from breast milk. In one week after they weaned from breast milk, bovine beta-lactoglobulin levels were found in the bloodstream among 38% of the infants. After two weeks, 21% retained beta-lactoglobulin in the bloodstream. The researchers concluded that: *"The gut may often be transiently permeable to BLG when cow's-milk-based formula is started."*

INSERM researchers from the Hospital Saint-Lazare (Heyman *et al.* 1988) studied intestinal permeability with milk allergy among infants. They tested 33 children ages one month to 24 months, which included 18 healthy infants and 15 with milk allergies, using the protein marker horseradish peroxidase and jejunal biopsies. No absorption permeability was seen in the control children over two months of age, illustrating that *"gut closure probably occurred earlier in life."* However, milk allergy children had about eight times the permeability levels than the control children.

The connection may lie in the health condition of the mother. French doctors (de Boissieu *et al.* 1994) reported that in one case, a 1-month-old breast-fed boy who had regurgitation, diarrhea, feeding difficulties, and malaise—typical of food sensitivities. They conducted intestinal permeability tests on mother and baby. These illustrated that the mother's breast milk induced intestinal permeability in the baby. The child's symptoms continued without improvement after the mother eliminated dairy products from her own diet. Then the mother withdrew egg and pork from her diet. This resulted in an almost immediate disappearance of allergy symptoms in the child. The doctors tested the child again for intestinal permeability after provocation with mother's milk (the same test done previously). Intestinal permeability levels were normal. The doctors concluded that allergens can be transferred from mother to baby through breast milk.

After extensive research, medical scientists from the Department of Internal Medicine at France's University Hospital suggest that the risk factors for severe anaphylaxis include agents that produce increased intestinal permeability—which they indicated include alcohol, aspirin, betablockers and angiotensin-converting enzyme (ACE) inhibitors.

Researchers from Rush University's Division of Gastroenterology and Nutrition and the Rush-Presbyterian-St. Luke's Medical Center in Chicago (DeMeo *et al.* 2002) has proposed that the gastrointestinal tract maintains one of the body's biggest areas that offers exposure to the outside environment. This is because everything we eat ends up at the intestinal wall. The Rush University researchers illustrated in their research that disruptions to the gut barrier follow injury to these mechanisms. They further explained that this injury takes place from a number of causes, including nonsteroidal anti-inflammatory drugs, free radical oxidation, adenosine triphosphate depletion (metabolic stress) and damage to the epithelial cell cytoskeletons that regulate tight junctions. They also pointed out evidence that associates gut barrier damage to immune dysfunction and sepsis—infection from microorganisms. This of course alludes to the defenses provided by our probiotic microorganisms, which keep populations of infective microorganisms minimized—as we'll discuss in detail later.

Medical researchers from the University of Southampton School of Medicine (Macdonald and Monteleone 2005) have suggested that this epidemic of intestinal permeability among industrialized nations has been creating genetic mutations that produce greater levels of permeability among successive generations. This of course, provides the link between greater levels of allergies among those with allergic parents.

Thus we can conclude that intestinal permeability is not simply a creative explanation for allergies made without substantiation. It is a scientifically proven fact.

Dietary Factors

As we will read in the studies below, our diet, our childhood diet, and the diet of our mother during pregnancy and breastfeeding plays a significant role in our risk of food sensitivities. The mechanisms, as we have been discussing, relate to the immune system and the health of our intestines. An exhausted immune system will inevitably react differently than a strong immune system to a perceived foreigner. Our diets directly affect our immune system strength and the health of our intestines. Let's look at the research supporting these conclusions:

Researchers from the University of Western Australia and the Princess Margaret Hospital (Jennings and Prescott 2010) reviewed the clinical data regarding diet and environmental changes with respect to autoimmunity and food allergies. They concluded that dietary factors such as omega-3 fatty acids, oligosaccharides, probiotics, vitamin D, retinoic acid and various antioxidants in foods stimulate and assist immune function and the development of the immune system; and inherently decrease the risk of food allergies.

In a study of 460 children and mothers on Menorca—a Mediterranean island in Spain—medical researchers from Greece's Department of Social Medicine and the University of Crete (Chatzi et al. 2008) found that children of mothers eating primarily a Mediterranean diet (a predominantly plant-based diet) had significantly fewer food and other allergies. In fact, the higher the adherence to the Mediterranean diet during pregnancy, the fewer the allergies among the children.

The same researchers (Chatzi et al. 2007) surveyed the parents of 690 children from ages seven through 18 years old in the rural areas of Crete. The children also were tested with skin prick tests for 10 common allergens. They found that consuming a Mediterranean diet reduced the risk of allergic rhinitis by over 65%. The risk of skin allergies and respiratory conditions (such as wheezing) also reduced, but by smaller amounts. They also found that a greater consumption of nuts among the children cut wheezing rates in half, while consuming margarine more than doubled the prevalence of both wheezing and allergic rhinitis.

Remember the research showing that food sensitivities directly relate to asthma occurrence. Asthmatic parents increase the risk of food sensitivities among their children. Children who outgrow their milk allergy are more likely to contract asthma a few years later. Those with early allergies have a greater likelihood of later food sensitivities than those who don't.

An international group of researchers from around the world (Nagel *et al.* 2010) reported in the International Study on Allergies and Asthma in Childhood (ISAAC) that asthma occurrence is related to diet. The group conducted cross-sectional studies between 1995 and 2005 in 29 locations within 20 different countries. In all, 50,004 children ages eight through twelve years old were analyzed.

This study revealed that those with diets containing large fruit portions had lower incidence of asthma. This link occurred among both affluent and non-affluent countries. Fish consumption in affluent countries (where vegetable intake is less) and cooked green vegetables among non-affluent countries were also associated with a lower asthma rates. In general, the consumption of fruit, vegetables and fish was linked with reduced rates of asthma throughout life. At the same time, frequent consumption of meat burgers was linked with higher rates of lifetime asthma.

Consuming the Mediterranean diet (a predominantly plant-based diet), has clear results: It is linked with lower allergy and asthma rates.

This also means that diets weighted too far towards animal proteins increase the likelihood of food sensitivities, whether among mothers and their infants, adults in general, or children as they are growing up.

These associations also confirm the well-researched relationship between a diet rich in antioxidants (plant-foods have more antioxidants) and strengthened immunity in general.

Pathogenic Enzymes

The research clearly indicates that diets rich in animal foods increase the risk and incidence of food sensitivities. How does this happen? As we investigate the connection between animal-based diets and allergies, we must also include dietary factors that produce increased intestinal permeability and damage to intestinal cells and mucosal membranes. These factors are certainly interwoven, because it is our food that has the most intimate contact with our mucosal membranes, our intestinal cells and our intestinal brush barrier in general.

In 1980, Dr. Barry Goldin, a professor at the Tufts University School of Medicine, led a series of studies that found that certain diets promoted a group of cancer-causing enzymes, including beta-glucuronidase, nitroreductase, azoreductase, and steroid 7-alpha-dehydroxylase. These enzymes had been linked with colon cancer in previous studies.

Furthermore, studies on vegetarians found lower levels of these enzymes, while those eating animal-based diets had greater levels. Apparently, these cancer-related enzymes originate from a group of pathogenic bacteria that tend to occupy the intestines of those with animal-based diets. It was discovered that the cancer-producing enzymes are actually the endotoxins (waste products) of these pathogenic bacteria.

Dr. Goldin and his research teams studied the difference between these enzyme levels in omnivores and vegetarians. In one study, the researchers removed meat from the diets of a group of omnivores for 30 days. A reduction of steroid 7-alpha-dehydroxylase was found. When the probiotic L. acidophilus was supplemented to their diets, this group also showed a significant reduction in beta-glucuronidase and nitroreductase. So there were now two dietary connections with these disease-causing enzymes: animal-based diets and a lack of intestinal probiotics. The two are actually related, because probiotics thrive in prebiotic-rich plant-based diets and suffer in animal-rich diets.

Two years later, Dr. Goldin and associates (Goldin et al. 1982) studied 10 vegetarian and 10 omnivore women. He found that the vegetarian women maintained significantly lower levels of beta-glucuronidase than the omnivorous women.

The association between colon cancer and red meat has been shown conclusively in a variety of studies over the years by the way. An American Cancer Society cohort study (Chao et al. 2005) examined 148,610 adults between the ages of 50 and 74 living in 21 states of the U.S. They found that higher intakes of red and processed meats were associated with higher levels of rectal and colon cancer after other cancer variables were eliminated.

Other studies have confirmed that vegetarian diets result in a reduction of these carcinogenic enzymes produced by pathogenic bacteria. Researchers from Finland's University of Kuopio (Ling and Hanninen 1992) tested 18 volunteers who were randomly divided into either a conventional animal products diet or an extreme vegan diet for one month. The vegan group followed the month with a return to the original omnivore diet. After only one week on the vegan diet, the researchers found that fecal urease levels decreased by 66%, cholylglycine hydrolase levels decreased by 55%, beta-glucuronidase levels decreased by 33% and beta-glucosidase levels decreased by 40% in the vegan group. These reduced levels continued through the month of consuming the vegan diet. Serum levels of phenol and p-cresol—also endotoxins of pathogenic bacteria—also significantly decreased in the vegan group.

Within two weeks of returning to the animal diet, the formerly-vegan group's pathogenic enzyme levels returned to the higher levels they had before converting to the vegan diet. After one month of returning to the omnivore diet, the serum levels of toxins phenol and p-cresol returned to their previously higher levels prior to the vegan diet. Meanwhile, no changes in any of these enzymes or toxin levels occurred among the conventional omnivore diet (control) group.

A study published two years earlier by Huddinge University researchers (Johansson *et al.* 1990) also confirmed the same results. The conversion of an omnivore diet to a lacto-vegetarian diet significantly reduced levels of beta-glucuronidase, beta-glucosidase, and sulphatase (two other tumor-implicated enzymes) from fecal samples.

Another study illustrating this link between vegetarianism, pathogenic bacterial enzymes and cancer was conducted at Sweden's Huddinge University and the University Hospital (Johansson *et al.* 1998) almost a decade later. Dr. Johansson and associates measured the effect of switching from an omnivore diet to a lacto-vegetarian diet and back to an omnivore diet with respect to mutagenicity: testing the body's fluid biochemistry to determine the tendency for tumor formation.

In this extensive study, 20 non-smoking and normal weight volunteers switched to a lacto-vegetarian diet for one year. Urine and feces were examined for mutagenicity (cancer-causing bacteria and their endotoxins) at the start of the study, at three months, at six months and at twelve months after beginning the vegetarian diet. Following the switch to the lacto-vegetarian diet, all mutagenic parameters significantly decreased among the urine and feces of the subjects. The subjects were then tested once more, three years after converting back to an omnivore diet. The mutagenic biochemistry levels returned to their previously higher levels.

One might wonder what the connection is between cancer-causing enzymes and food sensitivities. The connection is found examining intestinal permeability and intestinal health in general. A cancer-causing factor typically stimulates the immune system to begin the inflammatory immune response, in this case, against the intestinal cells. If the intestinal cells are becoming damaged by these enzymes, the immune system launches a response to remove those damaged cells. This would typically consist of a cytotoxic T-cell attack against those damaged cells—the same mechanism observed in much of the intestinal permeability research.

Arachidonic Acid

To add to these factors is the problem of consuming too much arachidonic acid in the diet. Arachidonic acid is an essential fatty acid naturally converted from other fatty acids by the body. However, animal-based diets can directly overload the body with arachidonic acid, producing a pro-inflammatory condition.

This subject has been studied extensively by researchers from Wake Forest University School of Medicine, led by Professor Floyd Chilton, Ph.D. Dr. Chilton has published a wealth of research data that have uncovered that foods high in arachidonic acid can produce a pro-inflammatory metabolism, especially among adults. As we've discussed, a pro-inflammatory metabolism is basically trigger-happy and hypersensitive: producing fertile ground for food sensitivities.

In research headed up by Dr. Darshan Kelley from the Western Human Research Center in California, diets high in arachidonic acid stimulated four times more inflammatory cells than diets low in arachidonic acid content. And this problem increases with age. In other words, the same amount of arachidonic acid-forming foods will cause higher levels of arachidonic acid the older we get (Chilton 2006).

According to the USDA's Standard 13 and 16 databases, animal meats and fish produce the highest amounts of arachidonic acid in the body. Diary, fruits and vegetables produce little or no arachidonic acid. Grains, beans and nuts produce none or very small amounts. Processed bakery goods produce a moderate amount of arachidonic acid.

As we saw in the intestinal permeability research, inflammation within the tissues and cells of the intestinal wall results in increased intestinal permeability, which in turn admits macromolecules into the intestinal tissues and bloodstream. This in turn invokes the IgE immune response.

Phytanic Acid

Another association we can make between intestinal wall health and animal-based diets relates to phytanic acid. Phytanic acid (tetramethyl-hexadecanoic acid) is a byproduct of plant-food digestion inside the intestinal tracts of bovine (cows and bulls). Phytanic acid is thus present in the meat of these animals. When this branched-chain fatty acid degrades, mammalian peroxisomes are generated. Thus phytanic acid is deposited in tissues, and accumulated around the body.

Otto-von-Guericke University (Germany) professor Dr. Peter Schönfeld has showed that nonesterified phytanic acid directly alters inner mitochondrial membrane permeability though the conductance of hydrogen ions (H+). These open the cell's permeability transition pores, and causes the release of magnesium ions through the cell membrane (Schönfeld 2004).

This mechanism damages the cell, stimulating an inflammatory response. Among intestinal cells, this scenario contributes to intestinal permeability and autoimmunity—consistent with the observations from the research among animal-based diets.

Plant-based Nutrients

The connection between plant-based diets and reduced food sensitivities is also confirmed as we investigate research associating plant-derived nutrients with allergies.

In a study by researchers from Korea's Kyung Hee University (Oh *et al.* 2010), atopic dermatitis among young children was studied together with antioxidant intake. One hundred eighty children at an average age of five years old were studied. Several antioxidant-related nutrients were found to lower the risk of allergic dermatitis. Beta carotene reduced the risk of atopic dermatitis by 56%. Vitamin E reduced the risk of atopic dermatitis by 67%. Folic acid reduced the risk by 63%. Iron reduced the risk of atopic dermatitis by 61%. Retinol and alpha-tocopherol reduced the risk by 26% and 36%, respectively. Vitamin C did not produce any reduction of risk.

Researchers from the Medical University of Vienna (Diesner *et al.* 2010) concluded after a study conducted inside a nursing home, that food sensitivities are under-diagnosed and under-estimated among elderly persons. They also recognized that deficiencies in certain micronutrients such as zinc, iron, vitamin D and others among the aging or elderly appear to contribute to allergy development. They commented that a less active digestive system resulting from gastritis or anti-ulcer medication could also be a contributing factor. Undigested or partially digested proteins may become subject to an immunoglobulin response. The researchers pointed out that anti-ulcer pharmaceuticals (commonly used by the elderly) tend to mediate (pro-allergy) Th2 levels among aged animal groups.

Processed Foods

Processing of a food typically consists of chopping or pulverizing the food, heating it to high temperatures, distilling or extracting its contents, or otherwise isolating some parts of the food by straining off, clarifying or refining. Food processing is typically considered by humans as a good thing, because humans like to focus on one or two characteristics or nutrients of a food as making up that food's intrinsic value. In the end it is a value proposition, because all the energy and work required to produce the final food product must equal or be greater than the increase in the processed food's value.

Typically this increase in value is due to the food being sweeter, smoother or simply easier to eat or mix with other foods. In the case of oils or flours, the food extract is used for baking purposes, for example. In the case of sugar, which is extracted from a number of whole plants, including cane and beets, it is added to nearly every processed food.

Ironically, what is left behind in this value proposition is the food's real value. The fiber and nutrients are typically stripped away during food processing. Plant fiber is a necessary element of our diet, because it renders sterols that aid digestion and reduce LDL cholesterol. Many nutrients are attached to food fiber. Once the fiber is stripped away, the food's nutrients can be easily damaged by the heat of processing.

What is being missed in the value proposition of food processing is that nature's whole foods have their greatest value, nutritionally, prior to processing. When a food is broken down, many of the molecular bonds that hold the food's fibers and polysaccharides are lost. As these bonds are lost, the remaining components can become unstable in the body. When they become unstable, they can form free radicals, requiring our bodies to neutralize them. This produces instability elsewhere in the body, and places a burden upon our immune system.

In other words, *whole foods* provide the nutrients our bodies need, in the combinations already provided by nature. In some cases, we might need to physically peel a food to get to its edible part. In other cases, such as in the case of grains, we may need to heat or cook the whole grains to soften the fibers to enable chewing and digestion. In the case of wheats, milling the whole grain (including the bran) will render a healthy flour.

Because many of our processed foods have been in our diet for many decades, it is difficult to prove that a diet of processed food produces more allergies. To test this hypothesis, French researchers (Fremont *et al.* 2010) studied the effects of processed flax. Foods containing processed flax are somewhat of a new phenomenon. So they studied the introduction of processed flax into the French diet. They found that, in a study of 1,317 patients with allergies, those who were allergic to flax could be identified by their sensitivity to *extruded, heated flax,* rather than raw flax seed. This of course indicates that the increase in flax allergies among the French is likely due to the increase in *processed flax* rather than the increased availability of flax. Certainly, over time, as flax allergies proceed, there will be more allergies to raw flax. But now, while flax exposure is fairly recent, allergies to processed flax indicate that processing very likely increases the risk of food allergies.

So what is it about food processing that increases sensitivity?

Eating a food with its plant fibers intact will yield a more molecularly-balanced food. This is because the fibers deliver molecules the body recognizes. Our digestive enzymes and probiotics have evolved to break down (or not) certain types of molecules. Imbalanced or broken-down molecules are considered foreign.

We can also see how processing increases diseases when we compare the disease statistics of developing countries with developed countries.

For example, like many developing countries, India has more heart disease because of increased consumption of processed and fried foods. These processed foods damage intestinal health and promote free radicals. They are nutrient-poor. They burden and starve our probiotics. Frying foods also produces a carcinogen called acrylamide (Ehling *et al.* 2005).

Is there any other evidence that food processing is a contributing cause for many food sensitivities? Let's consider the case of the huge increase in peanut allergies over the past two decades:

On the Trail of Peanut Allergies

As discussed earlier, the rates of peanut allergies nearly doubled during the late 1990s, and have continued to steadily rise since then among industrialized nations. In fact, allergies to peanuts among U.S. children doubled from 1997 to 2002 (Sicherer *et al.* 2003).

So what changed during this period? Did industrialized counties eat more peanuts during this period? There is no evidence of that.

What did change during this period was the way peanuts were produced and packaged. Dry-roasting and sugar-coating ("honey roasted") of peanuts became more popular among consumers in Western industrialized countries due to the fact that more manufacturers obtained the processing capability to roast. This of course eventually bled over to other consumer nations that imported from these manufacturers.

Illustrating this trend, researchers from the Mount Sinai School of Medicine (Beyer *et al.* 2001) determined that even though the Chinese eat a significant amount of peanuts, there are significantly fewer peanut allergies in China. Since the Chinese primarily eat boiled or minimally fried peanuts—while Western countries eat mostly roasted peanuts—the researchers decided to compare the allergenicity of roasted peanuts with boiled and fried versions.

First they found that the Ara h1 protein content in peanuts—a significant allergen—was significantly reduced when peanuts are fried or boiled, as compared with the roasted. Secondly, they found that the IgE binding ability of the Ara h2 and Ara h3 proteins was reduced when peanuts were boiled or fried—again as compared with roasting. This protein-IgE binding ability is directly associated with the allergenicity of a food, as we've discussed earlier.

A couple of years later, researchers from the USDA's Agricultural Research Service (Chung *et al.* 2003) confirmed these findings when their tests revealed that mature roasted peanuts produced an increase in IgE binding along with more glycation end products.

This research was also duplicated later by other USDA researchers (Schmitt *et al.* 2004). However, in this latter study, the researchers also established that all three methods—frying, boiling and dry-roasting—increase the allergenicity of peanuts when compared with raw peanuts.

One of the leading researchers in the 2001 Mount Sinai study was Dr. Hugh Sampson. Here is a comment by Dr. Sampson on this topic:

> *"The Chinese eat the same amount of peanut per capita as we do, they introduce it early in a sort of a boiled/mushed type form, as they do in many African countries, and they have very low rates of peanut allergies. All the countries that have Westernized their diet are now seeing the same problem with food allergy as we see. Countries that have introduced peanut butter are now starting to see a rise in the prevalence of peanut allergies akin to the high rates already found in the UK, Australia, Canada and some European countries."*

We would add to this last point regarding peanut butter that many peanut butter producers use roasted peanuts. Additionally, there are generally two ways to manufacture peanut butter. Many commercial peanut butters are produced through a complex heating and blending process that includes mixing the peanut butter with sugar and hydrogenated oils.

Alternatively, peanut butter can simply be made using a natural grinding process where the whole peanuts are ground and packed into jars without heating or blending. This process typically produces a separation of the oil on top, which is why so many manufacturers over-process and blend their peanut butters. However, the oil stirs back in quite easily.

Glycation

Researchers from France's University of Burgundy (Rapin and Wiernsperger 2010) have confirmed that protein or lipid glycation produced by modern food manufacturers is linked to food sensitivities.

Glycation is produced during the manufacturing of food products, specifically when sugars and protein-foods are heated to extremely high temperatures during cooking or filling. During glycation, sugars bind to protein molecules. This produces a glycated protein and glycation end products, both of which have been implicated in cardiovascular disease, diabetes, some cancers, peripheral neuropathy and Alzheimer's disease (Miranda and Outeiro 2010).

In Alzheimer's disease, one of the products of a glycation reaction is the amyloid protein. Glycation end products introduced to the cerebro-spinal fluid have been directly implicated in the process of amyloid plaque build up among brain cells.

Glycation also takes place within the body. This occurs especially in diets containing high levels of refined sugars combined with considerable amounts of cooked or caramelized proteins.

The Western diet contains an incredible amount of processed protein compared to traditional diets. Americans eat far beyond the amount of protein required for health. Studies indicate that Americans eat an average of 80-150 grams of protein a day. This is significantly higher than the 25-50 grams of protein consumed in most healthy traditional diets around the world (Campbell and Campbell 2006; McDougall 1999).

This amount of protein in the American diet is also significantly higher than even U.S. RDA levels. The U.S. recommended daily allowance for protein is 0.8 grams per 2.2 lbs of body weight. This converts to 54 grams for a person weighing 150 pounds. Americans eat on average nearly double that amount.

To this we can add the sugar-laden Western diet. Today, nearly every pre-cooked recipe found in the mass market grocery stores contains re-fined sugar. Even processed organic foods contain organic cane syrup—a form of sugar that may not be as refined as white sugar, but is definitely refined, and stripped of the natural plant fibers in cane or beets.

Today, many brands are trying to white-wash the massive sugar content of their products by calling their sugar content "all natural." This is a deception, because nature in the form of fiber has been unnaturally stripped away from their refined sugar. This is hardly a "natural" proposition. Nature attaches sugars to complex fibers and nutrients in such a way that prevents them from easily attaching to proteins. Sugars that are cooked and stripped of their fibers become immediate glycation candidates within the body.

As our digestive system combines these sugars with proteins, many of the glycated proteins are identified as foreign by IgA, or IgE antibodies in immune-burdened or inflammatory intestines. Why are they considered foreign? Because, as we've mentioned, glycated proteins and their AGE end products damage blood vessels, tissues, brain cells and also stimulate cancerous cells. So the immune system is simply trying to protect us from our own diet!

There is no surprise that glycation among foods—and the glycation that occurs within the body as a result of the heavy consumption of refined proteins and sugars—is connected with the increase of allergies among Western societies over the past few decades. This has occurred with the increased consumption of overly-processed foods and manufacturing processes that pulverize and strip foods of their fiber; and blend denatured proteins and sugars using heating processes.

We should note that a healthy type of natural glycation also takes place in the body to produce certain nutrient combinations. Unlike the glycation produced by food manufacturers, this type of glycation is driven by the body's enzyme processes, resulting in molecules and end products the body uses and recognizes. When glycation is driven by the body's own enzyme processes, it is technically called *glycosylation.*

Hydrolyzed Proteins

Proteins are composed of very long chains of amino acids. Sometimes hundreds and even thousands of amino acids can make up a protein. The body typically breaks apart these chains through an enzyme reaction called *proteolysis.*

Proteolysis breaks down proteins into amino acids and small groups of amino acids called polypeptides. This is also called *cleaving.* As enzymes break off these polypeptides or individual amino acids from proteins, they replace the protein chain linkages with water molecules to stabilize the peptide or amino acid. This process is called *enzymatic hydrolysis.* Breaking away the peptides or amino acids allows the body to utilize the amino acid or polypeptide to make new proteins within the body.

The body then assembles its own proteins from these amino acids and polypeptides. The body's protein assemblies are programmed by DNA and RNA. For this reason, the body must recognize the polypeptide combinations. Strange polypeptide combinations can burden the body, especially if the body does not have the enzymes to break those peptides apart. While some enzymes can break apart multiple proteins and polypeptides, some proteins, such as gliadins, require special enzymes to be properly broken down into body-friendly peptides and aminos. Protein-cleaving enzymes are called *proteases.*

Food manufacturers can synthetically break down proteins by extrusion, heating and blending with a variety of processing aids, including enzymes. These processes synthetically break apart the proteins in the food. As water is integrated into the process, synthetic hydrolysis results.

This produces hydrolyzed protein foods. These synthetically hydrolyzed protein foods may not be recognized by the body's immune system.

French laboratory researchers (Bouchez-Mahiout *et al.* 2010) found by using immunoblot testing that hydrolyzed wheat proteins from skin conditioners produced hypersensitivity, which eventually crossed over to wheat proteins in foods. In other words, hydrolyzed wheat proteins in skin treatments are not necessarily recognized by the immune system. Once the body becomes sensitized to these hydrolyzed wheat proteins from skin absorption, this sensitivity can cross over to sensitivity to similar wheat proteins in foods.

Researchers from France's Center for Research in Grignon (Laurière *et al.* 2006) tested nine women who had skin contact sensitivity to cosmetics containing hydrolyzed wheat proteins (HWP). Six were found to react with either skin hives or anaphylaxis to different products (including foods) containing HWP. The whole group also had IgE sensitivity to wheat flour or gluten-type proteins. The tests showed that they had become sensitive not only to HWP, but also to unmodified grain proteins. As they tested further, they found that reactions often occurred among larger wheat protein peptide aggregates. The researchers concluded that the use of HWP in skin products can produce hypersensitivity not only to HWP, but this sensitivity can crossover to sensitivities to seemingly unrelated wheat proteins in foods.

Spanish researchers (Cabanillas *et al.* 2010) found that enzymatic hydrolysis of lentils and chickpeas produced allergens for four out of five allergic patients in their research.

The commercial enzymes used by many food manufacturers may also stimulate allergic responses. Danish researchers (Bindslev-Jensen *et al.* 2006) tested 19 commercially available enzymes typically used in the food industry on 400 adults with allergies. It was found that many of the enzymes produced histamine responses among the patients.

Hydrolyzing proteins through manufacturing processes create epitopes that the immune system does not recognize. Once the immune system launches an immune response to the epitope, it will remember those as allergens, even if they are part of foods once accepted by the body.

Lipid Transfer Proteins

Remember the Italian study (Asero *et al.* 2009) of 25,601 allergy clinic patients throughout Italy. Almost 50% had allergic skin reactions and 8.5% had IgE-mediated allergic reactions to food. Of these, 64% were female. Most of these sensitivities were to lipid transfer proteins.

The Italian study showed that pollen-related food LTP sensitivities occurred in a whooping 55% of all allergy sufferers among Italians. LTP allergy rates are seemingly lower among Northern European countries and the U.S. This is no surprise, since Italy is a big agricultural producer. It is considered by some to be the breadbasket of Western Europe.

However, as we illustrated in research in the previous chapter, increasingly, research is illustrating that LTP crossover could very well be at the root of sensitivities to a number of foods, including wheat.

In addition, most pollen-related food sensitivities are related to lipid transfer protein sensitization. Furthermore, the research has indicated a link between diet, lifestyle and pollen exposure.

It should be noted that Italy is an industrialized nation, but most of its urban population lives in the South. Thus it is no surprise that 96% of Type I food allergies among the group in the Asero research lived in the urban areas of Southern Italy. So while pollen-crops are grown throughout Italy, the greater per-capita pollen-related food allergy rates occur among those from urban areas—where processed, convenient foods are more readily consumed.

In a study by German researchers from the Paul-Ehrlich-Institute (Hartz *et al.* 2010), those with allergies to peach, cherry or hazelnuts were significantly sensitized to non-specific lipid transfer protein. As the three groups were compared, it became evident that becoming sensitized to LTP together with the allergic protein of peaches (Pru p3), produced a stronger potential of becoming allergic to hazelnuts and cherries. This is apparently because LTPs exhibit stronger IgE-binding capacity, and greater crossover capability.

LTPs are proteins that are intrinsically and complexly combined with other elements of a particular food. How does one become allergic to an LTP? Certainly it is due to a stressed or weakened immune system being exposed to the LTP epitope. This exposure can begin with LTP penetration through a thinned, weakened mucosal membrane of the sinuses; or by penetrating a weakened intestinal barrier.

Let's consider lipid transfer protein one (LTP1). This protein can be derived from barley during refining, and it is the notable protein component in beer foam. The refined LTP1 in beer foam is not like the LTP1 found within the barley grain, however. In its modified state, LTP1 produces a higher foam capacity than natural LTP1 from barley grain would produce. So beer producers have developed a more appealing "head" of foam, possibly at the expense of making available a protein the body can become sensitive to.

But what else are beer drinkers getting? They are consuming a modified version of LTP1. Does the body consider this a foreigner? Likely, because it *is* foreign. It has been modified. This LTP1 will have a slightly different molecular and magnetic configuration. Thus the body won't consider it a part of the natural diet.

Does this mean that beer is causing LTP type allergies? While beer allergies are not commonplace, they are increasingly occurring.

Beer allergies and anaphylaxis were studied by Israeli doctors and published in the *Journal of the Israel Medical Association* (Nusem and Panasoff 2009). As they tested for related allergens, they found that the cause of the beer allergies was not the alcohol, as there was no sensitivity to other alcohol beverages—only beer. They eventually concluded that the LTP allergen related to the barley refinement discussed above was at the root of the allergy syndrome.

Furthermore, Researchers from Japan's Okayama Prefectural University (Hiemori *et al.* 2008) wanted to investigate the cause of the sudden rise in beer allergies among Japanese beer consumers. Again, they found that the LTP 18-kDa IgE-binding proteins found as allergens likely originated from the barley used in the beer.

In other words, refined or isolated LTPs are portions of pollen and food molecules that a weakened immune system can become sensitized to. Once a sensitization reaction occurs, these LTPs are then recognized by the immune system as being antigens, or invaders—effectively stimulating an allergic reaction every time a similar LTP-containing food is eaten. Worse, becoming sensitized to one type of LTP can also cross over to becoming sensitized to other LTPs in foods.

Food Additives

This is a large topic, because so many processed foods are chock full of many different artificial additives. These include hundreds of artificial food colors, preservatives, stabilizers, flavorings and a variety of food processing aids. A number of these additives have been found to cause sensitivities in some people.

Illustrating the effects that food additives can have, Australian researchers (Dengate and Ruben 2002) studied 27 children with irritability, restlessness, inattention and sleep difficulties. The researchers saw many of these symptoms subside after putting the children on the Royal Prince Alfred Hospital Diet, which is absent of food additives, natural salicylates, amines and glutamates.

Using preservative challenges, the researchers were also able to determine that the preservatives significantly affected the children's behavior and physiology adversely.

Researchers from Britain's University of Southampton (Bateman *et al.* 2004) screened 1,873 three-year old children for hyperactivity and the consumption of artificial food colors and preservatives. They gave the children 20 mg daily of artificial colors and 45 mg daily of sodium benzoate, or a placebo mixture. The additive group showed significantly higher levels of hyperactivity than the group that did not consume the artificial colors and preservative.

While these studies are not proof that these food additives are allergens, we can say that with confidence that they can cause food intolerances, as hyperactivity is considered a reaction to eating these "foods."

Once an additive has caused intolerance symptoms such as those from the research above, there is always the possibility that the immune system may begin to become sensitive to some of the foods these additives are associated with. This likelihood increases should the immune system become continually exposed to the foods together with the additives over a considerable period of time.

Sulfites

Sulfites provide a classic case. The sulfite ion will aggressively preserve a food. Sulfites can also produce wheezing, tightness of the throat and other symptoms almost immediately after eating foods preserved with them. However, the effects of sulfites may not be as significant as often portrayed. It may well be that many sulfite-sensitivities seen among wine drinkers are actually the product of the alcohol rather than the sulfites.

Illustrating this, researchers from Australia's Centre for Asthma (Vally *et al.* 2007) tested eight wine-sensitive subjects with sulfite wine and non-sulfite wine. The researchers found that the wine sensitivities were unlikely caused by the sulfites in the wine.

Today, sulfites are used to preserve many wines, dehydrated potatoes and numerous dried fruits. Sulfites include potassium bisulfite, sulfur dioxide, potassium matabisulfite and others. Often labels do not disclose the use of sulfites, because the preservative may have been used early in the processing of the raw ingredients instead of added into the finished product. In addition, under current U.S. labeling laws, if an ingredient such as sulfite is less than 10 parts per million, there is no requirement for putting the ingredient on the panel.

Sulfite sensitivity may be the result of B12 deficiency. In a study presented to the American Academy of Allergy and Immunology, 18 sulfite-sensitive persons were given sublingual B12. The B12 effectively blocked adverse reactions to sulfites in 17 of the 18 (Werbach 1996).

Monosodium Glutamate

Monosodium glutamate also gets a lot of attention for producing sensitivity symptoms. This has also been echoed among a number of studies.

To better understand this, Harvard researchers (Geha *et al.* 2000) set out to study the effects of MSG sensitivities in a multi-center study. They found that of 130 human volunteers who thought they were sensitive to MSG, 38% physically responded to MSG with allergic symptoms. However, 13% also responded to a placebo (they thought contained MSG). Subsequent retesting continued to show inconsistent responses among some of those who thought they were MSG-sensitive.

This led the researchers to conclude that people who believe they are sensitive tend to react more strongly to MSG, but their responses were not always consistent. This of course may be the result of differing levels of tolerance and periods of sensitivity—again depending upon immunity.

This research still confirms that MSG can cause sensitivity responses. Possibly MSG may be overhyped somewhat, but like so many other food additives, there is no doubt that it is not a natural part of our food supply.

Microparticles

Some researchers have suggested that substances with microparticles can lead to increased intestinal permeability and food sensitivities (Korzenik 2005).

Microparticles are particles smaller than 100 μm, but larger than 0.1 μm. (Smaller molecules, in the nanometer range, are called nanoparticles.) Products that are produced with microparticles include toothpaste and mouthwashes. Food products that contain microparticles include powdered sugars and some refined flours.

We might better classify microparticles in the same category as overly processed foods. The bottom line is that the body can become sensitive to unnaturally-processed constituents should they be exposed to intestinal tissues and bloodstream—and not be recognized by the immune system.

Genetically Engineered Foods

Speaking of unnatural: A genetically engineered food is a food whose genes have been modified in a laboratory. A gene from one species is synthetically inserted into the DNA of another species. More technically, genes from one seed are inserted into another seed utilizing a virus as the vehicle. This seed is then reproduced and sold to farmers.

Today about 70% of the packaged foods in a conventional supermarket contain ingredients grown from genetically modified seeds. Much of the U.S. supply of corn, soybeans, canola and cotton are now genetically modified. (Organic versions of these foods are not genetically modified.) A few other foods now are sometimes grown from GMO seed, such as squash and zucchini.

The main purpose of genetic modification in many cases is to yield plants that are tolerant to more pesticides. A few have been designed to produce their own pesticides.

So what does this yield in terms of food? For those tolerant to more pesticides, it typically means the food will have more pesticide residue. For others, it may be a food that contains a substance that repels insects. In either case, because the DNA is being modified, the food will contain some proteins that are not contained in natural versions of this food. These proteins may not be well-recognized by the immune system, and may spark sensitivities among some people.

This is because proteins are determined by the DNA of the plant. In other words, change the DNA, and you change some of the proteins.

Curiously, shortly after GMO soy was introduced to the U.K., soy allergies in England skyrocketed by 50%. GMO soy contains larger levels of a recognized allergen called trypsin inhibitor. It also contains a number of new proteins. In mice, GMO soy slowed down the production of pancreatic enzymes, which altered the breakdown of all foods. Mice also showed organ damage, sperm damage and embryo damage after consuming GMO soy (Dona and Arvanitoyannis 2009).

In another study, when rats were given GMO soy, they suffered increased damage amongst many organs, had greater levels of many diseases, and about 50% of the mice' offspring died within three weeks of feeding (Smith 2007).

It should also be noted that this topic is currently the subject of significant debate among scientists. Many believe that the risk of increased allergies is minimal. For example, a study of a GM soybean variety by Spanish researchers (Batista et al. 2007) found that there were two potential new allergens within the protein samples analyzed. But when they gave the GM soy to volunteers, none had an allergic response. While this study illustrated that new potential allergens were produced in the new soy species, it did not prove allergic response. However, when we consider that the rate of allergies to soy is less than 1% of the entire population, the rate of allergenicity to these new allergens might even be less—perhaps .1%. This would mean that they would have needed to feed the soy to 1,000 people before they should see one allergic response.

It should also be noted that based on the science, many governments have banned the use of genetically modified crops and foods.

The critical issue here is to what extent we really understand the consequences related to genetic modification. This concern typically lands people in one of two camps: Do we trust that humans have the inherent wisdom to be able to modify nature in such a way that will ultimately benefit humanity and the planet, and not result in disaster?

To this point we could consider the rise of petroleum use and synthetic plastics, which have transformed society in many ways. These have certainly led to monumental environmental and health disasters: Ones that have not only destroyed or endangered many species, but could actually destroy the earth's ability to support the human race altogether.

Many scientists have proposed that GM crops should be banned simply for their possible allergenicity. In addition, many scientists argue that GM crops may introduce new allergens into the environment (Bachas-Daunert and Deo 2009).

There are also other issues with GM crops: One is the fact that growers have to keep going back to the GM seed producers every year because the GM producers designed most seeds to not allow the plant to reproduce. This means that new seeds cannot be naturally produced by farmers—as they have for thousands of years.

Enzyme Deficiencies

If we are deficient in a particular enzyme, this can create a situation where the food is not properly broken down. This can create a macromolecule that may be exposed to the cells and tissues of the intestines. If the intestinal barrier is weakened, the immunoglobulins within the intestines can mark the macromolecule as an invader. Worse, the macromolecule can get into the internal tissues and bloodstream—where the immune system can launch an allergic attack against it.

The point is that the body has a very exacting way it breaks down proteins. As we discussed earlier, this requires specific protease enzymes and the process of natural enzymatic hydrolysis. This of course means that the body also needs to have plenty of water on hand as well.

Confirming the relationship between food allergies and digestive enzymes, researchers from the Medical University of Vienna (Untersmayr *et al.* 2007) studied the effects that incomplete digestion of fish proteins has on fish allergies. Healthy volunteers and those with diagnosed codfish allergies were challenged with codfish. They were also tested with fish proteins incubated with varying degrees of digestive enzymes. The subjects were tested for histamine release from fish allergen sensitivity with each type.

The researchers found that the inadequate breakdown of fish proteins produced more allergic responses, while a more complete breakdown by enzymes produced fewer allergic responses among both groups. Inadequate digestion produced allergens that the body sensitized to.

Here is a short list of the body's major digestive enzymes:

Major Digestive Enzymes

Enzyme	Foods it Breaks Down
Amylase	Starches
Bromelain	Proteins
Carboxypeptidase	Proteins (terminal)
Cellulase	Plant fiber (cellulose)
Chymotrypsin	Proteins
Elastase	Proteins and elastins
Glucoamylase	Starches
Isomaltase	Isomaltose and Maltose
Lactase	Lactose
Lipase	Fats
Maltase	Maltose
Nuclease	Protein nucleotides
Pepsin	Proteins
Peptidase	Proteins
Rennin	Milk
Steapsin	Triglycerides
Sucrase	Sucrose
Tributyrase	Butter Fat
Trypsin	Proteins
Xylanase	Hemicellulose (plant fiber)

We can see from this list that there are many different protein enzymes. This is because there are so many different types of protein molecules to break down. There are numerous enzyme sub-types and others that break down specific food constituents and particular foods. The body makes some of these; some are contained in a plant-based diet; and some are produced by our colonies of intestinal probiotics.

Breastfeeding

Research is increasing illustrating that breastfeeding is critical to the future possibility of food sensitivities. Plenty of research on breastfeeding has found that babies breast-fed from healthy mothers have a lower incidence of disease, higher rates of growth, and stronger immune systems. The reasons for these include not only that breast milk contains a variety of proteins, fatty acids, vitamins, nucleotides and colostrum (a special immune system-stimulator). Breast milk from a healthy mother also contains a variety of important probiotics.

Researchers from Japan's Shiga Medical Center for Children (Kusunoki *et al.* 2010) surveyed 13,215 parents of children aged from seven to 15 years old. The study compared allergic rates among three types of infant feeding histories: exclusive breastfeeding; mixed formula and breastfeeding; and exclusive formula feeding. The results showed conclusively that exclusive breastfeeding produced significantly fewer cases of bronchial asthma.

Researchers from University of Cincinnati's Department of Internal Medicine (Codispoti *et al.* 2010) studied 361 children, 116 who had allergic rhinitis. They found that prolonged breast-feeding among African American children decreased the allergy risk by 20%.

Researchers from Spain's University of Granada (Martínez-Augustin *et al.* 1997) studied intestinal permeability during the first month of life, along with antibody production to milk proteins. The study fed either cow's milk formula for low-birth weight or the same formula supplemented with nucleotides matching human breast milk. Blood and urine samples were obtained at one, seven and 30 days of age. They found that (low allergy risk) blood IgG antibodies to cow milk protein beta-lactoglobulin were higher among the babies that were fed the formula with the breast milk nucleotides.

Researchers from Sweden's Institute of Environmental Medicine (Kull *et al.* 2010) studied 3,825 children over a period of eight years to determine the role of breast feeding and food allergies. They determined that children who were exclusively breast-fed for four months or more experienced a significantly lower risk of asthma for the first eight years of their lives—as compared to those breast-fed for less than four months. The exclusively breast-fed group also were observed to have significantly better lung function.

Newborns and infants have under-developed intestinal epithelial barriers, and their immune system is still developing. For this reason, it is a sensitive time for the intestinal tract. Breast milk has been shown to stimulate greater levels of IgA within the intestinal tract—thereby reducing the risk of allergies (Brandtzaeg 2010).

However, this association between breast feeding and milk allergies is more complicated. University of Helsinki researchers (Saarinen *et al.* 2000) studied breast-fed and formula infants. From a sampling of 6,209 infants, 824 were found to be exclusively breast-fed. They found that the cumulative incidence of cow's milk allergies was higher in the cow's milk formula group than among the exclusively breast-fed group (2.4% versus 2.1%). This also illustrated that exclusive breast-feeding does not necessarily eliminate the potential for becoming allergic to milk. We would postulate that this rate of milk allergies was due to the mother's own IgE sensitivities to milk and passing these along, as we've discussed.

It also appears that some early exposure to cow's milk may reduce sensitivity. Israeli researchers (Katz *et al.* 2010) from the Assaf-Harofeh Medical Center studied 13,019 infants. The rate of IgE-mediated cow's milk allergy among the population was 0.5%. The average age that cow's milk feeding was introduced was significantly different between the allergic children and those not allergic. The healthy infants were started on milk an average of 62 days after birth. Those infants with cow's milk allergies were started on milk an average of 116 days after birth. Only 0.05% of those infants who were given cow milk formula within the first two weeks of life contracted milk allergies. This is compared to 1.75% of those children who took cow's milk formula between 105 and 194 days after birth contracting allergy to cow's milk.

No breast milk can result in other issues. Researchers from Italy's Siena University (Garzi *et al.* 2002) found that of the about-20% of infants given formula (not fed with breast-milk) suffered from gastroesophageal reflux (GERD), about a third also suffered from milk allergies.

Scientists from the Center for Infant Nutrition at the University of Milan (Arslanoglu *et al.* 2008) found that short-chain galactooligosaccharides (scGOS) and long-chain fructooligosaccharides (lcFOS) (both present in healthy breast milk) can reduce the incidence of atopic dermatitis (AD) and infections through six months of age. They fed 134 infants either a prebiotic-supplemented formula or a placebo-supplemented formula. Follow-ups continued until age two. Atopic dermatitis, asthma, and allergic urticaria rates were significantly higher among the infants given the placebo formula. Formula with oligosaccharide prebiotics lowers the risk of allergies. This of course relates to the fact that prebiotics increase probiotic populations within the intestines.

The bottom line: Exclusive breast-feeding for around the first four months reduces food allergy risk.

The Role of Obesity

The rates of obesity have increased as food sensitivities have increased among industrialized countries. This is not necessarily a direct association in itself, but it certainly is suspicious. Currently, about 72 million Americans—nearly one-third of the population—are obese according to the 2005-2006 National Health and Nutrition Examination.

As part of this National Health and Nutrition Examination study mentioned above, scientists from the University of North Carolina (Visness *et al.* 2009) directly correlated obesity with the prevalence of food allergies among children. They defined obesity as being over the 95th percentile of weight; and overweight as being over the 85th percentile of weight for children between the ages of two and nineteen years old.

The researchers found that obese children had greater levels of atopic sensitivities, allergen-specific IgE levels and allergy symptoms. They also found that obese children had a 31% greater risk of having allergies, and overweight children had a 25% greater risk of having allergies.

Incidentally, the researchers also found that allergies correlated with increased levels of C-reactive protein, which is known to reflect a status of inflammation within the body. As we have discussed, an overly inflammatory status leads to a lower tolerance of foods due to the heightened state of sensitivity within the immune system.

Anxiety, Stress and Depression

Mood and stress are critical to the intestinal barrier function. French researchers (Ducrotté 2009) have illustrated that food sensitization can occur from a dysfunction of afferent neurons, which can produce disturbances among the *"brain-gut axis."*

In other words, the interplay between stress and digestive responsiveness can stimulate immune response and increased intestinal permeability. Research has showed that chronic stress also plays a primary role in the occurrence and continuance of irritable bowel syndrome. This of course involves various neural and sensory relationships, as well as neurotransmitters and their receptors (Buret 2006).

Researchers from Norway's University of Bergen Medical School (Lillestøl *et al.* 2010) found that anxiety and depression are often associated in food intolerance. They studied 130 food sensitive patients with 75 healthy volunteers. They found that 57% of the food sensitive patients had at least one psychiatric disorder. Anxiety disorders were seen among 34% and depression disorders were seen among 16%. Meanwhile, 89% of the patients had irritable bowel syndrome. The researchers concluded that, *"anxiety and depression are common in patients with IBS-like complaints self-attributed to food hypersensitivity. Anxiety disorders predominate."*

The conclusion is that stress and anxiety induces intestinal hypersensitivity, and a higher risk of food sensitivities.

Sun Exposure

Multiple studies have found that allergies are significantly greater among regions further from the equator and those with less sunlight exposure. In both Europe and the U.S., those living in Southern regions have shown significantly lower incidence of food sensitivities and far fewer hospital visits for food allergies.

In the first chapter, we discussed the international European study of 17,280 adults from different countries by researchers from Australia's Monash Medical School (Woods *et al.* 2001). Among developed countries, 12% reported either having food allergies or food intolerances. Food allergy rates were higher among those living in Northern Europe as compared with Southern European countries.

Researchers from the Children's Hospital Boston (Rudders *et al.* 2010) studied allergic emergency room visits throughout the United States. They found that those living in Southern regions had significantly lower incidence of food allergies and far fewer hospital visits for food allergies. The Northeast region had 5.5 visits per thousand, while the South had 4.9 visits per thousand. This difference was even greater when the analysis was restricted to food sensitivities. The risk of food sensitivities was 33% higher for those living in the Northeast than those living in the sun-drenched South. The researchers concluded that: *"These observational data are consistent with the hypothesis that vitamin D may play an etiologic role in anaphylaxis, especially food-induced anaphylaxis."*

Researchers from Massachusetts General Hospital (Vassallo *et al.* 2010) researched the connection between the season of birth and the contraction of food allergies. The records of three Boston food allergy clinics were reviewed. In all, 1,002 patients with food allergies were studied. Forty-one percent of children with food allergies were born in the spring or the summer. Fifty-nine percent were born in the fall or the winter time. Children born in the fall or winter had a significantly higher risk of food allergies. The researchers proposed that the findings indicate that greater levels of UV-B exposure and subsequent vitamin D production might explain this occurrence.

(The author's book, *Healthy Sun* (2009) reveals other mechanisms involved in sunlight exposure.)

Ultra-Hygiene

Researchers from Finland's University of Turku (Kalliomäki and Iso-lauri 2002) concluded after a review of multiple studies that the sterile birthing environments among Western hospitals have reduced exposure to early microbes. This, they hypothesized, is a key reason that sensitivity and atopic diseases such as eczema, allergic rhinitis and asthma are on the rise among these Western nations. This has been called the *Hygiene Hypothesis of Allergy.*

The Finnish researchers supported their hypothesis with immunological data illustrating that the immune system responds to microbial antigens, both pathogenic and non-pathogenic ones, with the expression of cytokines that balance the T-helpers produced by the infants.

In other words, with an increase in exposure to available pathogens—to a degree—comes a strengthened immune system. This is to a degree because too many pathogens can overwhelm the immune system.

This is supported by a number of studies confirming that children born and raised on farms have a lower incidence of food allergies (Hamelmann *et al.* 2008).

For example, Finnish researchers (Metsälä *et al.* 2010) found that a lower family socioeconomic status lowered the risk of contracting milk allergies by 35%. Having given birth to five or more babies previous to the child (more siblings) reduced the risk of cow's milk allergies by 29%. Lower economic status is associated with more exposure to nature's microbes, soils and other elements. Lower socioeconomic status among the Fins is also associated with farmers, who tend to be poorer than their city-dwelling peers.

In a study mentioned earlier, University of Cincinnati researchers (Codispoti *et al.* 2010) found in a study of 361 children that multiple children in the home during infancy decreased the risk of allergic rhinitis by 60%.

Medical researchers from Switzerland's University of Basel (Waser *et al.* 2007) conducted a study of 14,893 children between the ages of five and 13 from five different European countries. The testing group included 2,823 children from farms and 4,606 children attending Steiner Schools (known for their farm-based living and instruction). They found that children on the farms—particularly those who drank farm milk—had significantly fewer allergies and asthma. The reason, as we'll discuss, stems from the increase in probiotics among raw farm milk.

Dr. Oner Ozdemir, M.D. at the SEMA Research and Training Hospital in Turkey, characterizes the issue with an understanding of immune and probiotic mechanisms:

> *"Development of the child's immune system tends to be directed toward a T-helper 2 (Th2) phenotype in infants. To prevent development of childhood allergic/atopic diseases, immature Th2-dominant neonatal responses must undergo environment-driven maturation via microbial contact in the early postnatal period. Lactic acid bacteria and bifidobacteria are found more commonly in the composition of the intestinal flora of nonallergic*

children. Epidemiological data also showed that atopic children have a different intestinal flora from healthy children. Probiotics are ingested with live health-promoting microbes that can modify intestinal microbial populations in a way that benefits the host; and enhanced presence of probiotic bacteria in the intestinal microbiota is found to correlate with protection against atopy."

Airborne Allergens

Once the immune system is compromised or burdened, any number of allergens can be met with an inappropriate and excessive response by the immune system. Once the immune system has overreacted to an airborne allergen, it can produce the same reaction should it meet that allergen within a food.

For this reason, Polish researchers (Swiderska-Kiełbik *et al.* 2010) found that those who have occupational contact working with birds in zoos, facilities that slaughter birds, or pet birds, are significantly more likely to develop allergies to eggs, feathers and other related allergens.

Spanish allergy researchers (Prieto *et al.* 2010) found that lupin inhalation from manufacturing facilities caused sensitization to lupin proteins, which carried over to food sensitivities to lupin-related foods and lupin flour-containing foods.

Researchers from France's Nancy Central Hospital Immunology Clinic (Moneret-Vautrin *et al.* 1996) estimated that while food allergy-related asthma is less common than food allergy-related atopic dermatitis, there is an 8.5% incidence of food allergies among asthma sufferers. This also connects airborne sensitivities with food sensitivities.

Furthermore, the researchers pointed out that occupational exposure to inhaled food proteins is increasing. They advised that egg protein or feather inhalation is particularly risky. Among adults, food allergies are common after bronchi become sensitized to either food allergen inhalation or cross-reactive pollen allergens. They also reported latex as a cross-allergen. They documented that intestinal permeability caused by viral infections, aspirin, alcohol, and other toxins is a typical precursor to these cross-reactive sensitizations.

This conclusion confirms the premise that immunosuppression caused by the exposure to the unnatural increase in synthetic toxins can produce increased sensitivity to food allergens, especially those available from abnormal situations.

Let's not forget the research from the University of Ferrara (Boccafogli *et al.* 1994), Japan's Yokohama City University Hospital (Maeda *et al.*

2010) and many others that indicated airborne allergens such as pollen can crossover to food allergies once sensitized.

We can conclude that the abnormal inhalation of proteins, either as pollens or from milled, cooked or ground foods, can increase the likelihood of food sensitivities related to those proteins or pollens (also proteins) inhaled. The risk is significantly higher among immunosuppressed people.

Tobacco

Tobacco smoke contains carbon monoxide, nicotine, aldehydes, ketones and other toxins. These can easily burden the immune system with toxin overload. This is especially when it pervades the oxygen environment of a child, or the bloodstream of the mother.

Illustrating this, researchers from the Respiratory Diseases Department of France's Hospital of Haut-Lévèque in Bordeaux (Raherison *et al.* 2008), studied 7,798 children from six cities in France. The research found that children from parents (especially mothers) who smoked, had a significantly greater likelihood of having asthma and allergies than children from families that did not smoke.

Mold

An undue amount of mold can also overwhelm the immune system. Mold is related to asthma and rhinitis, and as we showed earlier, research indicates that the risk of food sensitivities increases among those with asthma and rhinitis.

This was confirmed by researchers from the National University of Singapore (Tham *et al.* 2007), who found that home dampness and indoor mold is linked to an increase in allergies among children. They studied 4,759 children from 120 daycare centers. After eliminating other possible effects, home humidity was significantly associated with increased rates of allergic rhinoconjunctivitis. As discussed earlier, allergic rhinoconjunctivitis is the inflammation of the conjunctiva and sinuses as a result of histamine release following an allergic immune response. As mold burdens the immune system, the body responds with hypersensitivity.

Yeast Infections

Overgrowths of yeasts like *Candida albicans* can also contribute to or be a primary cause for food intolerances and even food allergies in progressive cases. *Candida albicans* can grow conjunctively with *Staphylococcus aureus*, resulting in the accelerated growth of both microorganisms. This can result in a tremendous burden for the immune and probiotic systems as they try to defend against the incursion of the combined yeast and bacteria infections. We see this lethal combination involved in many of the fatalities from swine flu and other influenza contagions. The deaths typically occur in immunosuppressed patients with concurrent bacteria infections. Immunosuppression is also related to food sensitivity.

As the immune system becomes overloaded with a microorganism invasion, it will often respond with an acute inflammatory response, simply because the system is already on alert mode. This produces a number of inflammatory-type symptoms.

We illustrated these associations in the previous chapter, with research from Australia's Ninewells Hospital and Medical School (McKenzie *et al.* 1990).

Mercury

Exposure to mercury has been suspected as a possible culprit in reducing immunity and thus increasing the risk of hypersensitivity.

This was illustrated in multicenter research from the Department of Medicine from Lavoro Medical Center in Bari, Italy (Soleo *et al.* 2002). Here researchers studied the effects of low levels of inorganic mercury exposure on 117 workers. They compared these with 172 general population subjects. There was no difference in the white blood cell count between the two groups. However, the exposed worker group had increased levels of CD4+ and CD8+ cytokines. CD4+ levels were significantly high. A significantly lower level of interleukin (IL-8) occurred among the exposed workers.

This research concluded that even low levels of environmental exposure to mercury (and likely other heavy metals) suppresses the immune system. As we've discussed, the increase in these cytokines and the burdening of the immune system in general increases the potential for an inflammatory intestinal response and subsequent food sensitivity.

C-Sections

Researchers from the Netherlands' National Institute for Public Health and the Environment (Roduit et al 2009) studied the allergic status of 2,917 children with respect to whether they were born with a cesarean section. They tested 1,454 of the children for IgE antibodies for inhalants and food allergens at age eight. They found conclusively that babies born with cesarean section had a significantly increased risk of asthma and food sensitivities.

Researchers from Finland's National Institute for Health and Welfare (Metsälä *et al.* 2010) studied all children born in Finland between 1996 and

2004 that were diagnosed with cow's milk allergies. In all, 16,237 allergic children were found. Children born of cesarean section had a 18% greater risk of contracting milk allergies.

Researchers from the Germany's National Research Centre for Environment and Health and the Institute of Epidemiology (Laubereau *et al.* 2004) studied 865 healthy infants whose parents had allergies. They tested the babies at one, four, eight and twelve months old. They found that babies (147) born with cesarean section had over double the risk of sensitivities to allergens than their peers without C-section birth.

No Proven Vaccination Connection

Many, especially parents of children with food allergies, have attributed childhood food allergies to vaccination—now given to children in most industrialized countries. This, however, is not supported by the research. In this case, we should detail the evidence concluding that vaccination does not necessarily predicate allergies.

Researchers from Australia's University of Melbourne (Matheson *et al.* 2010) studied the association between childhood immunizations and allergic atopic disease. They participated in the Tasmanian Longitudinal Health Study. The TAHS was begun in 1968. All Tasmanian school children born in 1961 took part in the study focused upon asthma. Over 45,000 individuals and 8,583 families, which included 16,267 parents and 21,036 siblings participated. These children and families were studied for over four decades. The TAHS subjects were followed through 44 yrs of age. Their childhood immunizations were compared with their asthma and atopic disease rates at 44 years old. Immunizations included Diphtheria, Tetanus, Pertussis, Polio, Smallpox vaccinations. The research found no association between childhood immunizations and asthma, eczema, food allergies, or hay fever.

In another study, conducted by medical researchers from Israel's Ben-Gurion University, 186,663 cases of pertussis vaccination and 41,479 cases of BCG vaccination were studied among others. In all groups, they found no statistical association between asthma and these vaccinations. Because of the close association between food sensitivities and asthma, we can conclude that this result should also relate food allergies as well.

This does not mean vaccinations might not be implicated in cases of food intolerance. It also does not mean that the cocktail of vaccinations now given to children might not heighten the immune system to the point of hypersensitivity. Today children receive more than thirty vaccinations for practically every type of infection with a history of risk to children. Adult vaccines are also on the increase. Today's vaccine lineups include polio, measles, mumps, rubella, chickenpox, rotavirus, tetanus, pertussis, meningitis, diphtheria, hepatitis A and B, influenza, and now the human papillomavirus vaccine.

There is good reason for many of these vaccines. And vaccination simply stimulates the body's own immune response. Still, the combined vaccine cocktails now given to infants and children could in some cases overload the immune system, resulting in food sensitivities, but this has yet to be proven scientifically. In this case, other toxins are likely involved.

Autoimmunity

Research indicates that the risk of developing (or already having) food sensitivities increases significantly for those with autoimmune diseases. There are many conditions now being defined as an autoimmune disease, and it appears that new ones are being added. Why?

About 3% of the U.S. population suffers from systemic or tissue-specific autoimmune disorders (Jacobson et al. 1995), with women making up about 85% (Walsh and Rau, 2000). A significant amount of research data confirms the conclusion that environmental exposures contribute significantly to autoimmune disease in general (Cooper et al. 2002; Hess 1997).

For example, researchers from Sweden's University Hospital in Upp-sala (Lidén et al. 2010) found that many rheumatoid arthritis (RA) patients have food allergies. They surveyed 347 RA patients, and found that 27% of the RA patients reported that they had food intolerances. These in-cluded sensitivities to cow's milk, meat and wheat gluten. Further testing using oral tolerance parameters found that 22% had cow's milk intoler-ance, and 33% had wheat gluten intolerance.

Swiss researchers from the University Hospital in Zurich (Bentz et al. 2010) studied 79 Crohn's disease patients with 20 healthy subjects. Food-activated IgG antibodies were found to be significantly increased among the Crohn's patients. The scientists tested 40 additional patients to con-firm the result. In total, they found that 83% of the patients maintained significant levels of IgG antibodies against processed cheese and yeast. When a diet that eliminated these foods was instituted, daily stool fre-quency (a common issue among Crohn's sufferers) significantly decreased compared with the control (sham) diet. Abdominal pain was reduced and Crohn's patients on the elimination diet reported increased well-being.

Intestinal diseases come with a variety of names, including intestinal hypersensitivity, inflammatory bowel disease, irritable bowel syndrome, Crohn's disease, colitis and many others. In practically every one of these conditions, there is a disruption of the intestinal barrier along the walls of the intestines. Because the intestinal barrier function responds to neural impulses from the vagus nerve and other sympathetic nerves, there is an association with stress.

As these neural impulses are activated by corticotrophin-releasing hormone (a stress response hormone), mucosal mast cells release tryptase, TNF-alpha, nerve growth factor and interleukins that directly disrupt the intestinal barrier function (Keita and Söderholm 2010).

As we've discussed, a dysfunctional barrier function causes permeability issues, which burden the immune system within the intestinal area and the body as a whole, as the body must respond to the entry of foreigners.

As the immune system responds to macromolecule entry into the epithelial layer, there are particular responses. The responses are similar between ulcerative colitis disease and Crohn's disease. Both show an increase in chloride and water secretion, which lead to an increase of intestinal wall permeability, along with a faster turnover (death) of intestinal wall cells. The cytokine that appears to stimulate this process in Crohn's disease in particular is tumor necrosis factor alpha (TNF-a). In ulcerative colitis, the same processes are stimulated by the cytokine interleukin-13 (IL-13) (Salim and Söderholm 2010).

Illustrating this, researchers from the Norway's University of Bergen Medical School (Lillestøl et al. 2010) studied 71 allergic patients. Of the group, 66, or 93%, had irritable bowel syndrome. Forty-three, or 61%, had atopic symptoms—primarily rhinoconjunctivitis. In addition, 43 were sensitized to inhalant allergens. Of the 71 patients, 41% (29) had food allergies. The researchers described the IgE-positive mast cells as *"armed."*

As we investigate autoimmunity in more detail, we unfold a number of relationships between autoimmunity and environmental factors. We also discover a strong link between autoimmunity and the viability of the immune system itself. This relationship becomes apparent as most autoimmune diseases occur during the middle age years or elderly years. The relationship between our environment and autoimmune disorders is also highlighted by the rise in autoimmune disease as our environment becomes increasingly contaminated with chemical toxins.

Recently, the Immunosciences Lab in California (Vojdani 2008) released a study that tested the fluids of 420 patients with a variety of autoimmune-type disorders. These were screened for 96 different antibodies to a variety of different infectious and proteins. A significant number of the autoimmune-patients tested positive to one or multiple *autoantibodies.* This leads to a thesis that some autoimmunity is related to a derangement of the immune system from previous infections, and/or the immune system has been overloaded with too many toxins.

We have discussed how the thymus can weaken with age, stress and toxic overload. The thymus is where T-cells are programmed with the antigen-programming called T-cell receptors or TCRs. These direct the T-cells to identify particular types of infected cells or toxins. The thymus accomplishes this through the major histocompatibility complex or the MHC as explained in the chapter on the immune system.

However, this MHC programming can be corrupted by stress and toxins. Over the years of toxic load bombardment and malnourishment, the thymus can begin to collapse and become increasingly unproductive. As this happens, the immune system's T-cells are not programmed with the most up-to-date instructions. Should the thymus not be productive, T-cells will not be appropriately programmed with the updated MHC and TCR information. They will become less tolerant and less adaptable.

Researchers are now suspecting that this lack of updated programming causes T-cells to begin attacking the body's own intestinal cells: Especially if those intestinal cells have become altered as a result of exposure to new toxins or macromolecules.

This is only logical, since over time the body's cells must adapt to all the stressors that we throw at them in order for our body to keep living in a toxic world. How else could we survive so many lethal toxic threats? As intestinal cells begin to adapt and change, they become increasingly unrecognizable if the immune system is working with older programming.

Today, our intestinal cells must learn to adapt to so many chemicals in our foods: preservatives, food dyes and overly processed and isolated ingredients. Our immune systems must learn to adapt to these plus chemicals in our immediate environment: formaldehyde, PCBs, plasticizers and petrochemicals. Our immune systems must learn to adapt to the stresses of our modern culture: not getting enough sleep, rushing for time, and dealing with money. For some of us, our intestinal cells must also learn to adapt to deficient water. For some of us, our cells must also learn to adapt to a lack of good nutrition. Any changing environmental element will require the cells and the immune system to adapt.

Over time, all these adaptations are reflected in our cells' gene sequences. These will also be reflected on the cell membrane.

In the case of the intrusion of a toxic chemical, for example, the immune system stimulates a detoxification event to clear the toxin. This may dispatch macrophages to take apart the toxin. Should the toxin not be cleared, the free radicals produced by the toxin or the toxin itself may enter and damage cells within the body. Once cells are invaded, the invaded cell genes adapt to the invasion in order to accommodate it.

Viruses are more specifically tuned to forcing genetic changes. In either case, the immune system will often initiate an inflammatory response and detoxification event the toxin and/or the invaded cells. This produces swelling, sneezing, coughing, watery eyes and so on.

However, should the cell adapt without a significant loss in function, the cell's genes make adjustments, which are communicated through to the thymus' MHC programming of T-cells. Since the T-cells have been given updated genetic information, the body is adapted to the intrusion.

We might compare this to how we adapt to weather. When there is hot weather, we will wear different clothes and move more slowly. During cold weather, we put on many more clothes and shiver more to create heat. During the wintertime, we adapt to the cold weather with many changes to our house and habits in order to stay warm.

As the cell adapts, it produces a reflective molecular signal on the cell membrane reflecting its change. This ligand can signal the TCR of the thymus that it is genetically different but functional.

This signal is comparable to a ship raising a flag that it has undergone change for other boats to see from far away. This 'flag' can be read by T-cells that are searching for cells that have been invaded. Should T-cells without updated programming 'read' such a signal on the surface, they dispatch the appropriate immune response. A large group of 'flagged' cells will likely cause a full-scale inflammatory attack against the region.

In the case of a lack of nutrients or water for extended periods, the DNA and RNA within the cell may be forced to adapt to a condition where the cell operates with less fuel. We could compare this to the ship raising a flag that it is trying to accommodate running out of fuel.

The first nutrient deficiency to damage the cell is oxygen. Without oxygen, our cells will starve for energy and will not be able to function. This can take place within minutes. The second most dangerous nutrient deficiency is water. Should the cell not have enough water, it will begin to deteriorate. We'll discuss this shortly.

Our DNA may also undergo direct damage from ionizing electromagnetism. This has been illustrated in the research on nuclear bomb victims. Electromagnetic ionizing waveforms originating from radiation from x-rays, CT-scans and so on will subtly stress the cell's ability to communicate within itself and with other cells. The cell must then adapt to these new environmental waveforms by making genetic accommodations. The need for chronic adjustment can result in the mutation of DNA. This mutation may also turn the cell into a cancerous cell.

In the same way, we find our bodies can accommodate many environmental toxins: Despite these toxins' ability to damage our cells and burden our immune system. Why have our bodies seemingly adapted to the avalanche of plastics and the plasticizers that come with them over the past three decades? The plethora of plastics have certainly increased our immune system burden, disrupted our hormones and damaged our livers. Yet many of us have little in the way outward allergies, sensitivities or other obvious symptoms of plastic use. The problem is that we cannot readily recognize the genetic accommodation to plasticizer toxicity. These may include hormone imbalances, chronic fatigue, reduced immunity, allergic reactions to natural elements like pollen and grass, and of course autoimmune conditions.

Our cells are adjusting to new environments all the time. For example, if we were to move to a warmer location—with greater UV radiation and contact with the sun's infrared rays—our cells will begin to operate with slower metabolism, allowing the body's core temperature to remain balanced. Though this might stress the cells somewhat, this sort of adapting mechanism is not considered harmful, because the sun's rays (except perhaps mid-day UV) are considered healthy to the body. However, should our body move into a 'sick' building—where it is exposed to toxic chemicals—our cells might react more violently, with allergies and physical stress, should our (burdened) cells be forced to adapt to a toxic environment. The same cells may have adapted to a change of weather nicely, but an overburdened cell can easily react negatively to a toxic environment.

As we will discuss further, conventional Western medicine's solution to autoimmune disorders is to try to stop the symptoms by interrupting the symptoms of inflammation and immune response. While this may temporarily slow the inflammatory response, this solution also can weaken the entire immune system by blocking the body's healing mechanisms. This puts more burdens on the body because the body cannot efficiently detoxify and heal itself from the offending toxins or pathogens. This chemical 'solution' ends up increasing the burden upon the body's already-overloaded immune system.

This pharmaceutical strategy would be analogous to punishing our dog because he barked at a thief who was invading our home.

Toxins and Immunosuppression

Clinical research by Professor John G Ionescu, Ph.D. has concluded that environmental pollution is clearly associated with the development of new sensitivities. Dr. Ionescu's research indicated that environmental noxious agents, including many chemicals, contribute to the total immune burden, producing increased susceptibility for intolerances.

Environmental toxins are also sensitizing in themselves, producing new trigger allergens. Professor Ionescu draws this conclusion from studying more than 18,000 atopic eczema patients:

"Beside classic allergic-triggering factors (allergen potency, intermittent exposure to different allergen concentrations, presence of microbial bodies dyand sensitizing phenols), the adjuvant role of environmental pollutants gains increasing importance in allergy induction."

According to Dr. Ionescu, toxic inputs such as formaldehyde, smog, industrial waste, wood preservatives, microbial toxins, alcohol, pesticides, processed foods, nicotine, solvents and amalgam-heavy metals have been observed to be mediating toxins for new sensitization of a variety of atopic allergies.

Research has concluded that allergen responses are accelerated by pharmaceutical use because they stimulate histamine and/or acetylcholine. These provoke smooth muscle neuromediators, which stimulate rapid nutrient absorption within the intestines (Liu *et al.* 1977).

This is also consistent with findings of other scientists—as discussed earlier—that pharmaceuticals can increase intestinal permeability.

Immunosuppression may be a long word, but it really is very simple: The immune system has been overburdened and compromised by the combination of unnatural, synthetic or deranged foods or toxins. The chart on the next page itemizes a few of these toxins that promote immunosuppression:

Major Modern Toxins

Source	Toxin
Antacids	Heavy Metals
Antiperspirant	Aluminum
Carpets, rugs	Molds, dander, lice, PC-4, latex
Cigarette Smoke	Carbon monoxide, nicotine, aldehydes, ketones
Cosmetics	Aluminum, phosphates and chemicals
Dental Fillings	Mercury, alloys, various chemicals
Dish soap	Perfumes, dyes, phosphates
Electric Blankets	EMFs, PC-4, various toxins

Food	Food colors, preservatives, trans-fats, pesticides, arachidonic acids, acrylamide, phytanic acid, artificial flavors
Soaps and Shampoos	Fragrances, chemicals, phosphates
House	Radon, formaldehyde, pollen, dust, mold, dander
Householder cleaners	Chlorine, various phosphates
Indoor Light	Blinking fluorescent lights
Industrial Plant or Freeway	Lead, mercury, carbon monoxide
IUDs	Copper
Laundry soaps	Perfumes, dyes, phosphates
Old pillows	Lice eggs, dander, molds
Paints	Lead, arsenic, cadmium, various toxins
Pesticides	Neurotoxins, poisons
Pets	240 infectious diseases & parasites (65 from dogs/39 from cats)
Pipes	Lead, copper, deposits
Plastics	Plasticizers (see also tap water)
Pools and spas	Chlorine, various carbonates
Appliances	Electromagnetic frequencies
Restaurants	Parasites, pesticides, trans-fats
Pans	Aluminum, copper, lead
Shampoo	Chemical fragrances, phosphates
Stoves, Fireplaces	Carbon monoxide, arsenic, soot
Tap Water	Chlorine, microorganisms, pesticides, nitrates, pharmaceuticals
Toothpaste	Propylene glycol, microparticles, synthetic sweeteners
Work environment	Various toxins
Microorganisms	Various species

For each of these toxins, the liver and immune system must launch a variety of macrophages, T-cells and B-cells to break them apart and escort them out of the body. This means that each toxin represents an additional load the immune system must carry.

We might compare this to moving dirt. A small handful of dirt can be carried around easily, and dispersed without much effort. However, a truckload of dirt is another matter completely. What do we do with a truckload of dirt? If we dumped it on our lawn, we'd have a hill of dirt that would bury the front of our house, preventing us from getting in or out of the house.

This is a useful comparison because while our bodies can handle a small amount of toxins quite easily, modern society is increasingly dumping toxic 'dirt' into our atmosphere, water and foods, effectively inundating our bodies by the 'truckload.'

With this increased burden, the research shows that the body's defenses are lowered. The mucosal membrane is thinned. The immune system is on alert. In this immunosuppressed state, the body is more likely to over-react to macromolecules, LTPs or other food proteins that it is exposed to.

Chapter Five

Probiotics and Food Sensitivities

As the reader will discover among the research provided here, probiotics provide not only a cause but a contributing solution to many food sensitivities. To emphasize the importance of probiotics, we've decided to devote an entire chapter specifically focused on how probiotic deficiencies can cause or contribute to food sensitivities; and how probiotics can be used to resolve intestinal damage. We'll also show how a lack of probiotics can directly cause or cause conditions that can promote food sensitivities—including Crohn's disease, irritable bowel syndrome (IBS), colitis and others.

Probiotics and Early Oral Tolerance

Our first major encounter with large populations of bacteria comes when our baby body descends the cervix and emerges from the vagina. During this birthing journey—assuming a healthy mother—we are exposed to numerous species of future resident probiotics. This first inoculation provides an advanced immune shield to keep populations of pathobiotics at bay. The inoculation process does not end here, however.

Because we get much of our bacteria as we pass through the vagina, cesarean section babies have significantly lower colonies of healthy bacteria. *Bifidobacterium infantis* is considered the healthiest probiotic colonizing infants. Some research has indicated that while 60% of vagina-birth babies have *B. infantis* colonies, only 9% of C-section babies are colonized with probiotics, and only 9% of those are colonized with *B. infantis*. This means that less than one percent of C-section babies are properly colonized with *B. infantis*, while 60% of vagina births are colonized with *B. infantis*. (The remaining 40% would indicate an unhealthy vagina.)

Our body establishes its resident strains during the first year to eighteen months. Following the inoculation from the vagina, these are accomplished from a combination of breast-feeding and putting everything in our mouth, from our parent's fingers to anything we find as we are crawling around the ground. These activities can provide a host of different bacteria—both pathobiotic and probiotic.

Mother's colostrum (early milk) can contain up to 40% probiotics. This will be abundant in bifidobacteria, assuming the mother is not taking antibiotics. Healthy strains of bifidobacteria typically colonize our body first and set up an environment for other groups of bacteria, such as the lactobacilli, to more easily become established.

Picking up a good mix of cooperative probiotic species is a crucial part of the establishment of our body's immune system. Some of the probiotic strains we ingest as infants may become permanent residents.

They will continue to line the digestive tract to protect against infection while learning to collaborate with our immune system.

As our digestive tracts begin to become fully functional, interstitial and intercellular lymphocytes build up around our intestinal walls and mucosal membranes. However, these immune defenses only become functional when they are stimulated by the colonizing bacteria we gained from mother and the world around us. This probiotic stimulation renders the production of regulatory cytokines and immunoglobulins such as IgA.

These work together with our probiotics to seal up and defend our intestinal tissues from macromolecules and other potential allergens. IgA coats our intestinal cells and quietly removes allergens before they can invade our intestinal cells.

In other words, oral tolerance is established early in life as the body begins to respond to probiotic bacteria. This is called *down regulation of systemic immunity*. Oral tolerance marks the beginning of the maturity of the digestive tract. In other words, in order to become independent of mother, the baby body's immune system must recognize the good guys from the bad guys. Probiotics are the mediators for this discernment.

Imagine moving to a new location among the U.S. territories during the 1800s in the United States. The territories were full of different threats of various kinds. As we build our new log home and begin to settle in, we begin to try to distinguish between the creatures that will hurt us and those that won't. Say we are lucky enough to meet up with a frontiersman before we start building. The frontiersman has lived in 'these parts' for several decades. He begins telling us about what to 'watch out for' among the region. He also shows us how to prevent the bears from coming around and how to defend ourselves from the bears should they invade our new home. With his assistance, we can go about building our home and prepare for those threats.

Without his assistance, it would become difficult to determine what we should be defend ourselves from. As a result, we might just shoot some very harmless (and even helpful) creatures, while allowing some dangerous creatures (such as bears) too much proximity.

Oral tolerance is like being able to distinguish between the good creatures and the bad ones. Our probiotics "show" our bodies what molecules are nutritious and what molecules should be blocked and destroyed by the immune system. How and why does this take place? Our probiotic bacteria are living beings. For millions of generations, these species have been living among our ancestors. Therefore, they have learned by experience what makes us healthy and what can make us sick. This information has been handed down through their generations through genetic evolution.

In fact, it is more practical than that: What makes us sick likely also makes them sick.

Therefore, our probiotics can properly guide our immune system in terms of what is good for us and what is bad for us. Our immune system will then "mark" those "bad guys" for future responses when it comes into contact with them.

Of course, this does not exist in a vacuum, as our body's own DNA and immune system cells also will help our bodies recognize the good guys and bad guys. But without healthy probiotics, which our immune system has relied on for millions of years, there is no training.

Should our family's probiotics not be available for this training, we are in trouble. Caesarian sections, for example, will prevent our bodies from coming into contact with mother's probiotics from the birthing canal. Should we then be deprived of her breast milk, we will also miss out on these important probiotics that help train our immune system.

This scenario can result in a variety of situations. Our immune system may launch against the wrong things, including "good" proteins that give us nourishment. It may also launch against even the slightest difference in our air or what we might touch. This is called *sensitization*. The body's immune system becomes overly sensitized to things it should become tolerant to.

The other thing that can happen without the right probiotics is that that baby's brush barrier will not form properly, with the right mix of tight junctions and desmosomes. The intestines may then let into the body large molecules and toxins that the immune system knows it cannot handle. Once the immune system "sees" these invaders, it will launch an inflammatory attack in order to purge them, while alerting the body that it has been invaded (Pierce and Klinman 1977).

Illustrating this, researchers from Finland's University of Tampere Medical School (Majamaa and Isolauri 1997) found that the probiotic *Lactobacillus* GG (ATCC 53103) promotes IgA immunity, prevents increased intestinal permeability, and helps control antigen absorption. They gave Lactobacillus GG with whey formula or whey without probiotics to 27 children with atopic eczema and cow's milk allergy. They also gave Lactobacillus GG to mothers of 10 breast-fed infants with atopic eczema and cow's milk allergy.

The atopic dermatitis symptoms improved significantly during the one-month study period among infants and mothers treated with the probiotics. Probiotic-treated infants also showed decreased levels of alpha 1-antitrypsin while the non-probiotic group did not. The probiotic-treated groups also had lower levels of intestinal permeability. The researchers concluded: *"These results suggest that probiotic bacteria may promote endogenous barrier mechanisms in patients with atopic dermatitis and food allergy, and by alleviating intestinal inflammation, may act as a useful tool in the treatment of food allergy."*

This role played by probiotics to mediate and moderate potential allergens appears critical during the first few months of life, when the mucosal epithelial layer, the intestinal barrier and the immune system are all still in development. Probiotics increase plasma levels IL-10 and total IgA in children with allergic predisposition. Both of these immunoglobulins are central to intestinal immunity and preventing intestinal permeability and the hypersensitive allergic response.

University of Helsinki researchers (Salmi *et al.* 2010) studied 35 infants with atopic eczema, of which 16 had milk allergies. They gave the infants Lactobacillus rhamnosus GG or a placebo. After four weeks, they found that the intestinal organic acids of the milk allergy children began to look more like the non-allergic infants.

Researchers from Germany's Royal Veterinary and Agricultural University (Rosenfeldt *et al.* 2004) wanted to find out if probiotics could reverse intestinal inflammation and strengthen intestinal barrier function in 41 allergic children. Probiotics *Lactobacillus rhamnosus* 19070-2 and *Lactobacillus reuteri* DSM 12246 were given to the children for six weeks—who displayed symptoms of moderate and severe allergic atopic dermatitis. Intestinal permeability was quantified using the lactulose-mannitol test. Gastrointestinal symptoms were also analyzed. Before the probiotic treatment, the researchers found that lactulose-to-mannitol ratios were high, indicating increased intestinal permeability. After the probiotic treatment, the probiotic group's lactulose-to-mannitol ratios were significantly lower. The probiotic group also experienced a significant decrease in gastrointestinal symptoms and eczema symptoms. The researchers concluded: *"The study suggests that probiotic supplementation may stabilize the intestinal barrier function".*

Remember the research from the University of Turku (Kalliomäki and Isolauri 2002) mentioned earlier. This clinical trial showed that probiotic supplementation reduced atopic eczema risk by 50% among children. They concluded by saying: *"Probiotics have also been shown to reverse increased intestinal permeability and to reduce antigen load in the gut by degrading and modifying macromolecules."*

As infants wean from breast milk, they can also pick up a host of probiotic colonies from drinking raw milk or by feeding on yogurt or kefir. These will introduce still new probiotics into the intestines. The probiotics will all help increase baby's oral tolerance and further develop the intestinal barrier.

Our Anti-Microbial Society

The parade of infective microorganisms and infectious diseases in our rather sterile society continues despite our dramatically-increased use of prescriptive and over the counter antibiotics, antifungals, antivirals, antiseptic soaps and cleaning disinfectants.

The use of antibiotics has soared over the past few decades—suspiciously over the same period that food sensitivities have also soared. Today, over 3,000,000 pounds of pure antibiotics are taken by humans annually in the United States. This is complemented by the approximately 25,000,000 pounds of antibiotics given to animals each year.

Meanwhile, many of these antibiotics either are given in vain or are ineffectual. The Centers for Disease Control states that, *"Almost half of patients with upper respiratory tract infections in the U.S. still receive antibiotics from their doctor."* This said, the CDC also warns that *"90% of upper respiratory infections, including children's ear infections, are viral, and antibiotics don't treat viral infection. More than 40% of about 50 million prescriptions for antibiotics each year in physicians' offices were inappropriate."*

Indeed, the growing use of antibiotics has also created a Pandora's box of *superbugs*. As bacteria are repeatedly hit with the same antibiotic, they learn to adapt. Just as any living organism does (yes, bacteria are alive), bacteria learn to counter and resist repeatedly utilized antibiotics. As a result, many bacteria today are resistant to a variety of antibiotics. This is because bacteria tend to adjust to their surroundings. If they are attacked enough times with a certain challenge, they are likely to figure out how to avoid it and thrive despite it.

This has been the case for a number of other new antibiotic-resistant strains of bacteria. They have simply evolved to become stronger and more able to counteract these antibiotic measures.

This phenomenon has created *multi-drug resistant organisms*. Some of the more dangerous MDROs include species of *Enterococcus, Staphylococcus, Salmonella, Campylobacter, Escherichia coli*, and others. Superbugs such as MRSA are only the tip of the bacterial iceberg.

Another growing infectious bacterium is *Clostridium difficile*. This bacterium will infect the intestines of people of any age. Among children, this is one of the world's biggest killers—causing acute, watery diarrhea. It is also a growing infection among adults. Every year *C. difficile* infects tens of thousands of people in the U.S. according to the Mayo Clinic. Worse, *C. difficile* are increasingly becoming resistant to antibiotics and infections from clostridia are growing in incidence each year.

Medical researchers from the Norwegian University of Science and Technology (Mai *et al.* 2010) found that early antibiotic use increased the likelihood of allergies at age eight. Over 3,300 children were studied for antibiotic use and respiratory conditions at the ages of two months, one year, four years and eight years old. Of all groups, 43% of the children received antibiotics. A third of the children had a respiratory infection, including pneumonia, bronchitis or otitis. The researchers found that those who used antibiotics during their first year of life had increased rates of wheeze and eczema by age eight.

Intestinal Dysbiosis

Dysbiosis is a state where the body has an imbalance between probiotic populations and pathogenic bacteria populations. In other words, the system is being overrun by the pathogenic bacteria and there are not enough probiotics in place to control their populations. When the body is lacking probiotics, or is overgrown with pathobiotic populations, there is typically an intestinal infection of some type. The extent of the infection, of course, depends upon the type of pathogenic bacteria present, and their populations in proportion to probiotic populations.

Many disorders can be traced back to dysbiosis. Some are direct and obvious, and some are not so obvious, and often appear as other disorders. In general, most digestive disorders are either caused by or accompanied by a lack of balanced intestinal probiotic populations. There are several types of dysbiosis.

We can usually detect *putrefaction dysbiosis* from the incidence of slow bowel movement. Symptoms of putrefaction dysbiosis include depression, diarrhea, fatigue, memory loss, numbing of hands and feet, sleep disturbances, joint pain and muscle weakness. Many of these disorders and others are often due directly to the overgrowth of pathobiotics and their endotoxins. The bacteria are burdening the blood stream with endotoxin waste products and neurotoxins; infecting cells, joints, nerves, brain tissues and other regions of the body.

Another overgrowth issue is *fermentation dysbiosis*. This is often evidenced by bloating, constipation, diarrhea, fatigue, and gas; and the faulty digestion of carbohydrates, grains, proteins and fiber. This is also a result of pathobiotic overgrowth, but in this type of dysbiosis, yeasts are prevalent among the overgrowth populations. As we know from baking bread, yeast will ferment quickly in warm, humid environments.

A body with low probiotic populations will create havoc for the immune system. *Deficiency dysbiosis* is related to an absence of probiotics, leading to damaged intestinal mucosa. This can lead to irritable bowel syndrome, food sensitivities, and intestinal permeability. The lack of probiotics allows the intestinal wall to come into contact with foreign molecules. This can open up the junctions between the intestinal cells. This can in turn lead to the entry of these toxins along with larger more complex food particles into the bloodstream—such as larger peptides and protein molecules—as we have discussed. Because these molecules are not normally found in the blood stream, the immune system identifies them as foreigners. The body then launches an inflammatory immune response, leading to *sensitization dysbiosis*. Linked to probiotic deficiency, sensitization dysbiosis causes food and chemical sensitivities, acne, connective tissue disease and psoriasis. Intestinal permeability has also been suspected in a variety of lung and joint infections.

The obvious signs of dysbiosis include hormonal imbalances and mood swings, high cholesterol, vitamin B deficiencies, frequent gas and bloating, indigestion, irritable bowels, easy bruising of the skin, constipation, diarrhea, vaginal infections, reduced sex drive, prostate enlargement, food sensitivities, chemical sensitivities, bladder infections, allergies, rhinovirus and rotavirus infections, influenza, and various histamine-related inflammatory syndromes such as rashes, asthma and skin irritation.

Illustrating the connection between probiotics and allergic skin response, Denmark children ages one to thirteen years old who were diagnosed with atopic dermatitis were given freeze-dried *L. rhaminosus* 19070-2 and *L. reuteri* DSM 122460 probiotics for six weeks. The children were then examined for symptoms. Among the probiotic groups, 56% reported improved eczema symptoms, compared to 15% among the control groups (Rosenfeldt *et al.* 2003).

Clinical Findings on Probiotics and Allergies

Probiotics mechanisms have been increasingly connected to inflammatory and allergic responses. They play a critical role in maintaining the epithelial barrier function of the intestinal tract. We've shown that allergies increase with intestinal permeability. Without an adequate intestinal barrier, larger food molecules, endotoxins and microorganisms can enter the bloodstream more easily. These increase the body's total toxin burden, making the immune system more sensitive.

Finnish researchers (Ouwehand *et al.* 2009) gave 47 children with birch pollen allergies *Lactobacillus acidophilus* NCFM and *Bifidobacterium lactis* Bl-04 or a placebo for four months, beginning before the birch pollen season. The probiotic group had significantly less sinus congestion, and lower numbers of nasal membrane eosinophils.

Researchers from Finland's University of Turku (Kirjavainen *et al.* 2003) gave 35 infants with milk allergies *Lactobacillus* GG or a placebo for 5.5 months. The researchers concluded that: *"Supplementation of infant for-*

mulas with viable but not heat-inactivated LGG is a potential approach for the management of atopic eczema and cow's milk allergy."

The British medical publication *Lancet* published a study (Kalliomäki *et al.* 2001) where 132 children with a high risk of atopic eczema were given either a placebo or *Lactobacillus rhamnosus* GG during their first two years of life. While 31 of 68 of the children receiving the placebo contracted atopic eczema, only 14 of 64 children receiving the probiotic developed atopic eczema by the end of the study.

University of Helsinki researchers (Viljanen *et al.* 2005) treated 230 milk-allergic infants *Lactobacillus* GG, four probiotic strains, or a placebo for four weeks. Among IgE-sensitized allergic children, the LGG provoked a reduction in symptoms while the placebo group did not.

Researchers from Sweden's Umeå University (West *et al.* 2009) fed Lactobacillus F19 or a placebo to 179 infants with allergic eczema from four months to 13 months old. The placebo group had double the incidence of eczema at 13 months than the probiotic group. The probiotic group as a whole also tested with more balanced Th1/Th2 ratios—with greater Th1 levels than the placebo group.

Allergy Hospital researchers from Helsinki University (Kuitunen *et al.* 2009) gave a probiotic blend of two lactobacilli, bifidobacteria, propionibacteria and prebiotics, or a placebo to mothers of 1,223 infants with a high risk of allergies during the last month of pregnancy term. Then they gave their infants the dose from birth until six months of age. They evaluated the children at five years of age for allergies. Of the 1,018 infants who completed the dosing, 891 were evaluated after five years. Allergies among the cesarean-birth children were nearly half in the probiotic group compared to the placebo group (24.3% versus 40.5%).

University of Milan researchers (Arslanoglu *et al.* 2008) found that a mixture of prebiotics galactooligosaccharides (GOS) and fructooligosaccharides (FOS) reduces allergy incidence. A mix of these or a placebo were given with formula for the first six months after birth to 134 infants. The incidence of dermatitis, wheezing, and allergic urticaria in the prebiotic group was half of what was found among the placebo group. The researchers concluded that: *"The observed dual protection lasting beyond the intervention period suggests that an immune modulating effect through the intestinal flora modification may be the principal mechanism of action."*

Researchers from Finland's National Public Health Institute (Piirainen *et al.* 2008) found that *Lactobacillus rhamnosus* GG fed to pollen-allergic persons for 5-½ months resulted in lower levels of pollen-specific IgE, higher levels of IgG and higher levels of IgA in the saliva. This is consistent with lower sensitivity, greater immunity, and a greater tolerance for pollens and foods.

Researchers from the Medical School at Finland's University of Tampere (Majamaa and Isolauri 1997) gave *Lactobacillus* GG (ATCC 53103) or placebo to 27 infants allergic to milk. The probiotic group showed significant improvement of allergic symptoms after one month of treatment. This and levels of fecal tumor necrosis factor-alpha gave cause for the researchers to conclude that: *"These results suggest that probiotic bacteria may promote endogenous barrier mechanisms in patients with atopic dermatitis and food allergy, and by alleviating intestinal inflammation, may act as a useful tool in the treatment of food allergy."*

Probiotics balance levels of pro and anti-inflammatory cytokines. They reduce antigens by digesting or otherwise modifying proteins and other food molecules. Probiotics can reverse increased intestinal permeability among children with food allergies. They enhance IgA responses, which are often dysfunctional in food allergy children. Probiotics also normalize the gut microenvironment (Laitinen and Isolauri 2006).

Probiotics improve the intestinal barrier function. They reduce the production of proinflammatory cytokines (Miraglia del Giudice and De Luca 2004).

Research from Sweden's Linköping University (Böttcher *et al.* 2008) gave *Lactobacillus reuteri* or a placebo to 99 pregnant women from gestational week 36 until infant delivery. The babies were followed for two years after birth, and analyzed for eczema, allergen sensitization and immunity markers. Probiotic supplementation lowered TGF-beta2 levels in mother's milk and babies' feces, and slightly increased IL-10 levels in mothers' colostrum. Lower levels of TGF-beta2 are associated with lower sensitization and lower risk of IgE-associated eczema.

German researchers (Grönlund *et al.* 2007) tested 61 infants and mother pairs for allergic status and bifidobacteria levels from 30-35 weeks of gestation and from one-month old. Every mother's breast milk contained some type of bifidobacteria, with *Bifidobacterium longum* found most frequently. However, only the infants of allergic, atopic mothers had colonization with *B. adolescentis*. Allergic mothers also had significantly less bifidobacteria in their breast-milk than non-allergic mothers.

Japanese scientists (Xiao *et al.* 2006) gave 44 patients with Japanese cedar pollen allergies *Bifidobacterium longum* BB536 for 13 weeks. The probiotic group had significantly decreased symptoms of rhinorrhea (runny nose) and nasal blockage versus the placebo group. The probiotic group also had decreased activity among plasma T-helper type 2 (Th2) cells and reduced symptoms of Japanese cedar pollen allergies. The researchers concluded that the results: *"suggest the efficacy of BB536 in relieving JCPsis symptoms, probably through the modulation of Th2-skewed immune response."*

Researchers from the Wellington School of Medicine and Health Sciences at New Zealand's University of Otago (Wickens *et al.* 2008) studied the association between probiotics and eczema in 474 children. Pregnant women took either a placebo, *Lactobacillus rhamnosus* HN001, or *Bifidobacterium animalis* subsp *lactis* strain HN019 starting from 35 weeks gestation, and their babies received the same treatment from birth to two years old. The probiotic infants given *L. rhamnosus* had significantly lower incidence of eczema compared with infants taking the placebo. There was no significant difference between the *B. animalis* group and the placebo group, however.

Researchers from Japan's Kansai Medical University Kouri Hospital (Hattori *et al.* 2003) gave 15 children with atopic dermatitis either *Bifidobacterium breve* M-16V or a placebo. After one month, the probiotic group had a significant improvement of allergic symptoms.

Japanese scientists (Ishida *et al.* 2003) gave a drink with *Lactobacillus acidophilus* strain L-92 or a placebo to 49 patients with perennial allergic rhinitis for eight weeks. The probiotic group showed significant improvement in runny nose and watery eyes symptoms, along with decreased nasal mucosa swelling and redness compared to the placebo group. These results were also duplicated in a follow-up study (2005) of 23 allergy sufferers by some of the same researchers.

Researchers from Tokyo's Juntendo University School of Medicine (Fujii *et al.* 2006) gave 19 preterm infants placebo or *Bifidobacterium breve* supplementation for three weeks after birth. Anti-inflammatory serum TGF-beta1 levels in the probiotic group were elevated on day 14 and remained elevated through day 28. Messenger RNA expression was enhanced for the probiotic group on day 28 compared with the placebo group. The researchers concluded that: *"These results demonstrated that the administration of B. breve to preterm infants can up-regulate TGF-beta1 signaling and may possibly be beneficial in attenuating inflammatory and allergic reactions in these infants."*

Scientists from Britain's Institute of Food Research (Ivory *et al.* 2008) gave *Lactobacillus casei* Shirota (LcS) to 10 patients with seasonal allergic rhinitis. The researchers compared immune status with daily ingestion of a milk drink with or without live *Lactobacillus casei* over a period of five months. Blood samples were tested for plasma IgE and grass pollen-specific IgG by an enzyme immunoassay. Patients treated with the *Lactobacillus casei* milk showed significantly reduced levels of antigen-induced IL-5, IL-6 and IFN-gamma production compared with the placebo group.

Levels of specific IgG also increased and IgE decreased in the probiotic group. The researchers concluded that: *"These data show that probiotic supplementation modulates immune responses in allergic rhinitis and may have the potential to alleviate the severity of symptoms."*

Researchers from the Skin and Allergy Hospital at the University of Helsinki (Kukkonen *et al.* 2007) studied the role of probiotics and allergies with 1,223 pregnant women carrying children with a high-risk of allergies. A placebo or lactobacilli and bifidobacteria combination with GOS was given to the pregnant women for two to four weeks before delivery, and their babies continued the treatment after birth. At two years of age, the infants in the probiotic group had 25% fewer cases of eczema and 34% few cases of atopic eczema.

The same researchers from the Skin and Allergy Hospital and Helsinki University Central Hospital (Kukkonen *et al.* 2009) studied the immune effects of feeding probiotics to pregnant mothers. In all, 925 pregnant mothers were given a placebo or a combination of *Lactobacillus rhamnosus* GG and LC705, *Bifidobacterium breve* Bb99, and *Propionibacterium freudenreichii* ssp. *shermanii* for four weeks prior to delivery. Their infants were given the same formula together with prebiotics, or a placebo for six months after birth. During the infants' six-month treatment period, antibiotics were prescribed less often among the probiotic group by 23%. In addition, respiratory infections occurred less frequently among the probiotic group through the two-year follow-up period (even after treatment had stopped) compared to the placebo group (an average of 3.7 infections versus 4.2 infections).

Finnish scientists (Kirjavainen *et al.* 2002) gave 21 infants with early onset atopic eczema a placebo or *Bifidobacterium lactis* Bb-12. Serum IgE concentration correlated directly to *Escherichia coli* and bacteroide counts, indicating the association between these bacteria with atopic sensitization. The probiotic group had a decrease in the numbers of *Escherichia coli* and bacteroides after treatment.

Sonicated *Streptococcus thermophilus* cream was applied to the forearms of 11 patients with atopic dermatitis for two weeks. This led to a significant increase of skin ceramide levels, and a significant improvement of their clinical signs and symptoms—including erythema, scaling and pruritus (Di Marzio *et al.* 2003).

Japanese researchers (Odamaki *et al.* 2007) gave yogurt with *Bifidobacterium longum* BB536 or plain yogurt to 40 patients with Japanese cedar pollinosis for 14 weeks. *Bacteroides fragilis* significantly changed with pollen dispersion. The ratio of *B. fragilis* to bifidobacteria also increased significantly during pollen season among the placebo group but not in the *B.*

longum group. Peripheral blood mononuclear cells from the patients indicated that *B. fragilis* microorganisms induced significantly more Th2 cell cytokines such as interleukin-6, and fewer Th1 cell cytokines such as IL-12 and interferon. The researchers concluded that: *"These results suggest a relationship between fluctuation in intestinal microbiota and pollinosis allergy. Furthermore, intake of BB536 yogurt appears to exert positive influences on the formation of anti-allergic microbiota."*

Scientists from the Department of Oral Microbiology at Japan's Asahi University School of Dentistry (Ogawa *et al.* 2006) studied skin allergic symptoms and blood chemistry of healthy human volunteers during the cedar pollen season in Japan. After supplementation with *Lactobacillus casei*, pro-inflammatory activity of cedar pollen-specific IgE, chemokines, eosinophils and interferon-gamma levels all decreased among the probiotic group.

Researchers from the School of Medicine and Health Sciences in Wellington, New Zealand (Sistek *et al.* 2006) gave *Lactobacillus rhamnosus* and *Bifidobacteria lactis* or placebo to 59 children with established atopic dermatitis. They found that food-sensitized atopic children responded significantly better to probiotics than did other atopic dermatitis children.

French scientists (Passeron *et al.* 2006) found that atopic dermatitis children improved significantly after three months of *Lactobacillus rhamnosus* treatment, based on SCORAD (symptom) levels of 39.1 before and 20.7 afterward.

Scientists from Finland's National Public Health Institute (Piirainen *et al.* 2008) gave a placebo or *Lactobacillus rhamnosus* GG to 38 patients with atopic eczema for 5.5 months—starting 2.5 months before birch pollen season. Saliva and serum samples taken before and after indicated that allergen-specific IgA levels increased significantly among the probiotic group versus the placebo group (using the enzyme-linked immunosorbent assay (ELISA)). Allergen-specific IgE levels correlated positively with stimulated IgA and IgG in saliva, while they correlated negatively in the placebo group. The researchers concluded that: *"L. rhamnosus GG displayed "immunostimulating effects on oral mucosa seen as increased allergen specific IgA levels in saliva."*

Children with cow's milk allergy and IgE-associated dermatitis were given a placebo or *Lactobacillus rhamnosus* GG and a combination of four other probiotic bacteria (Pohjavuori *et al.* 2004). The IFN-gamma by PBMCs at the beginning of supplementation was significantly lower among cow's milk allergy infants. However, cow's milk allergy infants receiving *L. rhamnosus* GG had significantly increased levels of IFN-gamma, showing increased tolerance.

The British medical publication *Lancet* published a study (Kalliomäki *et al.* 2003) where 107 children with a high risk of atopic eczema were given either a placebo or *Lactobacillus rhamnosus* GG during their first two years of life. Fourteen of 53 children receiving the probiotic developed atopic eczema, while 25 of 54 of the children receiving the placebo contracted atopic eczema by the end of the study.

In a study from the University of Western Australia School of Pediatrics (Taylor *et al.* 2006), 178 children born of mothers with allergies were given either *Lactobacillus acidophilus* or a placebo for the first six months of life. Those given the probiotics showed reduced levels of IL-5 and TGF-beta in response to polyclonal stimulation (typical for allergic responses), and significantly lower IL-10 responses to vaccines as compared with the placebo group. These results illustrated that the probiotics had increased allergen resistance among the probiotic group of children.

Researchers from the Department of Otolaryngology and Sensory Organ Surgery at Osaka University School of Medicine in Japan (Tamura *et al.* 2007) studied allergic response in chronic rhinitis patients. For eight weeks, patients were given either a placebo or *Lactobacillus casei* strain Shirota. Those with moderate-to-severe nasal symptom scores at the beginning of the study who were given probiotics experienced significantly reduced nasal symptoms.

Lactose Intolerance and Probiotics

Most nutritionists and physicians assume that lactose intolerance means the person is deficient in the body's production of *lactase*—an enzyme that breaks down milk sugar. New research, however, is indicating that probiotics are as important if not more important for the body's ability to digest milk and break down lactose.

For this very reason, both mother's breast milk and raw cow's milk contain important probiotics that not only furnish lactase: Probiotics also directly digest lactose as part of their own eating regimen. Let's look at the evidence from the research:

Scientists from the University of Buenos Aires (Gaón *et al.* 1995) studied 30 human subjects to see if lactose intolerance could be reduced with probiotics. Milks containing *Lactobacillus casei* and *Lactobacillus acidophilus* or no probiotics were given to the subjects. The subjects who drank the probiotic milk were significantly less likely to have bloating, diarrhea and other symptoms of lactose intolerance.

Scientists from the Chinese Center for Disease Control and Prevention in Beijing (He *et al.* 2004) gave live probiotic yogurt, heat-treated yogurt or acidified gelled milk (each containing 20 grams of lactose) to 45 lactose-intolerant men. Lactose digestion improved significantly among the live yogurt group compared to the other groups. The researchers concluded that: *"The live flora in dairy product could improve lactose digestion in male adult lactose malabsorbers."*

Researchers from the University Medical Center Groningen in The Netherlands (He *et al.* 2008) gave *Bifidobacterium longum* and a yogurt enriched with *Bifidobacterium animalis* to 11 lactose-intolerant persons. *Bifidobacterium* levels increased during and after supplementation. *B. animalis* and *B. longum* were not detected before supplementation, but both strains were present in feces during supplementation. They disappeared after supplementation ended. Lactose-intolerance symptoms decreased during supplementation, but resumed following supplementation. The researchers noted that, *"supplementation modifies the amount and metabolic activities of the colonic microbiota and alleviates symptoms in lactose-intolerant subjects."*

Scientists from the Department of Food Science and Human Nutrition at University of Missouri (Mustapha *et al.* 1997) determined that milk containing *L. acidophilus* was effective in improving lactose digestion and tolerance.

Beta-galactosidase from the yeast *Kluyveromyces lactis* eaten at mealtime with milk and cereal (cornflakes) and an unrefined cereal (bran) reduced lactose intolerance in a Guatemalan study (Solomons *et al.* 1985) of lactose intolerant patients. Exogenous betagalactosidases produced by the probiotic yeast effectively eliminated lactose malabsorption in those deficient in lactase.

Scientists from Alabama's A&M University (Onwulata *et al.* 1989) gave plain yogurt, sweet acidophilus milk, hydrolyzed-lactose milk, or a lactase tablet and whole milk to ten lactose-intolerant persons. They found that the lactase produced by the probiotics in yogurt was, *"superior to exogenous commercial lactase in alleviating lactose maldigestion."*

Scientists from University of Minnesota's Department of Food Science and Nutrition (Jiang *et al.* 1996) gave 15 lactose intolerant patients milk with lactose or the probiotics *Bifidobacterium longum* cultured in either lactose or lactose and glucose. The consumption of milk with lactose-grown *B. longum* resulted in significantly less hydrogen production and flatulence among the patients than the groups drinking the other milks. The researchers concluded that: *"Milks containing B. longum might reduce breath hydrogen response and symptoms from lactose malabsorption when the culture is grown in a medium containing only lactose to induce a higher beta-galactosidase level and increase rate of lactose uptake."*

Probiotics and Intestinal Permeability

We have discussed the mechanisms of increased intestinal permeability previously. We will summarize them here and relate the issue more closely with probiotics. Our probiotics line the walls of our intestines and move around our mucosal membrane. Here they police the intestinal cells and excrete acids that help manage the pH of the mucosal membrane. Should probiotic colonies be damaged by toxins, infection, antibiotics or poor dietary choices, their symbiotic relationship with our intestines can come to an end or become severely limited. This effectively thins the mucosal membrane and leaves the intestinal cells more exposed to food particles and toxins.

Should our probiotic colonies become scarce and our mucosal membrane thins, larger peptides, toxins and even invading microorganisms are allowed to have contact with the intestinal cells. This irritates the intestinal cells, producing an inflammatory immune response. This inflammatory immune response in turn damages the ability of the intestinal brush barrier to keep larger food proteins or toxins from invading our tissues and bloodstream.

Again, the intestinal brush barrier as a whole includes the mucosal layer of enzymes, probiotics and ionic fluid. This forms a protective surface medium over the intestinal epithelium. It also provides an active nutrient transport mechanism. It contains glycoproteins and other ionic transporters, which attach to nutrient molecules, carrying them across intestinal membranes. However, this mucosal membrane is supported and stabilized by the grooves between the intestinal microvilli.

This support is provided by four mechanisms existing between the intestinal microvilli: tight junctions, adherens junctions, desmosomes and probiotics. The tight functions form a bilayer interface between cells, controlling permeability. Desmosomes are points of interface between the tight junctions. The adherens junctions keep the cell membranes adhesive enough to stabilize the junctions. These junction mechanisms together regulate permeability at the intestinal wall.

In healthy intestines, the microvilli gaps are policed by billions of probiotic colonies. These perform a variety of maintenance tasks. They help process and break down incoming food molecules. They excrete acids to manage the environment. They secrete various nutrients. They control pathogenic bacteria that can threaten the region. They also communicate closely with the immune system to help signal invasions.

This symbiotic relationship gives the brush barrier its triple-filter mechanism that essentially screens for molecule size, ionic nature and nutrition quality. Before a molecule can come into contact with the intestines, tissues or bloodstream, it must pass through these filter mechanisms.

Should the probiotics become damaged, the entire mucosal brush barrier begins to break down. You might say that our probiotics provide the "glue" that keeps everything working smoothly.

The health of our probiotics and the health of the brush barrier can be threatened by a number of factors. Alcohol is one of the most irritating substances to our probiotics and the mucosal brush barrier in general (Bongaerts and Severijnen 2005).

In addition, many pharmaceutical drugs, notably NSAIDs, have been identified as damaging to probiotics and the mucosal brush barrier integrity. Foods with high arachidonic fatty acid capability (such as trans-fats and animal meats); low-fiber, high-glucose foods; and high nitrite-forming foods have been suspected for their ability to inhibit growth of our probiotics. They also can compromise the mucosal chemistry. Toxic substances such as plasticizers, pesticides, herbicides, chlorinated water and food dyes are also suspected. Substances that increase PGE-2 response also negatively affect permeability (Martin-Venegas et al. 2006).

In addition, the overuse of antibiotics can cause a die-off of our resident probiotic colonies. When intestinal probiotic colonies are reduced, pathogenic bacteria and yeasts can outgrow the remaining probiotic colonies. Pathogenic bacteria growth invades the brush barrier, introducing an influx of endotoxins (the waste matter of these microorganisms) into the bloodstream together with some of the microorganisms themselves.

Many distinguished scientists around the world have now attributed the breakdown of the mucosal brush barrier and the influx of macromolecules as the major cause for the increasing occurrence of food sensitivities in Western society. Healthy intestinal barriers prevent allergic response because they limit the entry of large food molecules into the body's tissues and bloodstream.

A food that has been a source of nutrition for many years can suddenly be identified by the immune system as a threat if its proteins get into the body's tissues before being properly broken down to size. This unfortunate circumstance results not only in the possibility of allergic response to some foods: Nutritional deficiencies can also result. Research is finally confirming these mechanisms (Laitinen and Isolauri 2005; Fasano and Shea-Donohue 2005).

Inflammatory responses resulting from increased intestinal permeability have now been linked to sinusitis, allergies, psoriasis, asthma, arthritis and other inflammatory conditions. Food sensitivities are simply one condition among others.

The research has also revealed a link between intestinal permeability and liver damage (Bode and Bode 2003). Alcohol consumption has also been associated with intestinal permeability (Ferrier *et al.* 2006).

Let's look at the research linking intestinal permeability to probiotics:

In a study by scientists from China's Qilu Hospital and Shandong University (Zeng *et al.* 2008), 30 irritable bowel syndrome patients with intestinal wall permeability were given either a placebo or a fermented milk beverage with *Streptococcus thermophilus, Lactobacillus bulgaricus, Lactobacillus acidophilus* and *Bifidobacterium longum.* After four weeks, intestinal permeability reduced significantly among the probiotic group.

Researchers from Greece's Alexandra Regional General Hospital (Stratiki *et al.* 2007) gave 41 preterm infants of 27-36 weeks gestation a formula supplemented with *Bifidobacterium lactis* or a placebo. After seven days, bifidobacteria counts were significantly higher, head growth was greater. After 30 days, the lactulose/mannitol ratio (marker for intestinal permeability) was significantly lower in the probiotic group as compared to the placebo group. The researchers concluded that, *"bifidobacteria supplemented infant formula decreases intestinal permeability of preterm infants and leads to increased head growth."*

Granada medical researchers (Lara-Villoslada *et al.* 2007) gave *Lactobacillus coryniformis* CECT5711 and *Lactobacillus gasseri* CECT5714 or a placebo to 30 healthy children after having received conventional yogurt containing *Lactobacillus bulgaricus* and *Streptococcus thermophilus* for three weeks. The supplemented yogurt significantly inhibited *Salmonella cholerasuis* adhesion to intestinal mucins compared to before probiotic supplementation. The probiotic supplementation also increased IgA concentration in feces and saliva.

German scientists (Rosenfeldt *et al.* 2004) gave *Lactobacillus rhamnosus* 19070-2 and *L. reuteri* DSM 12246 or a placebo to 41 children. After six weeks of treatment, the frequency of GI symptoms were significantly lower (10% versus 39%) among the probiotic group as compared to the placebo group. In addition, the lactulose-to-mannitol ratio was lower in the probiotic group, indicating to the researchers that, *"probiotic supplementation may stabilize the intestinal barrier function and decrease gastrointestinal symptoms in children with atopic dermatitis."*

Researchers from the People's Hospital and the Jiao Tong University in Shangha (Qin *et al.* 2008) gave *Lactobacillus plantarum* or placebo to 76 patients with acute pancreatitis. Intestinal permeability was determined using the lactulose/rhamnose ratio. Organ failure, septic complications and death were also monitored. After seven days of treatment, microbial infections averaged 38.9% in the probiotic group and 73.7% in the placebo group. Furthermore, only 30.6% of the probiotic group colonized potentially pathogenic organisms, as compared to 50% of patients in the control group. The probiotic group also had significantly better clinical outcomes compared to the control group. The researchers concluded that: *"Lactobacillus plantarum can attenuate disease severity, improve the intestinal permeability and clinical outcomes."*

Researchers from the Department of Medical Microbiology at the Radboud University Nijmegen Medical Centre in The Netherlands (Bongaerts and Severijnen 2005) studied the intestinal permeability connection in food allergies with great focus. They came to the conclusion that:

"Adequate probiotics can (i) prevent the increased characteristic intestinal permeability of children with atopic eczema and food allergy, (ii) can thus prevent the uptake of allergens, and (iii) finally can prevent the expression of the atopic constitution. The use of adequate probiotic lactobacilli, i.e., homolactic and/or facultatively heterolactic l-lactic acid-producing lactobacilli, reduces the intestinal amounts of the bacterial, toxic metabolites, d-lactic acid and ethanol by fermentative production of merely the non-toxic l-lactic acid from glucose. Thus, it is thought that beneficial probiotic micro-organisms promote gut barrier function and both undo and prevent unfavorable intestinal micro-ecological alterations in allergic individuals."

Probiotics, IBS and Crohn's

As we discussed earlier, the risk of food sensitivities increases substantially with irritable bowel syndrome (IBS), Crohn's disease, and other intestinal conditions. Most of these are considered autoimmune diseases. However, the concept that the body's immune system is attacking itself for no reason is illogical. There are reasons the immune system might target cells from within the body. These can range from the cells being damaged by environmental toxins, endotoxins, oxidative (free) radicals, viruses, to the immune system itself being damaged. How do probiotics intermix within these possibilities?

The research illustrates that probiotics directly attack foreign invaders like bacteria, viruses and fungi before they can damage the cells of the intestinal walls. Probiotics can also bind to oxidative radicals formed by many types of toxins. Probiotics will also line the intestinal cells, creating a barrier for toxins to enter the blood. They secrete lactic acid and other biochemicals that prevent endotoxin microorganisms from flourishing. Probiotics will also signal the immune system with the identities of pathogens, and then assist in their eradication.

Deficiencies of probiotics in the intestines usually result in overgrowths of pathogenic microorganisms like *Clostridia* spp., *E. coli*, *H. pylori* and *Candida* spp. These damage the cells of the intestinal wall and produce endotoxins that poison intestinal cells. These can damage the brush barrier of the intestines and result in intestinal permeability and an increased risk of food sensitivities.

Here is some research supporting these conclusions:

Researchers from the Medical University of Warsaw (Gawrońska *et al.* 2007) investigated 104 children who had functional dyspepsia, irritable bowel syndrome, or functional abdominal pain. They gave the children either placebo or *Lactobacillus rhamnosus* GG. for four weeks. The probiotic group had overall treatment success (25% versus 9.6%) compared to the placebo group. The IBS probiotic group had even more treatment success compared to the placebo IBS group (33% versus 5%). The probiotic group also had significantly reduced pain frequency.

French researchers (Drouault-Holowacz *et al.* 2008) gave probiotics or a placebo to 100 patients with irritable bowel syndrome. Between the first and fourth weeks of treatment, the probiotic group had significantly less abdominal pain (42% versus 24%) than the placebo group.

Researchers from Poland's Curie Regional Hospital (Niedzielin *et al.* 2001) gave *Lactobacillus plantarum* 299V or placebo to 40 IBS patients. IBS symptoms significantly improved for 95% of the probiotic patients versus just 15% of the placebo group.

Forty IBS patients took *Lactobacillus acidophilus* SDC 2012, 2013 or a placebo for four weeks in research at the Samsung Medical Center and Korea's Sungkyunkwan University School of Medicine (Sinn *et al.* 2008). The probiotic group had a 23% reduction in pain and discomfort while the placebo group showed no improvement.

Scientists from Italy's University of Parma (Fanigliulo *et al.* 2006) gave *Bifidobacterium longum* W11 or rifaximin (an IBS medication) to 70 IBS patients for two months. The probiotic patients reported a fewer symptoms and greater improvement than the rifaxmin patients. The researchers commented: *"The abnormalities observed in the colonic flora of IBS suggest, in fact, that a probiotic approach will ultimately be justified."*

Researchers from the University of Helsinki (Kajander *et al.* 2008) treated 86 patients with IBS with either a placebo or a combination of *Lactobacillus rhamnosus* GG, *L. rhamnosus* Lc705, *Propionibacterium freudenreichii* subsp. *Shermanii* JS and *Bifidobacterium animalis* subsp. *lactis*. After five months, the probiotic group had a significant reduction of IBS symptoms, especially with respect to distension and abdominal pain. The researchers concluded that: *"This multispecies probiotic seems to be an effective and safe option to alleviate symptoms of irritable bowel syndrome, and to stabilize the intestinal microbiota."*

Scientists from the Canadian Research and Development Centre for Probiotics and The Lawson Health Research Institute in Ontario (Lorea Baroja *et al.* 2007) studied 20 IBS patients, 15 Crohn's patients, five ulcerative colitis patients, and 20 healthy volunteers. All subjects were given a yogurt supplemented with *Lactobacillus rhamnosus* GR-1 and *L. reuteri* RC-14 for 30 days. IBS inflammatory markers were tested in the bloodstream. CD4(+) CD25(+) T-cells increased significantly among the probiotic IBS group. Tumor necrosis factor (TNF)-alpha(+)/interleukin (IL)-12(+) monocytes decreased for all the groups except the IBS probiotic group. Myeloid DC decreased among most probiotic groups, but was also stimulated in IBS patients. Serum IL-12, IL-2(+) and CD69(+) T-cells also decreased in probiotic IBS patients. The researchers also concluded that: *"Probiotic yogurt intake was associated with significant anti-inflammatory effects..."*

Researchers from the General Hospital of Celle (Plein and Hotz 1993) gave *Saccharomyces boulardii* or placebo to 20 Crohn's disease patients with diarrhea flare-ups. After ten weeks, the probiotic group had a significant reduction in bowel movement frequency compared with the control group. The control group's bowel movement frequency rose in the tenth week and then subsided to initial frequency levels—consistent with flare-ups.

In another study from Finland (Kajander *et al.* 2005), a placebo or combination of *Lactobacillus rhamnosus* GG, *L. rhamnosus* LC705, *Bifidobacterium breve* Bb99 and *Propionibacterium freudenreichii* subsp. *shermanii* JS was given to of 103 patients with IBS. The total symptom score (abdominal pain + distension + flatulence + borborygmi) was 7.7 points lower among the probiotic group. This represented a 42% reduction in the symptoms of the probiotic group compared with a 6% reduction of symptoms among the placebo group.

In a study from Yonsei University College of Medicine in Korea (Kim *et al.* 2006), 40 irritable bowel syndrome patients were given either a placebo or a combination of *Bacillus subtilis* and *Streptococcus faecium* for four weeks. The severity and frequency of abdominal pain decreased significantly in the probiotic group.

Researchers from Sweden's Lund University Hospital (Nobaek *et al.* 2000) gave 60 patients with irritable bowel syndrome either a placebo or daily rose-hip drink with *Lactobacillus plantarum* for four weeks. Enterococci levels increased among the placebo group but were unchanged in the test group. Flatulence was significantly reduced among the probiotic group compared with the placebo group. At a 12-month follow-up, the probiotic group maintained significantly better overall GI symptoms and function than the placebo group.

New York scientists (Hun 2009) gave 44 IBS patients either a placebo or *Bacillus coagulans* GBI-30 for eight weeks. The probiotic group experienced significant improvements in abdominal pain and bloating symptoms versus the placebo group.

Scientists at Ireland's University College in Cork (O'Mahony *et al.* 2005) studied 77 irritable bowel syndrome patients with abnormal IL-10/IL-12 ratios—indicating a proinflammatory, Th1 status. The patients were given a placebo, *Lactobacillus salivarius* UCC4331 or *Bifidobacterium infantis* 35624 for eight weeks. IBS symptoms were logged daily and assessed weekly. Tests included quality of life, stool microbiology, and blood samples to test peripheral blood mononuclear cell release of inflammatory cytokines interleukin (IL)-10 and IL-12. Patients who took *B. infantis* 35624 had a significantly greater reduction in abdominal pain and discomfort, bloating and distention, and bowel movement difficulty, compared to the other groups. IL-10/IL-12 ratios—indicative of Th1 proinflammatory metabolism—were also normalized in the probiotic *B. infantis* group.

Researchers from the Umberto Hospital in Venice in Italy (Saggioro 2004) studied probiotics on seventy adults with irritable bowel syndrome. They were given 1) a placebo; 2) a combination of *Lactobacillus plantarum* and *Bifidobacterium breve*; or 3) a combination of *Lactobacillus plantarum* and *Lactobacillus acidophilus* for four weeks. After 28 days of treatment, pain scores measuring different abdominal regions decreased among the probiotic groups by 45% and 49% respectively, versus 29% for the placebo group. The IBS symptom severity scores decreased among the probiotic groups after 28 days by 56% and 55.6% respectively, versus 14% among the placebo group.

Sixty-eight patients with irritable bowel syndrome were treated at the TMC Hospital in Shizuoka, Japan (Tsuchiya *et al.* 2004) with either placebo or a combination of *Lactobacillus acidophilus*, *Lactobacillus helveticus* and *Bifidobacteria* for twelve weeks. The probiotic treatment was either "effective" or "very effective" in more than 80% of the IBS patients. In addition, less than 5% of the probiotic group reported the treatment as "not effective," while more than 40% of the placebo patients reported their placebo treatment as "not effective." The probiotic group also reported significant improvement of bowel habits.

Researchers from Britain's University of Manchester School of Medicine (Whorwell *et al.* 2007) gave a placebo or *Bifidobacterium infantis* 35624 to 362 primary care women with irritable bowel syndrome in a large-scale, multicenter study. After four weeks of treatment, *B. infantis* was significantly more effective than the placebo in reducing bloating, bowel dysfunction, incomplete evacuation, straining, and the passing of gas.

Scientists from Denmark's Hvidovre Hospital and the University Hospital of Copenhagen (Wildt *et al.* 2006) gave 29 colitis-IBS patients either *Lactobacillus acidophilus* LA-5 and *Bifidobacterium animalis* subsp. *lactis* BB-12, or a placebo for twelve weeks. The probiotic treatment group had a decrease in bowel frequency from 32 per week to 23 per week. Furthermore, the probiotic group had an average reduction in the frequency of liquid stools from six days per week to one day per week.

Scientists at Poland's Jagiellonian University Medical College (Zwolińska-Wcisło *et al.* 2006) tested 293 ulcer patients, 60 patients with ulcerative colitis, 12 patients with irritable bowel syndrome and 72 patients with other gastrointestinal issues. Compared to placebo, *Lactobacillus acidophilus* supplementation resulted in a lessening of symptoms, a reduction of fungal colonization, and increased levels of immune system cytokines TNF-alpha and IL-1 beta.

Medical researchers from Finland's University of Helsinki (Kajander *et al.* 2007) sought to understand the mechanism of probiotics' proven ability to reduce IBS symptoms. They gave either a placebo or a combination of *Lactobacillus rhamnosus* GG, *Lactobacillus rhamnosus* Lc705, *Propionibacterium freudenreichii* subsp. *shermanii* JS and *Bifidobacterium breve* Bb99 to 55 irritable bowel syndrome patients. After six months of treatment, composition of feces and intestinal microorganism content illustrated a significant drop in glucuronidase levels in the probiotic group compared to the placebo group. The researchers concluded that there was a complexity of different factors, and so far unknown mechanisms explaining, *"the alleviation of irritable bowel syndrome symptoms by the multispecies probiotic."*

Probiotics and Other Digestive Problems

Chronic digestive problems, which include bloating, indigestion, and cramping are often symptoms of IBS, Crohn's disease or colitis. These diseases (IBS, etc.) are also typically accompanied by chronic pain and intestinal inflammation, however. Occasional indigestion, bloating and cramping is often associated with a developing case of dysbiosis caused by antibiotic use, poor diet, or an overgrowth of specific pathogenic microorganisms. Enzyme deficiency can be caused by probiotic deficiencies. Probiotics produce a number of enzymes, including protease and lypase—necessary for the break down of proteins and fats. Poor digestion is often the result of a lack of these and other enzymes. Gastrointestinal difficulties in general are often caused by dysbiosis. This can include an overgrowth of yeasts, pathogenic bacteria or both. Here are a few of the many studies showing that digestion can improve with probiotic use:

French researchers (Guyonnet *et al.* 2009) fed *Bifidobacterium lactis* DN-173010 with yogurt strains for two weeks to 371 adults reporting digestive discomfort. After two weeks, 82.5% of the probiotic group reported improved digestive symptoms compared to 2.9% of the control group.

Another group of French scientists (Diop *et al.* 2008) gave 64 volunteers with high levels of stress and incidental gastrointestinal symptoms either a placebo or *Lactobacillus acidophilus* Rosell-52 and *Bifidobacterium longum* for three weeks. At the end of the three weeks, the stress-related gastrointestinal symptoms of abdominal pain, nausea and vomiting decreased by 49% among the probiotic group.

Probiotics, Polyps, Diverticulosis and Diverticulitis

Polyps, diverticulosis and diverticulitis are abnormalities within the intestines or colon. They have been associated with Crohn's, IBS and ulcerative colitis, as well as increased food sensitivities. They also have been seen forming seemingly without other disease pathologies.

Diverticulosis is the bulging of sections of the intestines. When a bulging area weakens and bursts, that is called diverticulitis. A polyp, on the other hand, is a growth on the inside of the intestinal wall. These may be either benign or cancerous. All of these conditions are associated with intestinal probiotics, because healthy probiotic colonies are essential to the health of the intestinal wall. We can see the evidence from the research:

Scientists from Sweden and Ireland (Rafter *et al.* 2007) gave placebo or *Lactobacillus rhamnosus* GG and *Bifidobacterium lactis* Bb12 to 43 polyp patients (who also had surgery for their removal) for 12 weeks. The probiotics significantly reduced colorectal proliferation and improved epithelial barrier function (reducing intestinal permeability) among the polyp patients. Testing also showed decreased exposure to intestinal genotoxins among the probiotic polyp patient group.

Researchers from The Netherlands' University Hospital Maastricht (Goossens *et al.* 2006) gave *Lactobacillus plantarum* 299v or a placebo to 29 polyp patients twice a day for two weeks. Fecal sample examinations and biopsies were collected during colonoscopy. *L. plantarum* 299v significantly increased probiotic bacteria levels from fecal tests and from rectal biopsies. Ascending colon populations were not significantly greater, however.

Researchers from the Digestive Endoscopy Unit at Italy's Lorenzo Bonomo Hospital (Tursi *et al.* 2008) treated 75 patients with symptomatic diverticulosis. Mesalazine and/or *Lactobacillus casei* DG were given for 10 days each month. Of the 71 patients that completed the study, 66 (88%) were symptom-free after 24 months. The researchers concluded that mesalazine and/or *Lactobacillus casei* were effective in maintaining diverticulosis remission for an extended period, assuming continued treatment.

Probiotics and Ulcers

Ulcers often relate directly to food sensitivities because ulcer symptoms can worsen after eating certain foods. Also, some food sensitivities are a direct result of an ulcerated condition in the stomach or duodenum—allowing undigested food molecules access to upper intestinal cells. Some food intolerances are the direct result of an ulcer, as the food is rejected by the gastric cells. In allergies and other intolerances, the sensitivity may be the result of food molecules not being digested enough or not being correctly modified by probiotics, acids, bile, proteases and other biochemicals of the stomach and intestines.

Until only recently, medical scientists and physicians were certain that ulcers were caused by too much acid in the stomach and the eating of spicy foods. This assumption has been debunked over the past two decades, as researchers have confirmed that at least 80% of all ulcers are associated with *Helicobacter pylori* infections.

While acidic foods and gastrin produced by the stomach wall are also implicated by symptoms of heartburn and acid reflux, we know that a healthy stomach has a functional barrier that should prevent these normal food and gastric substances from harming the cells of the stomach wall. This barrier is called the mucosal membrane. This stomach's mucosal membrane contains a number of mucopolysaccharides and phospholipids that, together with secretions from intestinal and oral probiotics, protect the stomach cells from acids, toxins and bacteria invasions.

Helicobacter pylori damage the mucosal membrane that protects the stomach's gastric cells, and directly irritate the tissues. This damage produces the symptoms of heartburn.

As doctors and researchers work to eradicate *H. pylori*, which infects billions of people worldwide, they are finding that *H. pylori* is becoming increasingly resistant to many of the antibiotics used in prescriptive treatment. Research from Poland's Center of Gastrology (Ziemniak 2006) investigated antibiotic use on *Helicobacter pylori* infections: 641 *H. pylori* patients were given various antibiotics typically applied to *H. pylori*. The results indicated that *H. pylori* had developed a 22% resistance to clarithromycin and 47% resistance to metronidazole. Worse, a 66% secondary resistance to clarithromycin and metronidazole was found, indicating *H. pylori*'s increasing resistance to antibiotics.

H. pylori bacteria do not always cause ulcers. In fact, only a small percentage of *H. pylori* infections actually become ulcerative. Meanwhile, there is some evidence that *H. pylori*—like *E. coli* and *Candida albicans*—may be a normal resident in a healthy intestinal tract, assuming they are properly balanced and managed by strong legions of probiotics.

There is strong evidence that confirms the ability probiotics have in controlling and managing *H. pylori* overgrowths. We will also see that probiotics have the ability to arrest ulcerative colitis and even mouth ulcers:

Researchers from the Academic Hospital at Vrije University in The Netherlands (Cats *et al.* 2003) gave either a placebo or *Lactobacillus casei* Shirota to 14 *H. pylori*-infected patients for three weeks. Six additional *H. pylori*-infected subjects were used as controls. The researchers determined that *L. casei* significantly inhibits *H. pylori* growth. This effect was more pronounced for *L. casei* grown in milk solution than in the DeMan-Rogosa-Sharpe medium (a probiotic broth developed by researchers in 1960).

Mexican hospital researchers (Sahagún-Flores *et al.* 2007) gave 64 *Helicobacter pylori*-infected patients antibiotic treatment with or without *Lactobacillus casei* Shirota. *Lactobacillus casei* Shirota plus antibiotic treatment was 94% effective and antibiotic treatment alone was 76% effective.

Researchers from the Department of Internal Medicine and Gastro-enterology at Italy's University of Bologna (Gionchetti *et al.* 2000) gave 40 ulcerative colitis patients either a placebo or a combination of four strains of lactobacilli, three strains of bifidobacteria, and one strain of *Streptococcus salivarius* subsp. *thermophilus* for nine months. The patients were tested monthly. Three patients (15%) in the probiotic group suffered relapses within the nine months, versus 20 (100%) in the placebo group.

Italian scientists from the University of Bologna (Venturi *et al.* 1999) also gave 20 patients with ulcerative colitis a combination of three bifido-bacteria strains, four lactobacilli strains and *Streptococcus salivarius* subsp. *thermophilus* for 12 months. Fecal samples were obtained at the beginning, after 10 days, 20 days, 40 days, 60 days, 75 days, 90 days, 12 months and 15 days after the (12 months) end of the treatment period. Fifteen of the 20 treated patients achieved and maintained remission from ulcerative colitis during the study period.

British researchers from the University of Dundee and Ninewells Hospital Medical School (Furrie *et al.* 2005) gave 18 patients with active ulcerative colitis either *B. longum* or a placebo for one month. Clinical examination and rectal biopsies indicated that sigmoidoscopy scores were reduced in the probiotic group. In addition, mRNA levels for human beta defensins 2, 3, and 4 (higher in active ulcerative colitis) were significantly reduced among the probiotic group. Inflammatory cytokines tumor necrosis factor alpha and interleukin-1alpha were also significantly lower in the probiotic group. Biopsies showed reduced inflammation and the regeneration of epithelial tissue within the intestines among the probiotic group.

Scientists from Italy's Raffaele University Hospital (Guslandi *et al.* 2003) gave *Saccharomyces boulardii* or placebo to 25 patients with ulcerative colitis unsuitable for steroid therapy, for four weeks. Of the 24 patients completing the study, 17 attained clinical remission—confirmed endoscopically.

Researchers from Switzerland's University Hospital in Lausanne (Felley *et al.* 2001) gave fifty-three patients with ulcerative *H. pylori* infection milk with *L. johnsonii* or placebo for three weeks. Those given the probiotic drink had a significant *H. pylori* density decrease, reduced inflammation and less gastritis activity from *H. pylori*.

Lactobacillus reuteri ATCC 55730 or a placebo was given to 40 *H. pylori*-infected patients for four weeks by researchers from Italy's Università degli Studi di Bari (Francavilla *et al.* 2008). *L. reuteri* effectively suppressed *H. pylori* infection, decreased gastrointestinal pain, and reduced other dyspeptic symptoms.

Scientists from the Department of Internal Medicine at the Catholic University of Rome (Canducci *et al.* 2000) tested 120 patients with ulcerative *H. pylori* infections. Sixty patients received a combination of antibiotics rabeprazole, clarithromycin and amoxicillin. The other sixty patients received the same therapy together with a freeze-dried, inactivated culture of *Lactobacillus acidophilus*. The probiotic group had an 88% eradication of *H. pylori* while the antibiotic-only group had a 72% eradication of *H. pylori*.

Scientists from the University of Chile (Gotteland *et al.* 2005) gave 182 children with *H. pylori* infections placebo, antibiotics or probiotics. *H. pylori* were completely eradicated in 12% of those who took *Saccharomyces boulardii*, and in 6.5% of those given *L. acidophilus*. The placebo group had no *H. pylori* eradication.

Researchers from Japan's Kyorin University School of Medicine (Imase *et al.* 2007) gave *Lactobacillus reuteri* strain SD2112 in tablets or a placebo to 33 *H. pylori*-infected patients. After four and eight weeks, *L. reuteri* was significantly decreased *H. pylori* among the probiotic group.

In a study of 347 patients with active *H. pylori* infections (ulcerous), half the group was given antibiotics and the other half was given antibiotics with yogurt (*Lactobacillus acidophilus* HY2177, *Lactobacillus casei* HY2743, *Bifidobacterium longum* HY8001, and *Streptococcus thermophilus* B-1). The yogurt plus antibiotics group had significantly more eradication of the *H.*

pylori bacteria, and significantly fewer side effects than the antibiotics group (Kim *et al.* 2008).

Lactobacillus brevis (CD2) or placebo was given to 22 *H. pylori*-positive dyspeptic patients for three weeks before a colonoscopy by Italian medical researchers (Linsalata *et al.* 2004). A reduction in the UBT delta values and subsequent bacterial load ensued. *L. brevis* CD2 stimulated a decrease in gastric ornithine decarboxylase activity and polyamine. The researchers concluded: *"Our data support the hypothesis that L. brevis CD2 treatment decreases H. pylori colonization, thus reducing polyamine biosynthesis."*

Thirty *H. pylori*-infected patients were given either probiotics *Lactobacillus acidophilus* and *Bifidobacterium bifidum* or placebo for one and two weeks following antibiotic treatment by British researchers (Madden *et al.* 2005). Those taking the probiotics had a recovery of normal intestinal microflora, damaged during antibiotic treatment. The researchers also observed that those taking the probiotics throughout the two weeks showed more normal and stable microflora than did those groups taking the probiotics for only one out of the two weeks.

Researchers at the Nippon Medical School in Tokyo (Fujimori *et al.* 2009) gave 120 outpatients with ulcerative colitis either a placebo; *Bifidobacterium longum;* psyllium (a prebiotic); or a combination of *B. longum* and psyllium (synbiotic) for four weeks. C-reactive protein (pro-inflammatory) decreased significantly only with the synbiotic group, from 0.59 to 0.14 mg/dL. In addition, the synbiotic therapy resulted in significantly better scores on symptom and quality-of-life assessments.

Scientists from the Department of Medicine at Lausanne, Switzerland's University Hospital (Michetti *et al.* 1999) tested 20 human adults with ulcerative *H. pylori* infection with *L. acidophilus johnsonii*. The probiotic was taken with the antibiotic omeprazole in half the group and alone (with placebo) in the other group. The patients were tested at the start, after two weeks of treatment, and four weeks after treatment. Both groups showed significantly reduced *H. pylori* levels during and just following treatment. However, the probiotic-only group tested better than the antibiotic group during the fourth week after the treatment completion.

Medical scientists from the Kaohsiung Municipal United Hospital in Taiwan (Wang *et al.* 2004) studied 59 volunteer patients infected with *H. pylori*. They were given either probiotics (*Lactobacillus* and *Bifidobacterium* strains) or placebo after meals for six weeks. After the six-week period, the probiotic treatment *"effectively suppressed H. pylori,"* according to the researchers.

In the Polish study mentioned earlier (Ziemniak 2006), 641 *H. pylori* patients were given either antibiotics alone or probiotics with antibiotics. The two antibiotic-only treatment groups had 71% and 86% eradication of *H. pylori*, while the antibiotic-probiotic treatment group had 94% eradication.

Researchers from the Cerrahpasa Medical Faculty at Istanbul University (Tasli *et al.* 2006) gave 25 patients with Behçet's syndrome (chronic mouth ulcers) six *Lactobacillus brevis* CD2 lozenges per day at intervals of 2-3 hours. After one and two weeks, the number of ulcers significantly decreased.

Probiotics and the Inflammatory Response

As we've discussed earlier, when the immune system is prone to inflammatory response, it will respond with more hypersensitivity to macromolecules and other food elements that gain entry to the intestinal wall. In such a condition, the immune system is overreacting. Research has confirmed that these conditions are characterized by an increase in T-cell helper-2 cells (Th2); outside of their normal balance with Th1 cells. This sets up the hair-trigger immune system.

Research shows that probiotics produce a balance among the immune system. Let's see some of the evidence:

Researchers from the Department of Clinical Sciences at Spain's University of Las Palmas de Gran Canaria (Ortiz-Andrellucchi *et al.* 2008) studied the ability of *Lactobacillus casei* DN114001 to modulate immunity factors among lactating mothers and their babies. *L. casei* or a placebo was given to expecting mothers for six weeks. T helper-1 and T helper-2 (Th1/ Th2) levels were tested from breast-fed colostrum, early milk (10 days) and mature milk (45 days). Allergic episodes among the newborns were also observed throughout their first six months of life. Among the probiotic group, T-cell and B-cell levels were increased, and natural killer cells were significantly increased. Furthermore, Th1/Th2 ratios were more balanced (anti-inflammatory) among the probiotic group.. Levels of the proinflammatory cytokine TNF-alpha was decreased in maternal milk. Significantly fewer gastrointestinal issues occurred among the breast-fed children of the probiotic mother group as well.

Japanese scientists (Hirose *et al.* 2006) gave *Lactobacillus plantarum* strain L-137 or placebo to 60 healthy men and women, average age 56, for twelve weeks. Increased Con A-induced proliferation (acquired immunity), increases in IL-4 production by CD4+ T-cells, and a more balanced Th1:Th2 ratio was seen in the probiotic group. Quality of life scores were also higher among the probiotic group.

The Probiotic Conclusion

We conclude with a quote from a team of professors and researchers from Germany's Medical University of Charite in Berlin (Hamelmann *et al.* 2008), who commented on the state of allergy prevention with respect to probiotics:

> *"Primary prevention strategies of allergy so far have been aimed to fight allergy causes, by avoiding risk factors and inhibiting their mechanisms of action. The results of trials testing food or airborne allergen avoidance as a prevention strategy were, however, rather disappointing. A reverse approach for primary prevention of allergies aims to facilitate exposure to protecting factors which promote the induction of immunologic tolerance against innocuous antigens. These factors are associated with farming environment and a 'traditional lifestyle', but identification of these factors is quite difficult. Major candidates include food-borne microbes, helminths or their components, which are able to stimulate mucosal immunity, particularly in the gut. Similarly, new preventive and therapeutic strategies are being tested to induce specific food-allergen oral tolerance through the ingestion of progressively increasing doses of the offending food. This shifting of allergy prevention research from avoidance to tolerance induction will hopefully allow us to reverse the epidemic trend of allergy diseases."*

What does this mean as we look at the whole topic of food allergy causes? Yes, the Berlin researchers have identified that it is difficult to clearly detail precisely which parts of nature (the "farming environment") stimulate intestinal immunity. Rather, it is the environment of nature, *combined* with eating healthy foods and maintaining healthy probiotics that is most productive in preventing food sensitivities. While there are no absolutes in nature, we know by many scientific studies, including many mentioned in this text, that a natural environment, with healthy probiotics, fresh air, sunshine, plenty of clean drinking water, exercise, and a primarily plant-based diet will assure us of keeping a healthy immune system that breeds tolerance.

And how does a healthy immune system prevent food sensitivities? As we've discussed, a healthy, balanced immune system with strong probiotic populations will produce a *normal* response to any perceived invader. This response is typically an IgA response that surrounds and expunges the invader *before it gains access to the cells and tissues of the intestinal wall.*

Integral to this process is that the intestinal wall must have the proper mucous membrane layer. It must maintain this "moat" to prevent foreign bodies or large macromolecules from gaining access to the intestinal wall and blood stream. This is where the IgA antibodies and probiotics dwell, and protect our intestinal wall.

Should a foreigner gain access for any reason in a healthy, balanced immune system, the response will be immediate and *balanced*. The immune system will produce IgA, IgE and IgG antibodies to the foreigner, and will attach and break down the invader where ever it dwells, sending its parts out of the body. Once this is set up, the healthy immune system knows how to better prevent the invader from getting in. It will stimulate IgAs and probiotics to prevent a second incursion.

These responses will be localized within a healthy immune system. They will likely not stimulate the systemic response of a burdened immune system that must sound the alarm and turn on all the sirens just because a macromolecule got into the blood stream.

Chapter Six

Natural Solutions for Food Sensitivities

Dealing with a food sensitivity is no easy job. As any food-sensitivity sufferer will tell you, elimination diets are particularly difficult. They are wrought with danger. One slip up, be it accepting some unknown food from a friend (who doesn't know the allergen is in the food) or eating some restaurant food with unknown ingredients can lead to disaster, even death. We could compare this to walking on razorblades.

Illustrating how difficult elimination diets are, researchers from The Netherlands' University of Groningen Medical Center (Vlieg-Boerstra *et al.* 2006) assessed whether and to what degree children could actually eliminate a popular allergen food. Among 38 children who were practicing a strict allergen avoidance diet, allergenic foods were inadvertently in the diets of 34% of the children for sure, and likely in the diets of another 37%. Only 29% of the children were able to strictly avoid their respective allergens.

In another study, researchers from University of Southampton's School of Medicine (Monks *et al.* 2010) surveyed 18 teenagers with severe food allergies. They found that most of the teenagers ate foods labeled *"may contain"* their allergen, because they thought that it is unlikely the food actually contained the allergen. Furthermore, many only carried adrenaline in definite risk situations, and some did not even know how to deal with a reaction.

So we must ask: Is it more difficult to deal with a food sensitivity and do nothing to correct it than to undertake the necessary steps to reverse the sensitivity?

This of course bears another question: How likely is reversing the sensitivity? To this, many medical professionals simply dismiss any method as impossible.

This is despite the scientific evidence pointing to real solutions. This is despite thousands of years of traditional medicine's use of natural herbs to reverse food sensitivities. This is despite the many hypersensitive people who have been helped by some of these solutions.

This is also despite the fact that the majority of food-sensitive children outgrow their food sensitivities, and many adults outgrow their sensitivities. How can so many people outgrow them if reversing a food sensitivity is impossible? Is it simply chance? Is outgrowing a food sensitivity simply a random freak of nature?

This does not mean that these solutions are guaranteed to work for everyone. Each of us has an individual physiology. As such, it could be that a particular strategy will work for one person but not another. And the research supports this.

However, this doesn't mean that because one solution does not work, another won't. While one solution might correct a particular immunity weakness, another might correct another. Furthermore, just as a combination of events can bring on a food sensitivity (as we've shown), a combination of solutions can reverse the sensitivity.

This is evidenced by the many causes of allergies detailed in the previous chapters. We can see that different combinations of immunity, probiotics, diet, environment and so on can promote hypersensitivity. This means that different combinations of correction measures may be required to turn it around.

Could these methods be more difficult than a lifetime of walking on razorblades?

Many of the strategies here reflect the research we've discussed earlier showing the causes of hypersensitivity. To this we can reference nutrition researcher, Dr. Colin Campbell. Dr. Campbell has led numerous studies funded by many universities and government agencies. Dr. Campbell's sixth nutrition principle says:

> *"The same nutrition that prevents disease in its early stages (before diagnosis) can also halt or reverse disease in its later stages (after diagnosis)"*
> *(Campbell and Campbell 2006).*

In other words, many of the strategies to reverse food sensitivities are related to the causes of hypersensitivity. These relate directly to the status of our immune system. They relate to our probiotics, diet, environmental inputs and early feeding. Whether they are aware of them or not, those who outgrow their food sensitivities do so because of changes in one or more of these areas.

Remember that specific changes should accompany consultation from our physician or other health practitioner. We might even consider bringing in this book into our next consultation with our health professional.

Oral Immunotherapy

A natural solution that has proved successful in numerous studies is called *specific oral tolerance induction,* or SOTI. In SOTI, very small amounts of the offending food are periodically fed to the allergic subject, with gradual increases over time. This has shown to be successful in a majority of cases, as we'll see in the research that follows.

As we will see from the research, oral immunotherapy is a frequent treatment among European doctors for food sensitivity sufferers—and with great success. As of 2003, over a third of allergies were treated with immunotherapy in Europe (Canonica *et al.* 2003). Today that rate is significantly higher.

Sublingual immunotherapy is another method of SOTI. Here clinically-tested tablets that contain extracts of the allergic substance are given with exact dilution rates. The tablet is taken under the tongue until it dissolves.

Nasal immunotherapy has also been used with success, although it has been observed being primarily beneficial for rhinitis symptoms.

These methods are all considered safer than *subcutaneous injection*, because subcutaneous injection can sometimes produce acute responses, especially among children.

Doctors in the U.S. do not utilize immunotherapy anywhere near the degree that doctors do in Europe. Besides not being well-accepted by most physicians, the FDA does not recognize immunotherapy, and Medicare does not provide insurance for immunotherapy treatment. Many other insurers follow Medicare's lead in not insuring immunotherapy.

This is quite simply a disservice to the millions of food sensitivity sufferers in North America. Possibly this discussion might help change that.

Specific immunotherapy has been established for pollen-food sensitivities in many studies. Swiss researchers (Bucher *et al.* 2004) used specific immunotherapy for 27 birch pollen-allergic subjects that either had allergies to apple or hazelnut. Fifteen of the 27 volunteers were given immunotherapy and the others were controls. They were given increasing doses of one gram to 128 grams of either fresh apples or ground hazelnuts over a year's time. After the year, 87% of the immunotherapy group (13) increased tolerance of apple or hazelnuts with no adverse symptoms. The average amount of increase in the allergen food was about 20 grams—ranging from 12 grams to 32 grams.

Researchers from the Allergology Department of Rome's Catholic University (Patriarca *et al.* 2003) gave 59 food-allergy patients oral tolerance treatment (SOTI) with standard protocols. A randomized control group followed a strict elimination diet. Of the SOTI-treated patients, 83% completed the oral tolerance protocol and became tolerant to the foods they were sensitive to. During the protocol, 51% experienced some mild responses.

Researchers from Italy's University of Trieste (Longo *et al.* 2008) tested SOTI treatment with 60 children with severe milk allergies. The children were five years old or more. They were split into two groups of 30 children each. One group started SOTI immediately, starting with very small amounts of milk. The second group stayed on a milk-free diet for a year. After the year was finished, In other words, 90% of the SOTI group became tolerant of milk: 36% of the SOTI group were completely milk-tolerant and another 54% could drink limited amounts of milk. In the elimination diet group, every person in the group was still sensitive to cow's milk after the one year.

Researchers from France's University Hospital of Nancy (Morisset *et al.* 2007) tested SOTI with 60 milk allergy children, aged between 13 months and 6.5 years old; and 90 egg allergy children, ages 12 months to eight years old. They were randomized, and given either allergen elimination diets or gradual SOTI desensitization by feeding small amounts of the allergen. After six months, skin prick testing and IgE testing revealed that sensitivities continued in only 11% of the milk SOTI group, and 30% of the egg SOTI group, This means the success rates were 89% and 70%, respectively.

Allergy researchers from the University of Rome (Meglio *et al.* 2004) gradually desensitized (SOTI) 21 milk allergy children within six months by feeding increasing amounts of milk daily, with a goal of 200 ml per day of eventual tolerance. Within the six months, 71% of the children (15 of 21) accomplished the 200ml daily intake. Of the rest, three (14%) were able to tolerate 40-80 ml per day, and only three of the 21 children (14%) failed the SOTI treatment completely. This rendered a total success rate of 86%.

Researches from Italy's University of Trieste (Longo *et al.* 2008) found that even children with extreme allergic responses to milk could significantly benefit from oral immunotherapy protocol. They divided 60 severely-allergic (to milk) children five years old or higher into two groups. The first group of 30 was given immediate oral immunotherapy of gradually increasing amounts of milk for one year. The other group remained on a milk elimination diet throughout the year. After the year, 11 become completely tolerant to milk while 16 of the children became partially tolerant. That means that out of the 30 *severely allergic* children, 90% (27 out of 30) became tolerant to milk to one degree or another.

Researchers from Humboldt University in Berlin (Rolinck-Werninghaus *et al.* 2005) found that children given graduated doses of allergens achieved maximum dose tolerance after 37, 41 and 52 weeks using SOTI. They also found that those subjects put on a second elimination diet from the allergen had moderate systemic allergic responses when given the allergen again. This showed that while tolerance can be achieved with gradual dosing; the previously-sensitive food should be eaten periodically in order to maintain tolerance. The researchers concluded that: *"Regular allergen intake seems necessary to maintain the established tolerance."*

Allergy unit researchers from Italy's University of Messina (Caminiti *et al.* 2009) tested IgE-milk allergy children with the SOTI oral tolerance protocol. They gave 13 children either a randomized double-blind desensitization with milk or soy formula as placebo, or an open version of the protocol. The SOTI children were given one drop of whole milk diluted 1:25 the first week. The dose was doubled every week until they had achieved a 200 mL dose on week 18. Of the 13 children, 10 received the milk protocol in total. Seven of the ten achieved the 200 mL of milk tolerance. Only two children failed the protocol because of severe reactions, while one patient accomplished partial milk tolerance (64 mL) during the study. The soy children were still allergic to milk at the end of the study.

Researchers from Rome's Catholic University (Patriarca *et al.* 2007) conducted SOTI oral immunotherapy desensitization with 42 children who were as old as 16 years and had been diagnosed with a variety of food allergies. Ten patients—the control group—were treated with an elimination diet. The immunotherapy consisted of gradually increasing the dose of the allergen. Of the allergic children who started, 86% completed the protocol and became tolerant. Allergen-specific IgE levels decreased significantly, and allergen-specific IgG significantly increased among the entire immunotherapy group.

Spanish researchers (Fernández-Rivas eta l. 2009) found that after six months of sublingual SOTI therapy that peach allergy patients were able to tolerate from three to nine times the amount of peach they could tolerate before the trial.

Immunotherapy research has finally reached the Americas, with similar success:

Duke University Medical Center researchers (Hofmann *et al.* 2009) tested SOTI oral tolerance immunotherapy among 28 patients with peanut allergies. They guided and observed as patients gradually increased doses daily, and recorded symptoms after each dose increase. Twenty of the 28 allergy patients (71%) completed the study—becoming tolerant. In the beginning, 79% experienced mild upper respiratory tract symptoms, and 68% experienced abdominal symptoms. The initial escalation day resulted in the mild wheezing of 18% of the subjects. Mild symptoms on successive days fell to 46%, and only 3.5% had significant reactions during home dosing. Only 1.2% had upper respiratory tract symptoms and 1.1% had skin symptoms. *"Allergic reactions with home doses were rare,"* commented the researchers.

Cambridge University medical researchers (Clark *et al.* 2009) studied SOTI oral immunotherapy in four children allergic to peanuts. Peanut flour doses were increased from five mg to 800 mg of peanut protein using twice-weekly increases in doses. After six weeks, peanut dose maximum thresholds went from 1/40th to 1/4th of one peanut (5-50 mg) to at least 10 peanuts (approximately 2,380 mg) during challenges after the oral immunotherapy was completed. This translated to 48-times, 49-times, 55-times and 478-times the amount of peanuts tolerated by the four children than before the treatment.

Johns Hopkins University School of Medicine researchers (Skripak *et al.* 2008) tested 20 children (between the ages of six and 17 years old) who were allergic to milk with SOTI oral tolerance immunotherapy or placebo. They dosed using three phases: a build-up day with an initial dose of 0.4 mg of milk protein; gradually increased daily doses to 50 mg; which then continued daily but with eight weekly increases to a maximum of 500 mg per day. This dose was then continued daily for three to four months. Of the 12 patients who completed the SOTI treatment (12 of the milk dosing group completed along with seven in the placebo group):

The SOTI group went from a baseline of 40 mg of milk tolerance in the beginning of the treatment to a whopping 5,140 mg average (the range was 2,540 mg to 8,140 mg), while the placebo group remained at an average of 40 mg sensitivity. Their conclusion: *"Milk OIT appears to be efficacious in the treatment of cow's milk allergy."*

In earlier North American studies, researchers from Johns Hopkins University School of Medicine (Fleischer *et al.* 2004) evaluated 68 peanut allergy patients during a food elimination program followed by a gradual SOTI oral tolerance program. Out of the 68, 47 became tolerant to peanuts. After becoming tolerant, 23 of the 47 stayed in the study and continued consuming concentrated peanut foods at least once per month, and another 15 stayed in and ate peanuts infrequently. After some time, only three of 15 among the infrequent peanut consumers suffered peanut allergy rebounds. Of the 23 patients who remained in the study and ate peanuts at least monthly, none had a rebound of allergy.

University of Colorado Health Sciences Center researchers (Leung *et al.* 2004) gave 84 peanut allergy sufferers placebo or different doses of peanut subcutaneously once every four weeks for sixteen weeks. After the protocol, the tolerance levels among the peanut 'vaccine' group went from a low of 178 mg to 2,627 mg for the highest peanut 'vaccine' dose, compared to 710 in the placebo group. This translates to an increase in tolerance from about ½ a peanut (178 mg) to nearly nine peanuts (2,805 mg).

New strategies in immunotherapy have been gaining increasing attention in research over the past few years. These include *homologous protein immunotherapy*, which utilizes a homologous (or similar) protein to produce tolerance of a particular food. For example, soybeans have been used to increase tolerance to peanuts. Other targeted anti-IgE therapy strategies include *altered peptide immunotherapy* (Scurlock and Jones 2010).

Oral food challenge testing does sometimes result in a severe reaction and even the need to use epinephrine to quell the response. Researchers from New York's Mount Sinai School of Medicine (Järvinen *et al.* 2009) reviewed food challenges in New York between 1999 and 2007. They found that 34% involved reactions, 4% of which required epinephrine. This is a good reason for those with severe allergies to conduct SOTI under physician supervision.

Just because there are reactions does not mean SOTI treatment is not efficacious. Remember that the treatment alleviates *future* severe reactions. It can save many from future anaphylaxis and even death.

Researchers from the Mount Sinai School of Medicine (Nowak-Wegrzyn and Fiocchi 2010) reviewed the research on SOTI and concluded that tolerance is achieved in approximately 50-75% of children treated (although we can see that the European research reached levels closer to 85%-90%). They concluded that:

> *"Side effects are common both during the initial dose escalation and during home dosing. Most reactions are mild (oral pruritus, abdominal discomfort, and rashes) and decrease in frequency with the longer duration of OIT. Severe reactions treated with epinephrine have been reported during home dosing. Factors associated with increased risk of reactions to previously tolerated doses during home dosing include exercise, viral infection, dosing on empty stomach, menses, and asthma exacerbation."*

Even if a course of immunotherapy is not completely successful initially, immunotherapy also offers other benefits. According to much of the research, immunotherapy seems to substantially strengthen the immune system in general (Kamdar and Bryce 2010).

We should note that most of the research on oral tolerance immunotherapy was conducted with few changes to strengthen the immune system. As we will introduce throughout the remainder of this chapter, there are a number of strategies that can strengthen the immune system's tolerance. This increase in tolerance is also termed as *adaptogenic.*

These strategies, which include using diet, herbs, probiotics, sunshine and other means, have been shown by research to strengthen the immune system's adaptogenic capacities. As the immune system is strengthened, its ability to tolerate sensitive foods should grow. This occurs because the immune system can *modulate* its response when it is less burdened by other challenges. When the immune system is balanced and stabilized, it is less likely to respond with hypersensitivity.

This is illustrated by the increased tolerance that follows recovery from the common cold. During the detoxification stage of the cold, the immune system throws off much of its toxic burden through a massive toxin removal process. After recovery, the body's immune system is stronger. In this temporary state—at least until we dump more toxins on it—the immune system is more adaptogenic.

As we introduce these immune-stimulating strategies, consider them preparatory to eventual SOTI treatment, possibly conducted during an elimination period. Again, SOTI should be supervised by a health professional, especially if the person has experienced any severe reactions.

Early Diet Strategies

In the last two chapters, we laid out the science that illustrates the importance of breast feeding for the infant. The bottom line is that breast milk gives the child a host of immune cells, cytokines and immunoglobulins that fine tune the baby's immune system. Additionally, breast milk gives the child a host of probiotics that help colonize the intestinal tract and boost the immune system. Breast milk also delivers special nutrients to nourish both baby and its intestinal probiotics with prebiotic nutrition.

The combination of these elements feed and nurture the baby, helping the mucosal membrane and the intestinal barrier mature. At the end of the day, the child's immune system is handicapped without breast feeding. While there are some fine replacements for breast milk, nothing is quite as good as the real thing—from a healthy mother.

We might suggest that if the mother is unable to feed, there are breast milk banks that supply donated breast milk to mothers who cannot breast feed. Currently there are eleven banks in the U.S. and Canada. They require a prescription from a pediatrician, but this should not be difficult because most pediatricians advocate breast milk. These breast milk banks accept and store donated breast milk from lactating mothers under the rules and guidelines of the *Human Milk Banking Association of North America*. Breast milk providers are medically screened and the breast milk is also tested for diseases, alcohol and quality.

In addition, there are several natural lactation inducement strategies to consider. Unfortunately, these are outside the scope of this text.

When Should Cow's Milk be Introduced?

The research we laid out in Chapter Four illustrates that cow's milk or solid foods should not be introduced too early. This is because an infant's intestinal wall barrier has not matured enough, leaving the intestinal cells exposed to larger peptides and proteins that can stimulate a food sensitivity.

At the same time, some early exposure has benefits, especially when it comes to cow's milk. Early exposure can mean the immune system becomes more tolerant, but that is only if the intestinal barrier has matured to a point where the mucosal membrane, IgAs and desmosomes are all in place to prevent allergen exposure to the tissues and bloodstream.

For these reasons, many physicians suggest that mothers should wait four months before introducing cow's milk to their babies. Is this advice backed up with clinical evidence, however? Let's look at some of the research:

Researchers from Israel's Allergy and Immunology Institute and the Assaf-Harofeh Medical Center (Katz *et al.* 2010) surveyed the feeding history of 13,019 infants. Those children with apparent milk allergies were challenged and tested with skin prick testing. They found that .5% or 66 of the 13,019 children had active milk allergies. They also found that those children with milk allergies were introduced to milk at an average age of 116 days, while the infants without milk allergies were introduced to milk at an average age of 62 days.

Furthermore, the risk of becoming allergic to milk among infants who were introduced to milk in the first 14 days was .005%, while the risk of developing milk allergies when given milk between 105 days and 194 days was 1.75%. The researchers concluded that the early introduction of milk along with breast-feeding can prevent milk allergies.

We should add that these results did not include the effects of natural raw milk from grass-fed cows or even goats. These sources of milk might have significantly different results due to the fact that these milks contain natural probiotics and a host of immune factors that more closely match mother's breast milk. Extrapolating from the research we'll lay out later, raw cow's milk will likely do more to support the intestinal barrier than pasteurized cow's milk.

Early Milk Alternatives

This brings us to an often temporary, yet common problem for parents: Their infant or young child becomes sensitive to milk or other formula ingredient. Or perhaps their child has increased risk because the mother has food allergies or asthma.

Scientists around the world have focused a great amount of research upon this problem. This has resulted in several options, depending upon the sensitivity. Here we will lay out the research, and let the parent and their health professional apply the specific situation. Remember that parents should also consult their health practitioner prior to implementing any of these feeding strategies.

For children with milk sensitivities, there are several choices. Here are some of the choices we'll discuss in this section:

> ➤ Soy formulas
> ➤ Rice milk formulas
> ➤ Almond milk formulas
> ➤ Goat milk
> ➤ Donkey milk
> ➤ Sheep milk
> ➤ Hydrolyzed formulas (milk, soy, rice, casein)
> ➤ Partially-hydrolyzed formulas
> ➤ Amino acid formulas
> ➤ Omega-3 additives (with any formula)

Not all, but the majority of children with milk sensitivity will tolerate soy formula. Finish researchers (Klemola *et al.* 2002) found from testing 170 milk-allergic children that all but about 10% tolerated the soy formula. The other 10% tested sensitive to the soy formula.

Soy formulas are typically rich in protein. Still, some believe that they simply do not provide the nutrition for subtle brain development. The newest solution has been hydrolyzed formulations. Here the proteins are hydrolyzed in a way that approximates what is done in a healthy intestinal tract. Because larger macromolecules can seep through immature intestinal barriers and stimulate sensitivity, hydrolyzed proteins can provide a possible temporary feeding solution for an allergic child.

Hydrolyzed milk formulas are now recommended for babies with high allergy risk, especially if breast-feeding is impossible. Partially hydrolyzed formulas will also break down larger allergen-proteins like beta-LG into smaller peptides. When they are broken down enough, they become indistinguishable to the immune system because they are in amino acid or smaller peptide form. These partially hydrolyzed formulas appear to significantly reduce allergenicity to casein protein as well (Nentwich *et al.* 2001).

Hydrolyzed milk formulations may also reduce allergy risk in general, especially among those who are genetically susceptible. Researchers from the Marien-Hospital in Wesel, Germany (von Berg *et al.* 2003) studied 2,252 infants between 1995 and 1998 who had a genetic atopic risk for milk allergies. For one year, the infants were fed either cow's milk, a partially hydrolyzed whey formula, an extensively hydrolyzed whey formula, or an extensively hydrolyzed casein formula. Both the hydrolyzed casein formula and the partially hydrolyzed whey formula caused less allergies among the children compared to the cow's milk formula.

Finnish researchers (Seppo *et al.* 2005) gave 168 milk-allergic infants with an average age of eight months either hydrolyzed whey formula or soy formula. Both groups tolerated the two formulas quite well. They also found that both supported normal growth and nutritional status through two years old.

Spanish hospital researchers (Ibero *et al.* 2010) fed hydrolyzed casein milk formula to 67 milk-allergy children aged between one month and one year old. The formula was tolerated by 98.5% of the children.

Italian researchers (Fiocchi *et al.* 2003) found that children who were both allergic to cow's milk and soy tolerate and thrived from a hydrolyzed rice formula.

Another group of Italian researchers (D'Auria *et al.* 2003) studied 16 milk-allergic infants. They also found that rice hydrolysate formula renders normal growth and nutrition, along with *"adequate metabolic balance"* using standardized growth indices (Z scores) and biochemical nutrient testing.

Pediatrics researchers from The Netherlands' Wilhelmina Children's Hospital (Terheggen-Lagro *et al.* 2002) gave thirty milk-allergic children extensively hydrolyzed casein-based formula. They found that this was well tolerated by the children.

Italian researchers (Giampietro *et al.* 2001) found, in a two-center study of 32 milk-allergic children, that the majority successfully tolerated two extensively hydrolyzed whey-based formulas.

Researchers from Brazil's San Paolo Hospital (Agostoni *et al.* 2007) tested four different types of feeding with 125 infants with allergies. After being fed breast milk for four months or more, the infants were weaned to either soy formula, a casein hydrolysate formula, a rice hydrolysate formula, or were exclusively breastfed for the remainder of the year. Both the hydrolysates (casein- and rice-based) were accompanied by better weight compared to the soy formula—which fared the worst out of the feeding strategies.

In a recent review (Alexander and Cabana 2010), infants fed with partially hydrolyzed whey protein formula had a 44% reduced likelihood of developing allergic symptoms, as compared with children who fed with milk formula.

Hydrolyzed formulas have proved to reduce allergy risk better than partially-hydrolyzed formulas, however. In a study from Denmark (Halken *et al.* 2000), 595 children were either breast fed or given formula from June 1994 to July 1995. Of the 595, 478 children finished the study. Of these, 232 ended up being breast-fed; 79 were fed an hydrolyzed casein formula; 82 were fed an extensively hydrolyzed whey formula; and 85 were fed a partially hydrolyzed whey formula. Cow's milk allergy rates were highest among those fed partially hydrolyzed formula. Extensively hydrolyzed formula was more effective in preventing milk allergies.

Researchers from the University of Milan Medical School (Terracciano *et al.* 2010) tested 72 children with an average age of 14 months, and followed up over a 26 month period. They gave the children either hydrolyzed rice formula, extensively hydrolyzed milk formula or a soy formula. Surprisingly, they found that children not exposed to milk protein residue become tolerant to milk earlier than children fed hydrolyzed milk. The researchers felt that this was due to the substantial change in the protein among hydrolyzed milks.

Cow's milk hydrolysates can also produce allergens, however, French researchers (Ammar *et al.* 1999) discovered.

Researchers from Italy's University of Palermo (Carroccio *et al.* 2000) divided up a group of infants who were sensitive to cow's milk and/or hydrolyzed proteins into two groups. The 21 hydrolyzed protein-intolerant infants were fed donkey milk. The 70 cow's milk-intolerant infants were given casein-hydrolyzed milk.

The children were followed up after four years to see if either method produced more or less food sensitivities. All of the donkey milk infants suffered from multiple food sensitivities, whereas 28% (20) of the hydrolyzed-casein milk drinkers had food sensitivities. Four out of seven of the patients receiving donkey milk were also intolerant to sheep milk. Three of the 21 donkey milk drinkers became intolerant to the donkey milk. The good news is that 52% of the donkey milk drinkers became tolerant to milk over the four year period. Even better, 78% of the hydrolyzed-casein group became milk-tolerant over the four years.

Almond milk may also be a good alternative. Researchers from Italy's University of Messina (Salpietro *et al.* 2005) tested almond milk feeding on a group of 52 infants aged five to nine months who had milk allergies. They compared this to soy milk formula. They found that while supplementation with soy-based formula and hydrolyzed milk protein formulas both caused sensitivities in 23% and 15% respectively, none of the children developed sensitivities to almond milk. The researchers also found the almond milk to be safe and nutritious.

A newer option is amino acid formula. An amino formula contains an array of individual amino acids rather than hydrolyzed proteins. Amino acids are the fundamental building blocks for protein production. Mount Sinai School of Medicine researchers (Sicherer *et al.* 2001) tested 31 children with milk allergies with a pediatric amino acid-based formula and compared this with tolerance to hydrolyzed milk formula. Of the 31 children, 13 did not tolerate the hydrolyzed formula, while almost all of the children tolerated the amino acid formula. The amino formula also maintained normal growth rates among the children.

In addition, German researchers (Niggemann *et al.* 2001) found that among 73 milk-allergic infants, an amino acid-based formula fared better than extensively hydrolyzed cow's milk formula in terms of growth and health of the infants after six months.

A newer development is an amino acid-based formula combined with docosahexaenoic acid (DHA) and arachidonic acid—at levels that closely resemble those of breast milk. In a study of 165 allergic infants, Duke University Medical Center researchers (Burks *et al.* 2008) found that this amino acid/EFA formula was hypoallergenic, and provided a safe alternative to breast milk.

Swedish researchers (Furuhjelm *et al.* 2009) also found that consuming DHA during pregnancy decreases the risk of childhood allergy.

The American Academy of Pediatrics (AAP), the European Society of Pediatric Gastroenterology and Nutrition (ESPGAN) and the European Society of Pediatric allergy and Clinical Immunology (ESPACI) all concur that any of these alternative formulas should be tested using the double-blind placebo-controlled challenge tests on allergic children or children with a high risk of milk or other food allergies.

We should also note that once the infant's intestinal barrier matures, specific oral tolerance programs may be instituted to establish tolerance, again supervised by a health professional.

Solid Food Introduction Strategies

Introducing solid foods is an important milestone. This text will not profess the best method. Rather, we'll lay out some of the research. While some suggest that the order of foods introduced is important, others, including some researchers, have shown that the order is not important.

What is known is that most children are exposed to their sensitive foods at home or through breast feeding, and early solid food exposure can often lead to a sensitivity. This means that early solid foods are probably better being low-sensitivity, easily-digested plant-based foods such as squashes, fruits and other simple foods—rather than the more common allergen foods. This is supported by research. Also, introducing common allergenic solid foods into children's diets is best done a bit later, gradually and in small increments (Vlieg-Boerstra *et al.* 2008).

Illustrating this, Dutch researchers (Kiefte-de Jong *et al.* 2010) found that by two years of age, about 12% of children are constipated. Furthermore, those children with constipation were more likely to have been introduced to gluten prior to six months of age.

Feeding solid foods prior to three months old appears to increase allergies, but so does feeding any solid foods after seven months old. Researchers have confirmed, for example, that feeding grains before three months or after seven months increases the child's risk of celiac disease and/or wheat allergies (Guandalini 2007). From this we can assess from the research that a safe strategy is to gradually increase solid foods during the fifth or sixth month, accompanied by breast milk feeding through the first year.

Herbal Medicine for Food Sensitivities

There are numerous herbs that have been utilized in traditional medicine for modifying hypersensitivity and increasing the immune system's tolerance. Herbs that accomplish this are called *adaptogens*. Here we will discuss many adaptogens that have been shown among research and/or clinical use among traditional medicines, to alter hypersensitivity to foods and other allergens.

Here we will also lay out a wealth of clinical research that illustrates these effects along with other beneficial properties. This is generally because nature's herbs will typically contain tens if not hundreds of medicinal constituents, each one stimulating our metabolism and immune system in unique and even synergistic ways.

Herbal medicine works differently than pharmaceuticals designed to shut off a particular symptom. The proper use of herbal medicine can lead to changes in the way the immune system responds in general.

An ideal way to utilize herbal medicine by a person who has a food sensitivity is to dose with an appropriate herbal formulation during an elimination diet. After some time, oral tolerance therapy may be conducted, overseen by a health professional for those with severe reactions.

Here we will summarize some of the herbs that traditional doctors from different disciplines have utilized to curb allergic responses to foods, or in some way modify the immune system's responsiveness. In some cases, the herb will be utilized to strengthen the immune system. In other cases, the herb will be used to damper the nervous system or otherwise reduce hypersensitivity.

This presentation of the science and traditional use of medical herbs is not simply the personal opinion of the author. Rather, this discussion utilizes the medical science and research of numerous researchers, scientists and physicians trained in herbal medicines. Here the traditional clinical use of herbal medicine has been derived from a number of *Materia Medica* texts from various traditions or otherwise documented clinical uses of these herbs upon large populations over thousands of years. Unless otherwise noted in the text, this information utilized the following reference materials (see Reference section for complete citation):

Agarwal *et al.* 1999; Bensky *et al.* 1986; Chopra *et al.* 1956; Ellingwood 1983; Fecka 2009; Foster and Hobbs 2002; Frawley and Lad 1988; Gray-Davidson 2002; Griffith 2000; Gundermann and Müller 2007; Halpern and Miller 2002; Henih and Ladna 1980; Hobbs 2003; Hoffman 1990; Konrad *et al.* 2000; Lad 1984; LaValle 2001; Lininger *et al.* 1999; Mabey 1988; Mehra 1969; Melzig 2004; Miceli *et al.* 2009; Mindell and Hopkins 1998; Murray and Pizzorno 1998; Nadkarni and Nadkarni 1908/1975; Newall *et al.* 1996; Newmark and Schulick 1997; O'Connor and Bensky 1981; Potterton 1983; Schulick 1996; Schauenberg and Paris 1977; Schutz *et al.* 2006; Shi *et al.* 2008; Shishodia *et al.* 2008; Sung *et al.* 1999; Thieme 1996; Tierra 1992; Tierra 1990; Tiwari 1995; Tisserand 1979; Tonkal and Morsy 2008; Vila *et al.* 2002; Weiner 1969; Weiss 1988; Miceli *et al.* 2009; Wang and Huan 1998; Williard 1992; Williard and Jones 1990; Wood 1997.

The Food Allergy Herbal Formula (FAHF)

Mount Sinai School of Medicine researchers have been testing a traditional formula made of Chinese medicine herbs for about ten years now. The blend, dubbed the *Food Allergy Herbal Formula* (or FAHF), has undergone a variety of studies on mice, even though the formula and its derivatives have been used on humans for thousands of years in Chinese medicine. Recently, as we'll discuss, there has been one human phase I study using FAHF-2, focused on its safety. A phase II (drug) trial is now underway. The FAHF formula contains the following herbs:

> - Ling-Zhi (Chi) (*Ganoderma lucidum*)
> - Fu-Zi (Zhi) (*Radix lateralis aconiti*)
> - Wu-Mei (*Fructus pruni mume*)
> - Chuan-Jiao (*Pericarpium zanthoxyli bungeani*)
> - Xi-Xin (*Herba cum radice asari*)
> - Huang-Lian (Chuan) (*Rhizoma coptidis*)
> - Huang-Bai (*Cortex phellodendri*)
> - Gan-Jiang (*Rhizoma zingiberis officinalis*)
> - Gui-Zhi (*Ramulus cinnamomi cassiae*)
> - Ren-Shen (Hong) (*Radix ginseng*)
> - Dang-Gui (Shen) (*Corpus radix*)

FAHF-2 is the same formula, *minus* Fu-Zi and Xi-Xin.

As we discuss this formulation research, remember that traditional Chinese physicians have prescribed the complete FAHF formula or similar formulations using many of the same herbs for thousands of years—*and still do.*

The first Mount Sinai study (Li *et al.* 2001) sensitized mice to fresh whole peanuts by introducing the cholera toxin, followed by a boosting. They then fed the mice the FAHF-1 herbal formula for seven weeks. After the seven weeks, the FAHF-1 completely halted peanut-induced anaphylactic reactions in the mice. It also significantly reduced histamine release and lymphocyte proliferation, and reduced peanut-specific IgEs within two weeks of treatment. These tolerance levels remained for four weeks after the treatment was stopped. Cytokines IL-4, IL-5, and IL-13 synthesis were also decreased among the FAFH-1 mice.

The second published Mount Sinai study on FAFH (Srivastava *et al.* 2005) came four years later and also tested mice with induced peanut allergies. This used the revised FAHF-2 herbal formula, which removed two herbs, Fuzi and Xixin, as noted earlier. They found that the FAHF-2 also successfully blocked peanut allergy anaphylaxis, as well as rendered long term peanut tolerance. Among the FAHF-2 mice, there were no anaphylactic reactions, and histamine/body core temperatures decreased. They also observed a down-regulation of Th-2 response.

Another Mount Sinai study, this one two years later (Qu *et al.* 2007), found that, once again, peanut-specific IgE levels fell while IgG2a levels increased after dosing with FAHF-2. Reduced IL-4 and IL-5, and a modulation of the all-important inflammatory T helper Type I cell (Th1) and Th2 within the intestines, illustrated how this herbal combination modulated the immune system and increased tolerance.

Yet another FAHF-2 study by Mount Sinai Medical School researchers followed three years later (Kattan *et al.* 2008). Once again, the FAHF-2 formula proved successful in mice by reducing peanut anaphylaxis. This time, they also tested the individual herbs to see if they could isolate a single herb or constituent responsible for the activity.

This proved unsuccessful. Although most of the herbs had some positive effects upon histamine, cytokines and allergic symptoms, the formula worked in combination. In the end, the researchers admitted that the formula, *"may work synergistically to produce the curative therapeutic effects produced by the whole formula."* In other words, the herbs alone did not have the same synergistic effect the combination formula had.

Now let's think about this for a second. Here is a team of medical researchers from one of the world's most respected medical schools, failing to understand precisely what part of a formula—that has undergone ten years of laboratory and animal research—is the active element. What does this tell us about nature, and the wisdom of those Traditional Chinese medicine physicians who devised such a formula?

Furthermore, remember that these research teams did not fall off the turnip truck. They were experienced researchers with M.D. degrees and Ph.D.s. Some were professors of medicine at one of the world's most prestigious medical schools. Why did these physicians have to resort to an ancient Chinese herbal remedy? Perhaps these Traditional Chinese medicine physicians and healers had an understanding about the body and the application of herbal medicine that modern medicine has yet to comprehend.

The next Mount Sinai study focused on the *mechanisms* of the formulation (Srivastava *et al.* 2009). This time, mice with induced peanut allergies received FAHF-2 each day for seven weeks, while receiving periodic oral challenges with peanuts over a period of 36 weeks. They also gave some mice T-cell- or IFN-gamma- reducing antibodies during that period. Once again, they found that the FAHF-2 treatment protected mice from anaphylaxis, this time for more than 36 weeks after the treatment was stopped.

Furthermore, their testing revealed up to a 50% reduction of peanut-specific IgE levels, and up to a 60% increase in IgG levels, which continued long after the treatment period. In other words, the FAHF-2 formula modified their immune systems. The conclusion of the researchers:

> *"Food Allergy Herbal Formula-2 provides long-term protection from anaphylaxis by inducing a beneficial shift in allergen-specific immune responses mediated largely by elevated CD8(+) T-cell IFN-gamma production."*

Finally, nearly ten years after beginning research on the formula, human clinical studies have begun. Researchers from New York's Mount Sinai School of Medicine (Wang *et al.* 2010) tested 19 food allergy patients with FAHF-2. The herbal formula significantly decreased interleukin (IL-5) levels among the active treatment group after seven days of treatment. In culture, the herbal product also increased interferon gamma and IL-10 levels. The researchers determined that FAHF-2 was safe for humans—something that Chinese medicine has known for centuries.

One must wonder why these studies, for a combination of herbs that have been consumed by humans for thousands of years and are regularly taken as supplements, took ten years of mice research to achieve clinical testing? Could Chinese traditional healers be poisoning their patients?

Meanwhile, millions of people suffer from anaphylaxis and die each year of food allergies. Why has the research moved so slow?

One reason is that research such as this requires funding. Funding human studies in Western science research is not cheap. For this reason, researchers must typically follow a rigorous process of animal studies before human studies will be funded. These protocols are even more strict if the human studies aim to be approved by the FDA for distribution as drugs. It is one thing to study an herbal supplement on humans—as many are. But it is quite another protocol to be seeking clearance as a drug. As the researchers aimed to achieve drug clearance by the FDA for the FAHF formulation, FDA-approved phase one and phase two studies became necessary.

Note that a pharmaceutical developed by a billion-dollar drug company won't take ten years to get out of animal research. This is because there is significant investment and income at stake for a pharmaceutical company. Plus a pharmaceutical can be patented. Herbs cannot be patented. So there is a value proposition.

Certainly the efforts of the researchers who have promoted the research should be commended. They see the wisdom of applying for drug approval to allow the herbal formula to reach the mainstream of physicians and patients. At the same time, we must question the logic of the application of these protocols to products that already have thousands of years of application in traditional medicine. Furthermore, the herbal formulation and slight variations are already commercially available. Physicians could prescribe them today. While clinical testing is appropriate, there is little reason the research could not have gone to human testing immediately. Since the formulation is made up of herbs with a history of safety, the need for extended animal and drug testing is curious.

All of the herbs in the FAHF formulation, and combinations thereof, are also available for purchase without a prescription. However, because herbs are considered supplements and not medicines, suppliers cannot advertise that the formula treats any particular disease in many Western countries, including the United States. Supplement laws in the United States and most Commonwealth countries strictly regulate how herbs and herbal formulas can be labeled and advertised.

In the U.S., for example, this herbal formulation would be limited to descriptions that it provides support for the immune system. This follows "structure/function" statements required by dietary supplement act of 1994.

Furthermore, as we investigate (and demystify) the herbs in FAHF, we find that many of these have been quite commonly used elsewhere in Eastern and Western herbal medicine. Many are even commonly used as culinary herbs. Using the traditional texts mentioned and some recent research, let's review some of the FAHF herbs and their properties, beginning with the two eliminated from the formula by the Sinai researchers:

Xi-Xin

Xi-Xin's botanical name is *Herba asari*, and also called Chinese wild ginger (not to be confused with common ginger, which is also in the FAHF formula). The entire plant is used, but its roots have significant usefulness. It is pungent and warming, and widely used in Chinese and Ayurveda medicine to provide heat and help clear the body of phlegm and congestion. It is said to slow the histamine response while stimulating the immune system's detoxification routines. TCM doctors often prescribe it alone with aconitum to help relieve congestion. It is also sometimes combined with peppermint herb to help clear headaches and nasal congestion.

Fu-Zi

Fuzi's botanical name is *Aconitum carmichaelii*, and it is also referred to as *Radix Aconiti Carmichaeli Praeparata* among Chinese medicine. It is also commonly called aconitum, or monkshood by herbalists. It is a well-known herb among Chinese medicine and Ayurveda. There are many related species. The rationale for excluding this herb from the formula is likely because unprocessed aconitum can be lethally poisonous.

However, Ayurvedic and Chinese herbal formulations utilize aconitum only after it has been thoroughly steamed with ginger. This precise process of extraction makes aconitum a safe herbal medicine as prescribed by traditional doctors.

This toxin-extracted aconitum has been used for thousands of years for clearing obstructions and blockages among the organs and channels. It is used for chills, colds and congestion.

A number of traditional texts have documented its anti-inflammatory and anti-arthritic effects.

In its raw form, aconitum is used among herbalists strictly for external purposes. As a liniment, aconitum is considered useful for rheumatism and neuralgia.

It is also used in homeopathy in infinitesimal (significantly diluted) doses.

The type of aconitum utilized in the original FAHF formula is most certainly the processed version. It was also extremely diluted to reduce any potential of toxicity. Nonetheless, we should issue the appropriate warning about aconitum: *This is a lethal poison and should only be given by an health professional who is expert in its safe usage.*

Ling-Zhi

This is none other than *Ganoderma lucidum*, also known as reishi—a popular medicinal mushroom. It is known for significantly modulating the immune system.

Reishi contains many constituents, including steroids, triterpenes, lipids, alkaloids, glucosides, coumarin glycoside, choline, betaine, tetracosanoic acid, stearic acid, palmitic acid, nonadecanoic acid, behenic acid, tetracosane, hentriacontane, ergosterol, sitosterol, ganoderenic acids, ganolucidic acids, lucidenic acids, lucidone and many more.

Ling-Zhi strengthens the immune system and modulates the body's tolerance and responses to allergens. Reishi has been shown to increase production of IL-1, IL-2 and natural killer cell activity. A number of studies have shown that reishi significantly modulates IgE responses. It has been shown to lower IgE levels specific to allergens, and reduce histamine levels. It has also been shown to improve lung function and has been used traditionally for bronchitis and asthma.

Recently, researchers from Japan's University of Toyama (Andoh *et al.* 2010) found that reishi relieves skin itching and rash in several tests with mice.

Wu-Mei

Prunus mume (Seib et Zucc) is referred to as *Fructus pruni mume* in Chinese medicine. It is also called *omae* in Korea, *ume* or *umeboshi plum* in Japan, which translates, quite simply, to 'dark plum,' 'black plum,' or 'mume.' It is, quite simply, the fruit of a special variety of plums.

This plum is treasured for its immune-stimulating properties. The Chinese *Materia Medica* describes it as able to alleviate coughing and lung deficiencies. It has a strongly astringent property, and thus helps to cleanse the digestive tract and halt diarrhea. Research documented in the *Medica* has indicated that it stimulates bile production, is anti-microbial, and has been able to relieve fever, nausea, abdominal pain and vomiting.

Chuan-Jiao

This is the fruit from *Zanthoxylum simulans* which is also sometimes referred to as *Fructus Zanthoxyli Bungeani* or *Pericarpium zanthoxyli bungeani* in Traditional Chinese medicine. More precisely, this herb is also referred to as Sichuan pepper. The tree is also called prickly ash, and is grown around the world. The small peppers that come from the prickly ash tree can be dried and ground or used fresh.

Chuan-jiao is also referred to as fagara, sansho, Nepal pepper, Szechwan pepper, or even dried prickly ash. Some of these may simply be relatives of the Sichuan pepper.

Because it is very spicy and hot, it is often used in Sichuan dishes—known for their spiciness. Chuan-jiao contains limonene, geraniol and cumic alcohol, among with a number of other medicinal constituents.

In Traditional Chinese medicine, cuan-jiao is known to remove abdominal pain, vomiting, nausea and parasites—especially roundworm. It is also used as a skin wash for eczema, and has a mild diuretic effect.

Huang-Lian

This is from the species *Coptis chinnensis*. It is often referred to as *Rhizoma coptidis* in Chinese medicine. Its common names include gold thread or golden thread. In Ayurveda, other species of *Coptis* spp. are also considered gold thread.

Materia Medica of Traditional Chinese medicine document that gold thread removes heat associated with histamine responses that affect the eyes, throat and skin. It is also helpful for digestion. Applied topically, it has been used to calm skin rash, and has been used to treat boils and abscesses.

In Ayurveda, gold thread is considered a bitter and tonic herb that reduces fever (antipyretic). It is also reputed to belong in the same category as goldenseal.

Huang-Bai

This is from the plant with the botanical name *Phellodendron amurense* or *Phellodendron chinense*. It is also called *Cortex phellodendri* in Traditional Chinese medicine. One of huang-bai's most common Western names is the Amur cork tree. Others have simply called this tree the cork tree.

In a study by researchers from Taiwan's National Changhua University (Tsai *et al.* 2004), huang-bai in combination with another herb qianniuzi (Pharbitis) was found to significantly effect the ion transport mechanisms within the cells of the intestinal wall. Other clinical documentation has confirmed that it can reduce blood pressure, slow contraction reflexes within the intestines, and modulate the central nervous system. Ointments of huang-bai have been used traditionally for treating eczema as well.

Gan-Jiang

This is *zingiberis officinalis*, also called *Rhizoma zingiberis officinalis* in Traditional Chinese Medicine. It is quite simply common ginger root.

Ginger is extensively used in both Chinese and Ayurvedic medicine. It is also commonly used in Western herbalism and a number of other traditional medicines around the world.

Ginger is one of the most versatile food-spice-herbs known to humanity. In Ayurveda—the oldest medical practice still in use—ginger is the most recommended botanical medicine. As such, ginger is referred to as *vishwabhesaj*—meaning "universal medicine"—by Ayurvedic physicians.

An accumulation of studies and chemical analyses has determined that ginger has at least 477 active constituents. As in all botanicals, each constituent will stimulate a slightly different mechanism—often moderating the mechanisms of other constituents. Many of ginger's active constituents have anti-inflammatory and/or pain-reducing effects. These include a number of gingerols and shogaols.

Clinical evaluation has documented that ginger blocks inflammation by inhibiting lipoxygenase and prostaglandins in a balanced manner. This allows for a gradual reduction of inflammation and pain without the negative GI side effects that accompany NSAIDs. Ginger also stimulates circulation, inhibits various infections, and strengthens the liver.

Properties of ginger supported by traditional clinical use describe it as analgesic, anthelmintic, anticathartic, antiemetic, antifungal, antihepatotoxic, antipyretic, antitussive, antiulcer, cardiotonic, gastrointestinal motility, hypotensive, thermoregulatory, analgesic, tonic, expectorant, carminative, antiemetic, stimulant, anti-inflammatory, antimicrobial and more.

Ginger has therefore been used as a traditional treatment for bronchitis, rheumatism, asthma, colic, nervous disorders, colds, coughs, migraines, pneumonia, indigestion, respiratory ailments, fevers, nausea, colds, flu, ulcers, hepatitis, liver disease, colitis, tuberculosis and many digestive ailments to name a few.

Gui-Zhi

This is *Cinnamomum cassia*, also referred to as *Ramulus cinnamomi cassiae* in Traditional Chinese Medicine. It is commonly called cinnamon—a delicious culinary spice present in most kitchens.

Cinnamon is used in just about every traditional medicine. The bark is often used, although the twigs are also utilized. According to Western herbalism, Ayurvedic Medicine and Traditional Chinese Medicine, it is useful for colds, sinusitis, bronchitis, dyspepsia, muscle tension, toothaches, the heart, kidneys, and digestion. It is also thought to strengthen circulation in general. It is considered stimulant, expectorant, diuretic, analgesic and alterative. In other words, it is immune-system modulating.

It also apparently dilates blood vessels and warms the body according to these traditional disciplines.

Dang-Gui

This is *Angelica sinensis,* also referred to as *Corpus radix angelicae sinensis* in Traditional Chinese Medicine. In Western herbology it is sometimes referred to simply as angelica. It is also called dong quai.

This herb is considered antispasmodic, which means it reduces hypersensitivity. The root is usually used, and it is a very popular herb for balancing the female reproductive system and irregular menstruation. It is considered a tonic in general, and has been used in traditional medicine for colds, fevers, inflammation, arthritis, rheumatic issues and anemia.

Ren-Shen (Hong)

Panex ginseng is a traditional remedy for allergies with thousands of years of use. Panax ginseng will come in white forms and red forms. The color depends upon the aging or drying technique used.

The ginseng in the FAHF formula is termed *Radix* ginseng or *Ren Shen* because it is *Panex ginseng.* Depending upon how the ginseng is cured, there are several types of *Ren Shen.*

When ginseng is cultivated and steamed it is called 'red root' or *Hong Shen.* Ginseng root will turn red when it is oxidized or processed with steaming. Some feel that red root is better than white, but this really depends upon the age of the root and how it was processed. Soaking ginseng in rock candy produces a white ginseng that is called *Bai Shen.* This soaking seems odd, but it also has been known to increase some of its constituent levels such as superoxide and nitric oxide. When the root is simply dried, it is called 'dry root' or *Sheng Shaii Shen.* Korean red ginseng is soaked in a special herbal broth and then dried.

There are a number of species within the *Panax* genus, most of which also contain most of the same adaptogens, referred to as gensenosides. Most notable in the *Panex* genus is American ginseng, *Panax quinquefolius.*

Eleutherococcus senticosus, often called Siberian ginseng, is actually not ginseng. While it also contains adaptogens (eleutherosides), these are not the gensenoside adaptogens within *Panex* that have been observed for their adaptogenic properties.

Researchers from Italy's Ambientale Medical Institute (Caruso *et al.* 2008) tested an herbal extract formula consisting of *Capparis spinosa, Olea europaea, Panax ginseng* and *Ribes nigrum* (Pantescal) on allergic patients. They found that allergic biomarkers, including basophil degranulation CD63 and sulphidoleukotriene (SLT) levels were significantly lower after

10 days. They theorized that these biomarkers explain the herbal formulation's *"protective effects."*

Researchers from Japan's Ehime University Graduate School of Medicine (Sumiyoshi *et al.* 2010) tested *Panax ginseng* on mice sensitized to eggs. After the oral feedings, they found that the ginseng significantly reduced allergen-specific IgG Th2 levels. It also increased IL-12 production, and increased the ratio of Th1 to Th2 among spleen cells. In addition, it enhanced intestinal CD8, IFN-gamma, and IgA-positive counts. The researchers concluded that, *"Red Ginseng roots may be a natural preventative of food allergies."*

The Anti-Asthma Herbal Medicine Intervention Formula

Other adaptogenic herbs have been illustrated by research. The ASHMI herbal formulation is a blend of herbs studied by Dr. Xiu-Min Li and Dr. Hugh Sampson from New York's Mount Sinai School of Medicine. It is a derivative of another traditional Chinese formulation of fourteen Chinese herbs, named MSSM-002 by the Shandong Weifang Pharmaceutical Factory Co., Ltd of China. Like the FAHF formula, the ASHMI formula has undergone rigorous animal and laboratory testing, and some phase I safety testing with humans. ASHMI has also undergone human testing in China. The ASHMI studies have all shown great success in all of this research, primarily as an anti-asthma treatment.

This formula has been shown to modulate the TH1/TH2 balance and reduce hypersensitivity (Li *et al.* 2000). Mount Sinai researchers also found that ASHMI significantly reduced inflammatory cytokines IL-4 (Bolleddula *et al.* 2007).

Chinese researchers (Wen *et al.* 2005) gave the ASHMI formula or prednisone treatment to 91 allergic asthmatic patients, and compared the results. They found that after four weeks, the ASHMI group had significantly improved lung function. Furthermore, the ASHMI group's IgE levels, eosinophil levels and inflammatory cytokine levels dropped. Unlike the side-effects known in prednisone treatment, the ASHMI dosing produced no significant side effects.

One notable result as the two treatment groups were compared was that serum IFN-gamma and cortisol levels were significantly increased in the ASHMI group, while those two levels were lower in the prednisone group. This illustrates that the ASHMI actually strengthened the immune system while it was also lowering symptoms of allergic asthma among the patients.

This result is quite typical among herbal medicines by the way. Because herbs contain a wide variety of constituents that work in balance, they effect a number of physiological results in the body. They also typically have few adverse side effects, assuming they are properly prepared and recommended.

These results were enough for the FDA to approve phase I and phase II drug trials for the ASHMI herbal combination. In 2009, Mount Sinai researchers (Kelly-Peiper *et al.* 2009) reported that they had given ASHMI to 20 patients with allergic asthma in the phase I drug trial. This study proved ASHMI's safety. Its phase II trial is underway.

ASHMI contains three herbal extracts:
- ➤ Ling-Zhi (*Ganoderma lucidum*)
- ➤ Ku-Shen (*Sophora flavescens*)
- ➤ Gan-Cao (*Glycyrrhiza uralensis*)

We reviewed *Ganoderma lucidum* (reishi mushroom) earlier, as it was also part of the FAFH formula. Here is a quick survey of the other two herbs in this formulation:

Ku-Shen

The small shrub *Sophora flavescens* is known to substantially modulate the immune system. It has also been shown to slow tumor progression (Li *et al.* 2010).

Among other constituents, it contains prenylated flavonoids, quinolizidine alkaloids (such as matrine), dehydromatrine, flavascensine and a number of other alkaloids (Liu *et al.* 2010; Jung *et al.* 2010). Research has shown it to inhibit several cytokines involved in the inflammatory sequence, notably IL-6 and TNF-alpha. It also blocks the release of the pain precursor, substance P (Liu *et al.* 2007; Xiao et al 1999).

This co-opted Chinese herb has also been extensively used in Traditional Hawaiian herbal medicine for asthma. In further research, this Polynesian medicine, it has been shown to reduce allergy responses among the lung passages (Massey *et al.* 1994).

Gan-Cao

Glycyrrhiza uralensis is also called Chinese licorice. It is not the common licorice (*Glycyrrhiza glabra*) known in Western and Ayurvedic herbalism, however. It is known in Chinese medicine as giving moisture and balancing heat to the lungs. It has thus been extensively used to stop coughs and wheezing. It also is known to clear fevers. Either taken internally or topically, it is known to ease carbuncles and skin lesions. It is also soothing to the throat and eases muscle spasms. This makes the root antispasmodic.

One of Chinese licorice's active constituents is isoliquiritigenin. This has been shown to be a H2 histamine antagonist (Stahl 2008). Chinese licorice has been shown to prevent the IgE binding that signals the release of histamine. This essentially disrupts the histamine inflammatory process while modulating immune system responses (Kim *et al.* 2006).

Chinese licorice also contains glactomannan, triterpene saponins, glycerol, glycyrrhisoflavone, glycybenzofuran, cyclolicocoumarone, glycybenzofuran, cyclolicocoumarone, licocoumarone, glisoflavone, cycloglycyrrhisoflavone, licoflavone, apigenin, isokaempferide, glycycoumarin, isoglycycoumarin, glycyrrhizin and glycyrrhetinic acid (Li *et al.* 2010; Huang *et al.* 2010).

This combination of constituents gives Chinese licorice aldosterone-like effects. This means that the root stimulates the production of the steroidal corticoids. Animal research has confirmed that Chinese licorice is anti-allergic, and decreases anaphylactic response. It also balances electrolytes and inflammatory edema (Lee *et al.* 2010; Gao *et al.* 2009).

STA-1

STA-1 is another adaptogenic anti-asthmatic formula. There are several herbs in common with the other two formulas mentioned. This is not a coincidence, as Traditional Chinese medicine doctors will often formulate slightly different blends with many of the same herbs. Their precise action is determined by the symptoms and physiology of the patient. We bring up these anti-asthma formulas because they may be applicable to someone whose food sensitivities are expressed with lung symptoms.

The STA-1 formula, STA-2 formula (same herbs with slightly different extraction methods) or placebo was given to 120 patients with asthma for six months. After the six months, the STA-1 and the STA-2 groups exhibited significantly better symptoms and lung function as compared with the placebo group. The STA-1 group also showed significantly reduced allergen-specific IgE levels (Chang *et al.* 2006).

As mentioned, several of the herbs in this formulation are common with the previous formulas. This formula contains ten herbs:

> ➢ Gang-Cao (*Radix Glycyrrhizae*)
> ➢ Mai-Men-Dong (*Radix Ophiopogonis*)
> ➢ Xi-Yang-Shen (*Radix Panacis Quinquefolii*)
> ➢ Ban-Xia (*Tuber Pinellia*)
> ➢ Shu-Di-Huang (*Radix Rehmanniae Preparata*)
> ➢ Mu-Dan-Pi (*Cortex Moutan Radicis*)
> ➢ Shan-Zhu-Yu (*Fructus Corni Officinalis*)
> ➢ Fu-Ling (*Sclerotium Poriae Cocos*)

> Ze-Xie (*Rhizoma Alismatis Orientalis*)
> Shan-Yao (*Radix Dioscoreae Oppositae*)

Ding-Chuan-Tang Formula

This traditional Chinese Medicine formula is also focused upon asthmatics or bronchial symptoms. Pediatric medical researchers from Taiwan's Chang Gung University (Chan *et al.* 2006) gave this Ding Chuan Tang formula or a placebo to 52 asthmatic children for 12 weeks. At the end of the treatment period, symptoms improved among the asthmatic group; and serum inflammatory mediators also improved. Hypersensitivity also improved (decreased) among the herbal treatment group.

The formula contains nine herbs:

> Gang-Cao (*Radix Glycyrrhizae*)
> Ban-Xia (*Tuber Pinellia*)
> Ying-Xing (*Gingko Bilboae*)
> Ma-Huang (*Herba Ephedrae*)
> Kuan-Dong-Hua (*Flos Tussilaginis Farfarae*)
> Sang-Bai-Pi (*Cortex Mori Albae Radicis*)
> Su-Zi (*Fructus Perilla Frutescens*)
> Xing-Ren (*Semen Pruni Armeniacae*)
> Huang-Qin (*Radix Scutellariae Baicalensis*)

This formula also has several herbs in common with the FAFH formulation. Chinese scullcap (*Scutellariae baicalensis*), ginkgo and Ma-Huang (ephedra) are distinct in this formula.

Ma-Huang

Ephedra (*Ephedra sinica, E. vulgaris* and related species) has received some unfair restrictions and negative press over the past few years as a result of unscrupulous product formulators combining refined ephedra with caffeine and other inappropriate ingredients.

Ephedra in fact is a very popular herbal remedy in Traditional Chinese Medicine and Japanese Medicine—where it is called Mao. It grows all over the world, and thus has also been a part of North American Indian folk medicine and Western herbalism. In these disciplines, ephedra has been called Mormon tea, Desert tea, Brigham tea, Mexican tea and Nevada fir. It should be noted that some of these species of ephedra differ in constituents with the Asian variety, but still share some of the same effects.

Two primary constituents, ephedrine and norephedrine/pseudoephedrine, have been isolated and synthesized into decongestants and weight loss pharmaceutical drugs. These have been proven in multiple drug trials to curb allergic response, open the airways, and curb the appetite. However, these isolated constituents have also been known to cause side effects, which include nausea, flushing, insomnia, blood vessel constriction and restlessness. Whole herb ephedra in fact contains many other constituents that help balance and buffer these side effects. And for this reason, it has been used safely for thousands of years in these traditional medicines.

These other constituents include tannins, flavones, phosphorus, calcium and volatile oils. Ephedrine and pseudoephedrine make up anywhere from 30% to 90% of the alkaloid content of ephedra. These work synergistically with ephedrine and pseudoephedrine to reduce inflammation, dilate airways, clear the nasal passages, purify the bloodstream and increase urination.

Japanese researchers (Shibata *et al.* 2000) have found that these two constituents in ephedra inhibit mast/basophil/neutrophil cell degranulation. As we discussed in the immune chapter, mast/basophil/neutrophil cell degranulation releases histamine and other mediators that stimulate the allergic response.

Due to its side effects, natural ephedra should be prescribed by a knowledgeable herbalist or medical professional.

Modified Mai Men Dong Tang Formula

This formula, nMMDT, was modified from the traditional Chinese Mai Men Dong Tang formula used for centuries for allergic asthma in Chinese medicine. Researchers from Taiwan's China Medical University Hospital (Hsu *et al.* 2005) gave the mMMDT formula to 100 asthmatic patients for four months. After the treatment period, symptoms improved, lung capacity increased, and IgE levels decreased among the mMMDT group.

This formula contains five herbs:

➤ Gang-Cao, (*Radix Glycyrrhizae*)
➤ Mai-Men-Dong (*Radix Ophiopogonis*)
➤ Xi-Yang-Shen (*Radix Panacis Quinquefolii*)
➤ Ban-Xia (*Tuber Pinellia*)
➤ *Herba Tridacis procumbentis*

Ayurvedic Food Sensitivity Formulations

Ayurvedic doctors have been prescribing herbal medicine to their food-sensitive patients for thousands of years. There is a wealth of information provided in the Sanskrit and Materia Medica texts that have been passed down through the centuries. Texts that include tenets on Ayurveda include the Arshnashaka, Kricch-Hridroganashak, Mehnashaka, Kasa-swasahara, Pandunashaka, Kamla-Kushta-Vataraktanashaka, Rasayana, Sangrahi, Balya, Agnideepana, Tridoshshamaka, Dahnashaka, Jwarhara, Krimihara and Prameha. This information had a tradition of acceptance and clinical application among literally hundreds of millions of patients over the centuries. Ayurvedic doctors were highly esteemed and respected among Asia and the world for thousands of years. In fact, the medicines of Arabia, China, Europe, Greece and Rome borrowed many of their basic principles and uses of herbal medicines from Ayurveda. And of course, these medical traditions also practiced those principles on millions of patients over the centuries. We can conclude that Ayurveda has had a rich history of clinical use, success and safety.

Because of this history of safety, little thought was given to double-blind studies until recent years. This history of thousands of years of success and safety of Ayurvedic herbs did not indicate the need for clinical research until Ayurveda was challenged by modern medicine. The age of pharmaceuticals has challenged Ayurvedic formulations, just as they have challenged Chinese formulations. And just as Chinese formulations are proving successful in double-blind, placebo-controlled research, Ayurvedic medicine has also proved successful and safe in clinical research.

However, Ayurvedic medicine research has been trailing Chinese medicine over the past few years. Traditional Chinese medicine has enjoyed research funding over the past decade or so from the Chinese government, and more recently from a few Western medical schools. As a result, while Ayurvedic formulations have such a rich tradition of success, we must rely primarily upon the tradition texts for clinical documentation, with only a smattering of clinical research for additional substantiation.

For example, Indian researchers (Amit *et al.* 2003) tested an anti-food allergy botanical formula on rats. The combination proved to block histamine activity in this study.

This Ayurvedic formula contains the following seven herbs:

> ➢ Amalaki (*Phyllanthus emblica*)
> ➢ Haritaki (*Terminalia chebula*)
> ➢ Bihitaki (*Terminalia bellerica*)
> ➢ Sirisha (*Albizia lebbeck*)
> ➢ Black pepper (*Piper nigrum*)

> ➤ Ginger (*Zingiber officinale*)
> ➤ Long pepper (*Piper longum*)

Each of these have been used traditionally for inflammation and immune dysfunction. Let's discuss a few of these and other Ayurvedic herbs useful for food sensitivities. Note, however, that ginger was reviewed previously as Gan-Jiang.

Ayurvedic Triphala

Triphala is a combination of three Ayurvedic herbs: *Terminalia chebula, Terminalia bellirica* and *Emblica officinalis*. These three are also termed haritaki, bihitaki and amalaki, respectively. They are also called *"three fruits"* which is the direct translation of triphala. This combination has been utilized for thousands of years to rejuvenate the intestines, regulate digestion and create efficiency within the digestive tract.

The 'three fruits' also are said to produce a balance among the three doshas of *vata, pitta* and *kapha*. Each herb, in fact, relates to a particular *dosha:* haritaki relates to *vata,* amalaki relates to *pitta* and bibhitaki relates to *kapha*. The three taken together comprise the most-prescribed herbal formulations given by Ayurvedic doctors for digestive issues.

This use has been justified by preliminary research. For example, in a study by pharmacology researchers from India's Gujarat University (Nariya *et al.* 2003), triphala was tested on rats that had suffered intestinal damage and intestinal permeability from methotrexate. After being given the triphala, the researchers found that the triphala *"significantly restored the depleted protein level in brush border membrane of intestine, phospholipid and glutathione content and decreased the myeloperoxidase and xanthine oxidase level in intestinal mucosa of methotrexate-treated rats."* The triphala also produced a *"significant decrease in permeation clearance."* This of course means that the triphala significantly reduced intestinal permeability.

The traditional texts and the clinical use of triphala today in Ayurveda has confirmed these types of intestinal effects in humans.

We might want to elaborate a little further on Haritaki in particular. *Terminalia chebula* has been used by Ayurvedic practitioners specifically for conditions related to asthma, coughs, hoarseness, abdominal issues, skin eruptions, itchiness, and inflammation. It is also called He-Zi in traditional Chinese medicine.

Research has found that haritaki contains a large number of polyphenols, including ellagic acids, which have significant antioxidant and anti-inflammatory properties (Pfundstein *et al.* 2010).

Black Pepper

While *Piper nigrum* is considered Ayurvedic, it is probably one of the most common spices used in Western foods. In fact, the world probably owes its use of black pepper in foods to Ayurveda.

Black pepper is used in a variety of Ayurvedic formulations because of its anti-inflammatory action. Ayurvedic doctors describe black pepper as a stimulant, expectorant, carminative (expulsing gas), anti-inflammatory and analgesic. It has been used traditionally for rheumatism, bronchitis, coughs, asthma, sinusitis, gastritis and other histamine-related conditions. It is also thought to stimulate a healthy mucosal membrane among the stomach and intestines.

Black pepper used as a spice to increase taste is certainly not unhealthy, but it takes a significantly greater and consistent dose to produce its anti-inflammatory effects.

A traditional Ayurvedic prescription for gastroesophageal reflux or GERD, for example, is to take black pepper in a warm glass of water first thing in the morning. This initial dose of black pepper, according to Ayurveda, stimulates mucosal secretion, and thickens the mucosal membranes of the stomach and intestines.

Long Pepper

The related Ayurvedic herb, *Piper longum* has similar properties and constituents as black pepper. It is used to inhibit the inflammation and histamine activity that results in lung and sinus congestion. Like *P. nigrum*, *P. longum* is also known to strengthen digestion by stimulating the secretion of the mucosal membrane within the stomach and intestines. It is also said to stimulate enzyme activity and bile production.

Sirisha

Albizia lebbeck has been used in Ayurveda for allergies for thousands of years. It comes from the Siris tree, and contains a variety of glycosides, flavonoids, tannins and saponins. It has also been used in Ayurveda to treat inflammation, lung issues and skin issues.

Guduchi

Guduchi's botanical name is *Tinospora Cordifolia*. This climbing shrub, at home in tropical regions of India and China, has been utilized for thousands of years to modulate the immune system and increase tolerance. In other words, it is an adaptogen. Among Western herbalists this herb is referred to as heartleaf moonseed.

The guduchi plant contains a number of alkaloids, aliphatic compounds, diterpenoid lactones, glycosides, sesquiterpenes, phenolics, steroids, and various polysaccharides. Ayurvedic physicians report that the medicinal properties of guduchi are anti-allergic, antispasmodic, anti-arthritic, anti-inflammatory, antioxidant, anti-stress and hepato-protective (protects the liver).

Guduchi contains two researched constituents called tinosporide and cordioside. These have been shown to significantly modulate the immune system, including NK cells, B-cells, T-cells. It was shown to increase the production of cytokines IL-1Beta, IL-6, IL-12, IL-18 INF-alpha and TNF-alpha (Kapil and Sharma 1997; Nair et al. 2004).

Guduchi has been used extensively for asthma, chronic coughs, allergic respiratory conditions and allergic rhinitis. Researchers from India's Indira Gandhi Medical College (Badar et al. 2005) gave T. cordifolia extract or placebo to 75 allergic rhinitis patients for eight weeks. Of the guduchi extract-treated group, 83% reported complete relief from sneezing associated with allergies. The guduchi treatment also produced complete relief of nasal discharges in 69% of the group, and relief of nasal obstruction in 61%. There was no relief in most of the placebo group. The researchers also found that pro-inflammatory eosinophil and neutrophil counts decreased, and inflammatory goblet cells were absent in nasal smears among the guduchi-treated group.

Additionally, numerous animal and laboratory studies over recent years have confirmed the immune-modulating, liver-protective, antioxidant and anti-inflammatory effects of guduchi (Upadhyay et al. 2010).

Boswellia/Frankincense

Boswellia species include *Boswellia serratta, Boswellia thurifera,* and *Boswellia spp.* (other species). Boswellia contains a variety of active constituents, including a number of boswellic acids, diterpenes, ocimene, caryophyllene, incensole acetate, limonene and lupeolic acids.

The genus of *Boswellia* includes a group of trees known for their fragrant sap resin that grow in Africa and Asia. Frankincense was famously used in ancient Egypt, India, Arabia and Mesopotamia thousands of years ago as an elixir that relaxed and healed the body's aches and pains. The gum from the resin was applied as an ointment for rheumatic ailments, urinary tract disorders, and on the chest for bronchitis and general breathing problems. It is classified in Ayurveda as bitter and pungent.

Over the centuries, boswellia has been used as an internal treatment for a wide variety of ailments, including bronchitis, asthma, arthritis, rheumatism, anemia, allergies and a variety of infections. Its properties are described as stimulant, diaphoretic, anti-rheumatic, tonic, analgesic, antiseptic, diuretic, demulcent, astringent, expectorant, and antispasmodic.

In two studies, boswellic acids extracted from boswellia were found to have significant anti-inflammatory action. The trials revealed that boswellia inhibited the inflammation-stimulating LOX enzyme (5-lipoxygenase) and thus reduced the production of inflammatory leukotrienes (Singh *et al.* 2008; Ammon 2006).

Another study (Takada *et al.* 2006) showed that boswellic acids inhibited cytokines and suppressed cell invasion through NF-kappaB inhibition.

In an animal study by researchers from the University of Maryland's School of Medicine (Fan *et al.* 2005), boswellia extract exhibited significant anti-inflammatory effects. The report also concluded that, *"these effects may be mediated via the suppression of pro-inflammatory cytokines."*

In an *in vitro* study also from the University of Maryland's School of Medicine (Chevrier *et al.* 2005), boswellia extract proved to modulate the balance between Th1 and Th2 cytokines. This illustrated boswellia's ability to strengthen the immune system and increase tolerance.

Turmeric

Turmeric, or *Curcuma longa,* has been extensively used as a medicinal herb for many centuries, and this predicated its use as a curry food spice—as Ayurveda has long incorporated healing herbs with meals. Turmeric is a root (or rhizome) and a relative of ginger in the *Zingiberaceae* family.

Just as we might expect from a medicinal botanical, turmeric has a large number of active constituents. The most well known of those are the curcuminoids, which include curcumin (diferuloylmethane, demethoxycurcumin, and bisdemethoxycurcumin). Others include volatile oils such as tumerone, atlantone, and zingiberene; as well as polysaccharides and a number of resins.

As stated in a recent review from the Cytokine Research Laboratory at the University of Texas (Anand 2008), multiple studies have linked turmeric with *"suppression of inflammation; angiogenesis; tumor genesis; diabetes; diseases of the cardiovascular, pulmonary, and neurological systems, of skin, and of liver; loss of bone and muscle; depression; chronic fatigue; and neuropathic pain."*

Indeed, turmeric has been used for centuries for arthritis, inflammation, gallbladder problems, diabetes, wound-healing, liver issues, hepatitis, menstrual pain, anemia, and gout. It is described as alterative, antibacterial, carminative and stimulating. It also is known for its wound-healing, blood-purifying and circulatory powers. Studies have illustrated that curcumin has about 50% of the effectiveness of cortisone, without its damaging side effects (Jurenka 2009).

A number of studies have proved over the past decade that turmeric and/or its key constituents such as curcumin halt or inhibit both inflammatory COX and LOX enzymes. Curcumin has specifically been shown to inhibit IgE signaling processes, and slow mast cell activation (Aggarwal and Sung 2009; Thampithak *et al.* 2009; Sompamit *et al.* 2009; Kulka 2009).

In a study by researchers at the UK's University of Reading (Bundy 2004), 500 human volunteers with irritable bowel syndrome took either one or two tablets of a standardized turmeric extract for eight weeks. After the eight-week period, the prevalence of IBS dropped by 53% for the one-tablet group and reduced by 60% for the two-tablet group. Pain severity scores also dropped significantly.

In another study on 45 patients with peptic ulcers (Prucksunand 2001), ulcers were completely resolved and absent in 76% of the group taking turmeric powder in capsules.

Other studies have also shown similar positive gastrointestinal effects of turmeric. We can conclude from the evidence that turmeric strengthens the mucosal membranes within the digestive tract.

Coriander/Cilantro/Parsley

Coriandrum sativum is documented in Ayurvedic medicine as an antiallergy herb. This is also cilantro, which is also sometimes called Chinese parsley. It is related to Italian parsley, with many of the same constituents. Coriander is taken as fresh or juiced fresh, and it has been used by Ayurvedic practitioners primarily for allergic skin rashes and hay fever.

Fresh Italian parsley can readily be found in supermarkets and farmers' markets. While often used as a garnish (for looks and/or to clean the breath), a therapeutic quantity of parsley is about a *bunch*. A bunch of parsley is about two ounces or about ten stalks together with their branches and leaves. A bunch can be added to a salad or put into a soup. Parsley can be delicious with tomatoes, vinegar and olive oil. And of course, it can also freshen the breath.

Fennel Seed

Fennel (*Foeniculum vulgare*) contains anetholes, caffeoyl quinic acids, carotenoids, vitamin C, iron, B vitamins, and rutins. Ayurvedic and traditional herbalists from many cultures have used fennel to relieve digestive discomfort, gas, abdominal cramping, bloating and irritable bowels; and to treat food sensitivities. Fennel stimulates bile production. Bile digests fats

and other nutrients. Inadequate fat breakdown can result in macromolecules, including larger protein combinations.

The constituent anethole is known to suppress the inflammatory
TNF alpha, slowing excessive immune response. The combination of
anethole and antioxidant nutrients such as rutin and carotenoids are
known to strengthen immune response while increasing tolerance.

Fennel is not appropriate for pregnant moms, because it has been
known to promote uterine contractions. As with any herbal supplement,
fennel should be used under the supervision of a health professional.
Anyone with a birch allergy should also be aware that they may be sensitive to fennel. (The same goes for cumin, caraway, carrot and others).

Cumin

Cuminum cyminum has a long history of use among European and
Asian herbalists. It is described as antispasmodic and carminative, so it
tends to soothe inflammatory responses. Like fennel, cumin has been
used traditionally to ease indigestion, abdominal cramping and gas.

Cumin contains mucilage, gums and resins, which appear to give it its
ability to stimulate and strengthen the mucosal membrane of the digestive
tract. This may well be its central benefit for food sensitivities. Those
sensitive to celery should avoid cumin.

Bishop's weed or Khella

Bishop's weed (*Trachyspermum ammiis*) is also called khella or khellin
among Middle-Eastern herbalists. It is also referred to as Ajwain weed or
Ammi visnaga among Ayurvedic practitioners and traditional herbalists.
Some also refer to it as *Carum copticum,* Spanish toothpick, toothpick weed,
Daucus visnaga and honeyplant. The plant is related to celery and parsley,
and blooms with clusters of fragile white flowers. From the flower heads
come a fruit and seeds known for their medicinal properties.

Bishop's weed has a long tradition of use among Ayurvedic medicine
and Egyptian medicine, especially for coughs, bronchitis and hypersensitivity. It's use was mentioned in the *Ebers Papyrus*, written more than 3,000
years ago.

Often the fruit and seeds are crushed to produce a brown oil, which
is called omam. The oil can also be infused into creams and tinctures.
Omam water is also produced from Bishop's weed. To make omam water,
the seeds are simply soaked in water.

Bishop's weed has been shown to inhibit histamine release (Weiss
1988). It also opens the bronchi and is considered spasmolytic (stops

spasms), anti-cholinergic (blocks acetylcholine), and vagolytic (inhibits vagus nerve responses).

It most important constituents include thymol, isothymol, pinene, cymene, cromoglycate, terpinene and limonene. The fruits contain coumarins and furocoumarins. Khellin and visnagin are considered the more active compounds in bishop's weed.

Bishop's weed is also antimicrobial. Its antispasmodic traits may be due to its ability to dilate the bronchial passages and blood vessels without stimulation. These actions make it useful for allergies and inflammation response.

Khella's traditional uses thus include coughing, asthma, bronchitis, heart pain and muscle spasms. It has also been used for wound healing, headaches and urinary conditions. While side effects are few, Bishop's weed has been said to increase the skin's sensitivity to the sun.

There is little research on bishop's weed proving its usefulness. However, sodium cromoglycate—thought to be one of its more active anti-allergic constituents—has been extensively studied and proven effective for allergies and asthma.

Disodium cromoglycate was developed by Dr. Roger Altounyan, an asthma sufferer. It is used in many cases as a drug for asthma and allergy patients as an alternative to steroids. Dr. Altounyan derived the drug by isolating sodium cromoglycate from khella. Disodium cromoglycate has undergone extensive clinical drug studies, and is considered one of the more effective anti-allergic pharmaceutical drugs—and probably the most prescribed drug for allergies behind prednisone. Disodium cromoglycate stabilizes mast cells and smooth muscle fibers. This is effected through modulation of calcium and other ions involved in cell membrane permeability. This effect also alters the degranulation process, thus inhibiting histamine (González Alvarez and Arruzazabala 1981).

Job's Tears

Job's tears' genus-species name is *Coix lachryma-jobi* (L. var. ma-yuen Stapf). Job's tears are an ancient grain known to grow primarily in Asia. This grass is native to the tropical regions of Southern Asia, but has been increasingly cultivated as an ornamental grass around the world.

Researchers from National Taiwan University (Chen *et al.* 2010) tested the anti-allergic activity of Job's tears in the laboratory. They found that an extract of Job's tears suppressed mast cell degranulation and inhibited histamine release. It also suppressed the release of inflammatory mediators IL-4, IL-6 and TNF-A. The researchers concluded that Job's tears inhibited the body's physiological allergic response.

Pine Bark

The bioflavonoid-rich extract from French maritime pine bark (*Pinus pinaster*) called pycnogenol® has been the subject of numerous studies showing anti-allergy, antioxidant and anti-inflammatory effects.

In a German study (Belcaro *et al.* 2008), pycnogenol lowered C-reactive protein levels—known to increase during inflammation and allergies—after 156 patients were given 100 milligrams of pycnogenol or placebo for three months. The average CRP decrease was from 3.9 to 1.1 after treatment. This is 300%+ reduction in this inflammation marker.

Researchers from Loma Linda University's School of Medicine (Lau *et al.* 2004) gave 60 asthmatic children from 6-18 years old pycnogenol or placebo for three months. The pycnogenol group experienced a significant reduction of asthma symptoms, and an increase in pulmonary function. Pycnogenol also allowed the patients to reduce or discontinue the use of inhalers significantly more than the placebo group.

In a study of allergic rhinitis to birch pollen, 38 allergic patients were given pycnogenol several weeks before the start of the 2009 birch allergy season. The pycnogenol reduced allergic eye symptoms by 35% and sinus symptoms by 20%, compared to the placebo group. Better results were found among those who took pycnogenol 7-8 weeks before the birch pollen season began (Wilson *et al.* 2010).

Researchers from Ireland's Trinity College (Sharma *et al.* 2003) found that pycnogenol inhibited the release of histamine from mast cells. This effect appeared to come from the significant bioflavonoid content of the pycnogenol.

Dandelion

Dandelion species include *Taraxum officinale*, *Taraxum mongolicum*, and *Taraxum spp.* Dandelion contains hundreds of active constituents, which include beta-carboline alkaloids, beta-sitosterol, boron, caffeic acid, calcium, coumaric acid, coumarin, four steroids, furulic acid, gallic acid, hesperetin, hesperidin, indole alkaloids, inulin, iron, lupenol, lutein, luteolin, magnesium, mannans, monoterpenoids, myristic acid, palmitic acid, potassium, quercetins, rufescidride, sesquiterpenes, silicon, steroid complexes, stigmasterol, syringic acid, syringin, tannins, taraxacin, taraxacoside, taraxafolide, taraxafolin-B, taraxasterol, taraxasteryl acetate, taraxerol, taraxinic acid beta-glucopyranosyl, benzenoids, triterpenoids, violaxanthin, vitamin A (7,000 IU/oz), Bs, C, D, K and zinc among others (Williams *et al.* 1996; Hu and Kitts 2003; Hu and Kitts 2004; Seo *et al.* 2005; Trojanova *et al.* 2004; Leu *et al.* 2005; Kisiel and Michalska 2005; Leu *et al.* 2003; Michalska and Kisiel 2003; Kisiel and Barszcz 2000).

Taraxum is derived from the Greek words *taraxos* meaning 'disorder' and *akos* meaning 'remedy.' Dandelion is a common weed with a characteristic beautiful yellow flower that assumes a globe of seeds to spread its humble yet incredible medicinal virtues. Its hollow stem is full of milky juice, with a long, hardy root; and leaves that taste good in a spring salad. Dandelion is one of the most well known traditional herbs for all sorts of ailments that involve toxicity within the blood, liver, kidneys, lymphatic system and urinary tract. Dandelion has been listed in a variety of herbal formularies around the world for many centuries.

Dandelion's use was expounded by many cultures from the Greeks to the Northern American Indians—who used it for stomach ailments and infections. It is also used for the treatment of viral and bacterial infections as well as cancer. The latex or milky sap that comes from the stem has a mixture of polysaccharides, proteins, lipids, rubber, and metabolites such as polyphenoloxidase. The latex has been used to heal skin wounds and protect those wounds from infection—also the sap's function when the plant is injured.

Dandelion is known to protect and help rebuild the liver. The famous herbalist Culpeper documented that it *"has an opening and cleansing quality and, therefore, very effectual for removing obstructions of the liver, gall bladder and spleen and diseases arising from them, such as jaundice."* It is known to stimulate the elimination of toxins and clear obstructions from the blood and liver. This is thought to be the reason why dandelion helps clear stones and scarring from kidneys, gallbladder and bladder. It has also been used to treat stomach problems, and is thought to reduce blood pressure.

In ancient Chinese medicine, it has been recommended for issues related to the imbalance between liver enzymes and pancreatic enzymes. It has been used in traditional treatments for hypoglycemia, hypertension, urinary tract infection, skin eruptions, breast cancer, appetite loss, flatulence, dyspepsia, constipation, gallstones, circulation problems, skin issues, spleen and liver complaints, hepatitis and anorexia.

Dandelion is also thought to increase the flow of bile, necessary for the digestion of fats and other food constituents.

A study by researchers at Canada's University of British Columbia (Hu and Kitts 2004) found that dandelion extract suppressed the inflammatory mediator prostaglandin E2 (PGE2) without causing cell death. Further tests indicated that COX-2 was inhibited by the luteolin and luteolin-glucosides in dandelion.

In another study by Hu and Kitts (2005), nitric oxide was inhibited. Reactive oxygen species—free radicals—were also significantly reduced by dandelion—attributed to the plant's phenolic acid content. This in turn prevented lipid oxidation—one of the mechanisms in heightened LDL (bad cholesterol) levels and artery inflammation.

In a 2007 study from researchers at the College of Pharmacy at the Sookmyung Women's University in Korea (Jeon *et al.* 2008), dandelion was found to reduce inflammation, leukocytes, vascular permeability, abdominal cramping, pain and COX levels among exudates.

Dandelion was also found to stimulate fourteen different strains of bifidobacteria—important components of the intestinal immune system as we've discussed at length (Trojanova *et al.* 2004).

Another study found that dandelion extract significantly prevented cell death in Hep G2 (liver) cells, while stimulating TNF and IL-1 levels—illustrating its ability to arrest or slow liver disease and stimulate healing (Koo *et al.* 2004).

Other studies have illustrated that dandelion inhibits both interleukin IL-6 and TNF-alpha—both inflammatory cytokines (Seo *et al.* 2005).

Dandelion was shown to stimulate the liver's production of glutathione (GST)—an important antioxidant (Petlevski *et al.* 2003).

Dandelion increased the liver's production of superoxide dismutase and catalase, increasing the liver's ability to purify the blood of toxins and allergens (Cho *et al.* 2001).

Pro-inflammatory leukotriene production was decreased with an extract of dandelion (Kashiwada *et al.* 2001).

Dandelion illustrated the ability to inhibit inflammatory IL-1 cytokines (Kim *et al.* 2000) and Takasaki *et al.* (1999).

In a study of 24 patients with chronic intestinal colitis, pains in the large intestine vanished in 96% of the patients by the 15th day after being given a blend of herbs including dandelion (Chakŭrski *et al.* 1981).

Goldenrod

Goldenrod includes several varieties, including *Solidago virgaurea, Solidago altissima* and *Solidago canadensis*. Goldenrod's constituents include quinine, dictyopterol, cadinene, caffeic acid, caffeoylquinic acids, entgermacra, kaempferols, limonene and methyl caffeoyl, neochlorogenic acid, quercetin, quercetrin, quinate, rutin, saponins, sesquiterpenes, solicanolide, and several tannins among others. (Bradette-Hébert *et al.* 2008; Choi 2004; Vila *et al.* 2002; Sung *et al.* 1999; Bader *et al.* 1996; Bongartz and Hesse 1995)

Belonging to the daisy family, goldenrod is a perennial bushy plant indigenous to North America and many other places in the world. Its Latin name is derived from *solido* which means to 'make whole or strengthen.' The leaves and flowers are used for medicinal purposes.

Goldenrod has been used for many centuries for inflammatory conditions. It was used by early Americans and North American Indians for rheumatism, colds, headaches, sore throats, and neuralgia (pain). American Indians also used a mouthwash of goldenrod for toothaches. The flowers were chewed for sore throats.

Traditional herbalists have documented goldenrod's anti-inflammatory effects and wound-healing abilities. It has also been used traditionally for rheumatism, flatulence, arthritis, gout, prostatitis and eczema. Goldenrod has also been observed increasing glomerulus filtration and decreasing albumin levels. Thus it has been used for issues of nephritis, unuria and oliguria.

Goldenrod's medicinal properties are considered anti-inflammatory, antimicrobial, diaphoretic, antidiarrhoeic, carminative, stimulant, diuretic (increases urine output), analgesic, antiseptic, antispasmodic (reduces spasms), antioxidant, antifungal and antiedematous (reduces swelling). The flowers are typically used for medicinal purposes.

A German review of multiple clinical studies indicated that significant anti-inflammatory and pain-relieving effects were accomplished when dosages of goldenrod were comparable to NSAID use—with few of the adverse effects of NSAIDs (Klein-Galczinsky 1999).

In several randomized, placebo-controlled and double-blind clinical studies, goldenrod significantly reduced pain and inflammation in rheumatic diseases (Gundermann and Müller 2007).

Goldenrod was also found to boost immune response and promote cytotoxicity to tumor cells (Wu *et al.* 2008, Plohmann *et al.* 1997).

Goldenrod proved spasmolytic (reduced spasms), antihypertensive and diuretic in other investigations (von Kruedener *et al.* 1995).

Goldenrod proved to be a potent free radical scavenger in a study from Canada's McGill University (McCune and Johns, 2002).

A 60% ethanol extract of goldenrod showed anti-inflammatory activity similar to diclofenac (a well-known NSAID).

Goldenrod also stimulates glutathione activity (Apáti *et al.* 2006). The essential oil from goldenrod produced antimicrobial activity against a number of bacteria and yeasts (Morel *et al.* 2006).

Plant Corticoids

Corticosteroids systemically reduce allergic symptoms and response by blocking histamine release. For this reason, prednisone and similar cortisone drugs are the most-prescribed drugs for allergies. Prednisone and methylprednisone mimic the actions of cortisol produced by the adrenal gland. Cortisol's and cortisone's main mechanism is to slow or shunt the inflammatory response and suppress the immune system. Thus it is used for a wide range of inflammatory conditions.

However, because prednisone acts like a hormone, it significantly alters moods. This may begin with mild frustration or annoyance over trivial things. With consistent use, this can turn into rage, depression, mania, personality changes and psychotic behavior. Other side effects include weight gain, high blood pressure, sodium retention, headaches, ulcers, cataracts, irregular menstruation, elevated blood sugar, growth retarding, osteoporosis, wound healing impairment, moon face (puffiness of the face), glaucoma, bruising, buffalo hump (rounded upper back), and thinning of the skin.

In addition, over time, prednisone dosing can reduce the body's own production of cortisol. Furthermore, increased doses are usually required to maintain the same suppression of symptoms. This can result in an inflammatory and immunosuppressed situation should the prednisone dosing be reduced or withdrawn (Todd *et al.* 2002).

The body produces cortisol and other corticoids using a complex adrenal process that begins with the body's production of cholesterol (not the same as the dietary cholesterol obtained from animal diets). The body uses plant-based phytosterols to produce the steroidal compounds that stimulate cortisone production through the adrenal glands. In other words, the best raw materials for cortisone production come from a healthy plant-based diet of phytosterols. Let's discuss some of the many plants that provide these natural raw materials.

For many years, the pharmaceutical industry utilized wild yam (*Dioscorea floribunda* and *D. floribunda*) to produce the raw corticoid ingredient diosgenin. Diosgenin was utilized to produce progesterone and other steroid drugs. In the human body, the diosgenin in wild yam is a steroid, and is converted into progesterone and DHEA.

As wild yam production could not keep pace with pharmaceutical steroid demand, stigmasterols and sitosetrols from soy and solasodine from *Solanum dulcamara* became the preferred source of corticoid precursors for the pharmaceutical industry.

Many foods, especially those containing seeds, are good sources of phytosterols.

Bittersweet

Solanum dulcamara, a creeping shrub that grows along streams and bogs, has been used extensively in traditional Western herbal medicine for all varieties of allergic skin issues and inflammatory conditions. It has been used for rheumatism and circulatory problems. The alkaloid solamine and the glucoside dulcamarin have been recognized as its active constituents, but as discussed, solasodine appears to be intricately involved in stimulating corticoid production.

Perhaps it is for this reason that many traditional herbalists have recommended bittersweet in cases of allergic skin conditions. We should note that another constituent, solanine, can be poisonous in significant amounts. Therefore, as in all herbal products, consultation with a health professional is suggested before use.

Mallow

As long as we are discussing allergic skin responses, we should mention *Malva sylvestris*, also called mallow. This herb has been used in decoctions in European herbalism for allergic skin responses and eczema. For this reason, Swiss doctors during the World Wars were known to apply compresses onto skin rashes with good success.

Evening Primrose

Another herb known by traditional herbalists to be beneficial for allergic skin responses is evening primrose, or *Oenothera spp.* The seeds are rich in gamma-linolenic acid (GLA)— a fatty acid known to slow inflammatory responses of prostaglandins, especially those relating to skin hypersensitivity. The oil from evening primrose can be applied directly onto the skin and taken internally. Evening primrose oil has thus been used successfully in cases of allergic eczema, for example.

Wild Pansy

This herb, botanical name *Viola tricolor*, has been used traditionally in Western herbal medicine for eczema. Its wonderful colorful flowers are difficult to miss in grasslands across North America and Europe. Wild pansy is known to be high in saponins, as many other anti-allergic herbs are.

Saponins are the glycosides such as triterpenes—active compounds in many of the medicinal plants we've discussed in this chapter. Ginseng is a rich source of saponins, for example.

Wild pansy's saponins are drawn out via simple tea infusion. This can be applied externally onto skin rashes, as well as taken internally.

Red seaweed

Red seaweed has been used for thousands of years to treat inflammation-oriented conditions, including bronchitis and hypersensitivity. Researchers from the National Taiwan Ocean University (Kazłowska *et al.*

2010) studied the ability of the red seaweed *Porphyra dentata*, to halt allergic responses. The researchers found that a *Porphyra dentata* phenolic extract suppressed nitric oxide production among macrophages using a NF-kappa-Beta gene transcription process. This modulated the hypersensitivity immune response on a systemic level. The phenolic compounds within the red algae have been identified as catechol, rutin and hesperidin.

Other Anti-inflammatory Herbs

A number of other herbs also contain anti-inflammatory properties. These work in different ways, and while they may or may not specifically modulate food sensitivities, they can help strengthen the immune system, and thus reduce the inflammatory process the provokes hypersensitivity. Thus they can contribute to the modulation of the immune system, allowing us to begin tolerating foods that were not previously tolerated. Here is a quick overview of some of the most well-known (and most available) of these anti-inflammatory herbs:

Basil (*Osimum basilicum*) contains ursolic acid and oleanolic acid, both shown in laboratory studies to inhibit inflammatory COX-2 enzymes.

Rosemary (*Rosmarinus officinalis*) contains ursolic acid, oleanolic acid and apigenin—a few of the many constituents in this important botanical—shown to inhibit inflammatory enzymes in laboratory studies.

Oregano (*Origanum vulgare*) contains at least thirty-one anti-inflammatory constituents, twenty-eight antioxidants, and four significant COX-2 inhibitors (apigenin, kaempherol, ursolic acid and oleanolic acid).

Garlic (*Allium sativum*) probably deserves a larger section, but that information could easily encompass a book in itself (as was well documented by Paul Bergner: *The Healing Power of Garlic*, 1996). Garlic is an ancient medicinal plant with a wealth of characteristics and constituents that stimulate the immune system, protect the liver, purify the bloodstream, reduce oxidative species, reduce LDL cholesterol, reduce inflammation, and stimulate detoxification systems throughout the body. This is supported by a substantial amount of rigorous scientific research.

Garlic is also one of the most powerful antibiotic-antimicrobial plants known. A fresh garlic bulb has at least five different constituents known to inhibit bacteria, fungi and viruses. This antibiotic capability, however, is destroyed by heat and oxygen. Therefore, eating freshly peeled bulbs are the most assured way to retain these antibiotic potencies.

Cooked, aged or dehydrated garlic powder also has a variety of powerful antioxidants, but little of its antibiotic abilities. Garlic is also a tremendous sulfur donor as well. The combination of garlic's antibiotic, antioxidant, anti-inflammatory and immune-building characteristics make it a *must* food for any inflammatory condition.

The Herbal Conclusion

This of course is a long list of herbs and herbal formulations that have been shown in research and clinical use among traditional medicines to have adaptogenic properties. Choosing the right herb and/or formula for a particular sensitivity can thus be a little tricky. For this reason, a seasoned expert in herbal formulations can offer specific suggestions relating to ones constitution and precise level of sensitivities.

That said, one of the strategies that many traditional physicians have utilized is to select those herbs that target the symptoms of the patient. While this might be compared to "treating the symptoms," as some pharmaceutical strategies are accused of, herbal medicines work on a much deeper level as we've discussed. While an herb's primary constituents might be productive with particular symptoms, the rest of the herb's constituents will likely also modulate the immune system's tolerance. This is its adaptogenic ability. These are the effects we have also seen among the research on herbal medicines. This *"from the outside in"* strategy produces a deeper correction of the systemic immunity issues often at the root of the problem.

We also see in many of these herbs, their ability to stimulate a healthy mucosal membrane and strengthen the intestinal barrier. These illustrate a strategy of treating from both directions: *outside-in* and *inside-out*.

Therefore, in the case of a food allergy where the primary reaction is respiratory—coughing, lung congestion, and so on—the traditional herbalist might select those anti-allergic herbs listed above that are known for their respiratory responses. Likewise, a person with allergic skin reactions would be given those herbs known to help atopic skin responses. Concurrently, the herbalist would select those herbs discussed above that modulate and strengthen the intestinal barrier and intestinal mucosal membranes to reduce the exposure of the allergen on the intestinal tissues and bloodstream.

Proteolytic Enzymes

Enzymes are critical components in breaking down macromolecule proteins that can cause food sensitivities. While we are increasing our probiotics, strengthening the immune system and reviving our digestive system, mucosal membranes and intestinal brush barriers; we can also take some of the heat off our immune system by supplementing with naturally-produced proteolytic enzymes to help break down some of the proteins and peptides that our bodies have become sensitized to.

Proteolytic enzymes are produced by plant-based foods, probiotics, and our own gastric, liver and bile system. For those with compromised digestive systems, these enzymes may not be as available as they should. In these cases, the supplementation of natural enzymes can be extremely productive.

For example, chemical engineering researchers from Stanford University (Ehren *et al.* 2009) evaluated the breakdown of gluten-related proteins using two enzymes produced by probiotic microorganisms. Aspergillopepsin (ASP) produced from *Aspergillus niger* and dipeptidyl peptidase IV (DPP-IV) produced from the probiotic *Aspergillus oryzae* were tested. The two enzymes were tested on gluten-type peptides in a simulation of conditions that would resemble the digestion of whole gluten and whole-wheat bread. They found that ASP and DPP-IV collectively and effectively cleaved (broke down) the gluten-type proteins in the study.

A leading enzyme-producing company, Specialty Enzyme Biotechnology, Ltd., has led the way in the natural production of enzymes that break down gluten-foods, casein-foods and other food proteins in the digestive tract. This is a fifty year old company that produces its enzymes from natural plant sources or probiotic microorganism sources. The company and their branded subsidiary, *AST Enzymes*, now distribute a supplement geared towards gluten and casein sensitivities. According to company information and standardized independent laboratory assays, here is a list of the enzymes and their function within the body:

Enzyme	Function
Dipeptidyl Peptidase IV SEB-Pro GR™	Blend of five proteases that help digest proteins. DPP-IV focuses on proline component of gliadin (glutens) and casein proteins.
Amylase I, II & Glucoamylase	Breaks down carbohydrates and starches into dextrins and sugars
Cellulase	Digests cellulose, a complex polysaccharide found in all plant material.
Hemicellulase and Xylanase (HemiSEB® cellulose)	Break down carbohydrates and plant polysaccharides such as hemicellulose, a major component of plant cell walls.
Alpha-Galactosidase	Breaks down complex carbohydrates such as raffinose and stachyose

Lactase	Breaks down lactose into simple sugars
Lipase	Helps break-down fats into essential fatty acids

This combination provides a ready supply of enzymes that can assist a food-sensitive person in breaking down those macromolecule proteins they may be sensitive to. As we saw in the hydrolyzed protein feeding research among infants, when large sensitized proteins were broken down, most of the children were able to consume the hydrolyzed formula. In the same way, supplemented enzymes can break down proteins the body may be sensitive to, such as gluten-related proteins, soy, milk and others.

As mentioned some plant-based foods supply enzymes that are considered proteolytic. These include bromelain, papain and nattokinase. These have also been shown to have anti-inflammatory properties.

Papain is derived directly from papayas. It is a rich source of proteolytic enzymes. The nattokinase enzyme is produced by *Bacillus natto,* the bacterium used to ferment soy. Bromelain is another botanical enzyme with proteolytic and anti-inflammatory properties. Bromelain is derived from pineapple.

Probiotics also produce a significant number of our body's digestive enzymes. This is one reason why probiotics are so helpful for digestive issues, as we've discussed.

Magnesium, Sulfur, and Other Minerals

Magnesium deficiency has been found to be at the root of a number of conditions. Allergies appear to be one of them. This is because magnesium is a critical element used by the immune system. A body deficient in magnesium will likely be immunosuppressed. Animal studies have illustrated that magnesium deficiency leads to increased IgE counts, and increased levels of inflammation-specific cytokines. Magnesium deficiency is also associated with increased degranulation among mast/basophil/neutrophil cells, which stimulates the allergic response.

Clinical studies have confirmed that magnesium salts appear to improve allergic skin reactions (Błach *et al.* 2007).

Other research have reported that dietary sulfur can significantly relieve allergy symptoms. In a multi-center open label study by researchers from Washington state (Barrager *et al.* 2002), 55 patients with allergic rhinitis were given 2,600 mg of methylsulfonylmethane (MSM)—a significant source of sulfur derived from plants—for 30 days. Weekly reviews of the patients reported significant improvements in allergic respiratory symptoms, along with increased energy. Other research has suggested that sulfur blocks the reception of histamine among histamine receptors.

Good sources of sulfur include avocado, asparagus, barley, beans, broccoli, cabbage, carob, carrots, Brussels sprouts, chives, coconuts, corn, garlic, leafy green vegetables, leeks, lentils, onions, parsley, peas, radishes, red peppers, soybeans, shallots, Swiss chard and watercress.

The other macro- and trace-minerals should not be ignored, however. For example, research has shown that zinc modulates T-cell activities (Hönscheid *et al.* 2009).

Numerous holistic doctors now prescribe full-spectrum mineral combinations for food sensitivities. Many have attested to the ability of these minerals to balance the inflammatory response and stimulate healthy mucosal membranes.

Good sources of the full spectrum of trace and macro minerals include mineral water, whole rock salt, spirulina and vegetables.

Diet Strategies for Food Sensitivities

As we've discussed, much of the literature on food sensitivities gears the dietary discussion towards the elimination of sensitive foods. The author is basically telling the reader to *avoid those foods at any cost,* and *get used to it.* In other words, *learn how to avoid those foods that we are sensitive to by reading labels and menus carefully, and make sure that no speck of protein of foods we are sensitive to gets into our foods.*

While this might be important during a food elimination phase, this also presents a slippery slope. Once we begin traveling this path over the long term, we will find that it is full of danger. We find that the more we try to avoid those foods, the more possible contamination issues we face. Problems can come from the wrong spatula being used. Or maybe people are shelling peanuts around us at a baseball game. Or maybe fellow airplane passengers are chomping on nuts. Or maybe we pass by a peanut-butter machine in the grocery store. How bad can it get? Pretty bad.

While there is certainly a time and a place for avoiding foods we are sensitive to during an elimination period, this is not the subject matter of this book. In fact, many other authors have done a pretty good job on this subject. We have little to add with regard to food avoidance strategies.

At the same time, the focus on food avoidance strategies typically misses strategies that can resolve food sensitivities. Furthermore, they have produced a hyper-awareness that has caused many people to conclude they have a food allergy when they merely have a dietary intolerance possibly caused by a temporary digestive imbalance. It is for this reason that so many more people report having food allergies than actually do.

So let's have a conversation about diet that focuses on the foods that can strengthen our immune system and help us resolve our sensitivities.

In Chapter Four, we laid out the clear research that concludes that our choice of diet has everything to do with food sensitivities. What we eat is presented to the mucosal membranes and walls of our intestinal tract for absorption. Foods that our digestive tract, probiotics and immune system can easily manage with the least amount of toxic byproducts will help us rebuild our intestinal barrier and digestive immune systems.

On the other hand, those foods or drinks that are either over-processed, denatured, mixed with synthetic toxins or otherwise not intended for our body will damage our probiotic systems, damage our mucosal membranes, damage the brush barrier of our intestines—creating increased intestinal permeability—and stimulate the exaggerated immune response characteristic of food sensitivities.

So what should we be eating then?

As we summarize this information, the reader should remember that significant dietary changes done too quickly or otherwise incorrectly can have negative health consequences and even dangerous effects on a person with food sensitivities. Also note that a person may very well be sensitive to some of the foods discussed here. Therefore, it is suggested that new foods and dietary changes be made gradually, and under the supervision of a health professional knowledgeable in diet and food sensitivities.

Increasing Plant-Based Foods

As we covered in detail earlier, animal-based diets discourage the colonization of our probiotics, and encourage the growth of pathogenic microorganisms that can damage our intestines and brush barrier. Animal-based diets also produce byproducts such as phytanic acid and beta-glucuronidase that can damage our intestinal cells and mucosal membranes within the intestines.

Furthermore, the research clearly shows that people eating predominantly plant-based diets have significantly lower risks of allergies of any type. This is because plant-based foods discourage inflammatory responses. Plant-based foods are wholesome and nutritious. They feed our probiotics with complex polysaccharides called prebiotics. They are also a source of fiber (there is no fiber in meat)—critical for intestinal health.

Plant-based foods also contain many antioxidants, anti-carcinogens and other nutrients that strengthen the immune system.

Research on vegetarians has revealed that vegetarians tend to live longer, have less cancer (especially colon cancer) and heart disease, and have fewer food sensitivities and intestinal problems. Every nutrient is available in a vegetarian diet. And plant-based protein is a more digestible source of protein than animal-based proteins. This is because animal-based proteins are more complex and difficult to break down into amino acids. The body utilizes aminos and small peptides, not complex proteins. Plants provide aminos and smaller peptides in more digestible form.

Why isn't meat considered a common food allergen then? This actually may be a misnomer. We've shown that seafood allergies are in combination the most common allergens among many countries. Beef allergies have been shown in a number of studies. The complexities of digesting animal proteins produce increased levels of beta-glucuronidase, nitroreductase, azoreductase, steroid 7-alpha-dehydroxylase, ammonia, urease, cholylglycine hydrolase, phytanic acid and others. These enzymes and toxins deter our probiotics and produce intestinal inflammation.

Furthermore, as we investigated the causes of food sensitivities, intestinal inflammation and reduced levels of probiotics stood as scientifically established reasons for break down of the intestinal barrier and subsequent hypersensitivity to foods. So a predominantly animal-based diet may be implicated in food sensitivities more than most will want to accept.

Certainly this is not to say everyone can immediately accept a completely meatless diet. This is to say that a diet that contains more plant-based foods than is currently the norm among Western industrialized countries will likely assist the immune system in becoming more tolerant.

Whole Foods and Antioxidants

Some of the botanical constituents known to be significantly antioxidant, immunity-strengthening and blood-purifying include *lecithin* and *octacosanol* from whole grains; *polyphenols* and *sterols* from vegetables; *lycopene* and other phytochemicals from tomatoes; *quercetin* and *sulfur/allicin* from garlic, onions and peppers; *pectin* and *rutin* from apples and other fruits; *phytocyanidins* and antioxidant *flavonoids* such as *apigenin* and *luteolin* from various greenfoods; and *anthocyanins* from various fruits and even oats.

Some sea-based botanicals like kelp also contain antioxidants as well. Consider a special polysaccharide compound from kelp called *fucoidan*. Fucoidan has been shown in animal studies to significantly reduce inflammation (Cardoso *et al.* 2009; Kuznetsova *et al.* 2004).

Procyanidins are found in apples, currants, cinnamon, bilberry and many other foods. The extract of *vitis vinifera* seed (grapeseed) is one of the highest sources of bound antioxidant proanthrocyanidins and leucocyanidines called *procyanidolic oligomers*, or "PCOs." Pycnogenol also contains significant levels of PCOs.

Research has demonstrated that PCOs have protective and strengthening effects on tissues by increasing enzyme conjugation (Seo *et al.* 2001). PCOs also increase vascular wall strength (Robert *et al.* 2000).

Oxygenated carotenoids such as *lutein* and *astaxanthin* also have been shown to exhibit strong antioxidant activity. Astaxanthin is derived from the microalga *Haematococcus pluvialis*, and lutein is available from a number of foods, including spirulina.

Nearly every plant-food has some measure of some of these botanical constituents. They alkalize the blood and increase the detoxification capabilities of the liver. They help clear the blood of toxins. Foods that are particularly detoxifying and immunity-building include fresh pineapples, beets, cucumbers, apricots, apples, almonds, zucchini, artichokes, avocados, bananas, beans, leafy greens, berries, casaba, celery, coconuts, cranberries, watercress, dandelion greens, grapes, raw honey, corn, kale, citrus fruits, watermelon, lettuce, mangoes, mushrooms, oats, broccoli, okra, onions, papayas, parsley, peas, radishes, raisins, spinach, tomatoes, walnuts, and many others.

For example, the flavonoids *kaempferol* and *flavone* have been shown to block mast cell proliferation by over 80% (Alexandrakis *et al.* 2003). Sources of kaempferol include Brussels sprouts, broccoli, grapefruit and apples.

Diets with significant fiber levels also help clear the blood and tissues of toxins to support the immune system. Fiber in the diet should range from about 35 to 45 grams per day according to the recommendations of many diet experts. Six to ten servings of raw fruits and vegetables per day should accomplish this—which is even part of the USDA's recommendations. This means raw, fibrous foods can be at every meal.

Good fibrous plant sources also contain healthy *lignans* and *phytoestrogens* that help balance hormone levels, and help the body make its own natural corticoids. Foods that contain these include peas, garbanzo beans, soybeans, kidney beans and lentils.

Garlic, cayenne and onions can be added to any cooked dishes to add inflammation-inhibiting *quercetin* and other antioxidants. Cooked beans or grains can be spiced with turmeric, ginger, basil, rosemary and other anti-inflammatory spices such as cayenne.

Over the past few years, research has discovered that red, purple and blue fruits have tremendous antioxidant and anti-inflammatory benefits. Continued studies have concluded that oxidative species—free radicals—are at the root of much of the damage that burdens the immune system and triggers allergic inflammatory responses. Oxidative species come from poor diets and chemical toxins—exacerbated by stress.

The greatest and most efficient way to neutralize these oxidative radicals comes from fresh botanical foods. The method scientists and food technologists have used to measure the ability a particular food has to neutralize free radicals is the *Oxygen Radical Absorbance Capacity Test* (ORAC). This technical laboratory study is performed by a number of scientific bodies, including the USDA and specialized labs such as Brunswick Laboratories in Massachusetts.

Research from the USDA's Jean Mayer Human Nutrition Research Center on Aging at Tufts University has suggested that a diet high in ORAC value may protect blood vessels and tissues from damage that can result in inflammation (Sofic *et al.* 2001; Cao *et al.* 1998). These tissues, of course, include the intestines.

This research and others have implicated that damage from free radicals also contributes to many disease mechanisms, which burden the immune system and result in hypersensitivity. Although antioxidants cannot be considered treatments for any disease, many studies have suggested that increased antioxidant intake supports immune function and detoxification, allowing the body to better respond with greater tolerance. Many researchers have agreed that consuming 3,000 to 5,000 ORAC units per day can have protective benefits.

ORAC Values of Selected (Raw) Fruits (USDA, 2007-2008)

Cranberry	9,382		Pomegranate	2,860
Plum	7,581		Orange	1,819
Blueberry	6,552		Tangerine	1,620
Blackberry	5,347		Grape (red)	1,260
Raspberry	4,882		Mango	1,002
Apple (Granny)	3,898		Kiwi	882
Strawberry	3,577		Banana	879
Cherry (sweet)	3,365		Tomato (plum)	389
Gooseberry	3,277		Pineapple	385
Pear	2,941		Watermelon	142

There is tremendous attention these days on two unique fruits from the Amazon rain forest and China called *acai* and *goji berry* (or wolfberry) respectively. A recent ORAC test documented by Schauss *et al.* (2006) gives acai a score of 102,700 and a test documented by Gross *et al.* (2006) gives goji berries a total ORAC of 30,300. However, subsequent tests done by Brunswick Laboratories, Inc. gives these two berries 53,600 (acai) and 22,000 (gogi) total-ORAC values.

In addition, we must remember that these are the dried berries being tested in the later case, and a concentrate of acai being tested in the former case. The numbers in the chart above are for fresh fruits. Dried fruits will naturally have higher ORAC values, because the water is evaporated—giving more density and more antioxidants per 100 grams. For example, in the USDA database, dried apples have a 6,681 total-ORAC value, while fresh apples range from 2,210 to 3,898 in total-ORAC value. This equates to a two-to-three times increase from fresh to dried. In another example, fresh red grapes have a 1,260 total-ORAC value, while raisins have a 3,037 total-ORAC value. This comes close to an increase of three times the ORAC value following dehydration.

One of the newest additions to the new high-ORAC superfruits is the maqui superberry. This is small purplish fruit grown in Chile. It is about the size of an elderberry (another good antioxidant fruit).

Part of the equation, naturally, is cost. Dried fruit and concentrates are often more expensive than fresh fruit. High-ORAC dried fruits or concentrates from açaí, gogi or maqui will also be substantially more expensive than most fruits grown domestically (especially for Americans and Europeans). Our conclusion is that local or in-country grown fresh fruits with high total-ORAC values produce the best value. Local fresh fruit offers great free radical scavenging ability, support for local farmers, and pollen proteins we are most likely more tolerant to.

By comparison, spinach—an incredibly wholesome vegetable with a tremendous amount of nutrition—has a fraction of the ORAC content of some of these fruits, at 1,515 total ORAC. It should be noted, however, that some (dehydrated) spices have incredibly high ORAC values. For example, USDA's database lists ground turmeric's total ORAC value at 159,277 and oregano's at 200,129. However, while we might only consume a few hundred milligrams of a spice per day, we can eat many grams—if not pounds—of fruit per day.

Quercetin

A number of studies have shown that quercetin inhibits the release of the inflammatory mediator histamine (Kimata *et al.* 2000). Foods rich in quercetin include onions, garlic, apples, capers, grapes, leafy greens, tomatoes and broccoli. In addition, many of the herbs listed earlier contain quercetin as an active constituent.

In other words, quercetin stimulates and balances the immune system and immune response. In a recent study, quercetin was given to Wistar rats after they were sensitized to peanuts. After a week, the rats were given either the quercetin or a placebo for four weeks. After the treatment period, the rats' histamine levels and allergen-specific IgE levels fell. More importantly, the quercetin completely inhibited anaphylaxis among the treated rats, while the untreated rats experienced no change (Shishehbor *et al.* 2010).

Over the past few years an increasing amount of evidence is pointing to the conclusion that foods with quercetin slow inflammatory response and autoimmune derangement. Researchers from Italy's Catholic University (Crescente *et al.* 2009) found that quercetin inhibited arachidonic acid-induced platelet aggregation. Arachidonic acid-induced platelet aggregation is seen in allergic inflammatory mechanisms.

Researchers from the University of Crete (Alexandrakis *et al.* 2003) found that quercetin can inhibit mast cell proliferation by up to 80%.

Organic foods contain higher levels of quercetin. A study from the University of California-Davis' Department of Food Science and Technology (Mitchell *et al.* 2007) tested flavonoid levels between organic and conventional tomatoes over a ten-year period. Their research concluded that quercetin levels were 79% higher for tomatoes grown organically under the same conditions as conventionally-grown tomatoes.

Methylmethionine

One of the more productive whole foods applicable to food sensitivities is cabbage. Cabbage contains a unique constituent, s-methylmethionine, also referred to as vitamin U. Through a pathway utilizing one of the body's natural enzymes, called Bhmt2, s-methylmethionine is converted to methionine and then to glutathione in a series of steps.

In this form, glutathione has been shown to stimulate the repair of the mucosal membrane within the stomach and intestines. This rebuilding of the mucosal membrane is critical to replenishing the intestinal barrier that is depleted in many food sensitive people. Glutathione has also been shown to increase liver health.

Raw cabbage or cabbage juice has been used as a healing agent for ulcers and intestinal issues for thousands of years among traditional medicines, including those of Egyptian, Ayurvedic and Greek systems. The Western world became aware of raw cabbage juice in the 1950s, when Garnett Cheney, M.D. conducted several studies showing that methylmethionine-rich cabbage juice concentrate was able to reduce the pain and bleeding associated with ulcers.

In one of Dr. Cheney's studies, 37 ulcer patients were treated with either cabbage juice concentrate or placebo. Of the 26-patient cabbage juice group, 24 patients were considered "successes," achieving an astounding 92% success rate.

In another study, medical researchers from Iraq's University Department of Surgery (Salim 1993) conducted a double-blind study of 172 patients who suffered from gastric bleeding caused by nonsteroidal anti-inflammatory drugs (NSAIDs). They gave the patients either cysteine, methylmethionine sulfonium chloride (MMSC) or a placebo. Those receiving either the cysteine or the MMSC stopped bleeding. Their conditions became *"stable"* as compared with many in the control group, who continued to bleed.

Research has showed that this effect is due to the fact that s-methylmethionine stimulates the healing of cell membranes among the leaves and stems of plants that have been damaged. This is a similar story as most antioxidants. Plants produce antioxidants to help to protect them from damage from the sun, insects and diseases. It just so happens that what protects plants also helps heal humans.

Fatty Acid Strategies

The types of fats we eat relate directly to food sensitivities because some fats are pro-inflammatory while others are anti-inflammatory. This doesn't mean that the pro-inflammatory fats are necessarily bad. Rather, we must have a *balance* of fats between the pro- and anti-inflammatory ones, with the balance teetering on the anti-inflammatory side.

The fat balance of our diet is also important because our cell membranes are made of different lipids and lipid-derivatives like phospholipids and glycolipids. An imbalanced fat diet therefore can lead to weak cell membranes, which leads to cells less protected and more prone to damage by oxidative radicals—and increased intestinal permeability.

Illustrating this, Danish researchers (Willemsen *et al.* 2008) tested the intestinal permeability/barrier integrity of incubated human intestinal epithelial cells with different dietary fats. The different fats included individual omega-6 oils linolenic acid (LA), gamma linolenic acid (GLA), DGLA, arachidonic acid (AA); a blend of omega-3 oils alpha-linolenic acid (ALA), eicosapentaenoic acid (EPA), docohexaenoic acid (DHA); and a blend of fats similar to the composition of human breast milk fat. The DGLA, AA, EPA, DHA and GLA oils reduced interleukin-4 mediated intestinal permeability. LA and ALA did not. The blend with omega-3 oils, *"effectively supported barrier function,"* according to the researchers. They also concluded that DGLA, AA, EPA and DHA—all long chain polyunsaturated fats—were *"particularly effective in supporting barrier integrity by improving resistance and reducing IL-4 mediated permeability."*

Arachidonic acids in moderation are important for nutrition, and we all need them, especially in early feeding as infants. They are important factors in the inflammatory process—but in the right quantity. For this reason, our bodies convert linoleic acid to arachidonic as needed.

As we showed with the research earlier, a meat-heavy diet can over-supply arachidonic acid. Because arachidonic acid stimulates the production of pro-inflammatory prostaglandins and leucotrienes in the enzyme conversion process, too much leads to a tendency for our bodies to over-respond during an inflammatory event. Worse, a system overloaded with arachidonic acid makes halting the inflammatory process more difficult.

Interestingly, carnivorous animals cannot or do not readily convert linoleic acid (found in many common plants) to arachidonic acid, but herbivore animals do convert linoleic acid to arachidonic acid, as do humans. This conversion—on top of an animal-protein heavy diet—produces high arachidonic acid levels. On the other hand, a diet that is balanced between plant-based monounsaturates, polyunsaturates and some saturates will balance arachidonic acids with the other fatty acids.

Here is a quick review of the major fatty acids and the foods they come from:

Major Omega-3 Fatty Acids (EFAs)

Acronym	Fatty Acid Name	Major Dietary Sources
ALA	Alpha-linolenic acid	Walnuts, soybeans, flax, canola, pumpkin seeds, chia seeds
SDA	Stearidonic acid	hemp, spirulina, blackcurrant
DHA	Docosahexaenoic acid	Body converts from ALA; also obtained from certain algae, krill and fish oils
EPA	Eicosapentaenoic acid	Converts in the body from DHA
GLA	Gamma-linolenic acid	Borage, primrose oil, spirulina

Major Omega-6 Fatty Acids (EFAs)

Acronym	Fatty Acid Name	Major Dietary Sources
LA	Linoleic acid	Many plants, safflower, sunflower, sesame, soy, almond especially
AA	Arachidonic acid	Meats, salmon
PA	Palmitoleic acid	Macadamia, palm kernel, coconut

Major Omega-9 Fatty Acids

Acronym	Fatty Acid Name	Major Dietary Sources
EA	Eucic acid	Canola, mustard seed, wallflower
OA	Oleic acid	Sunflower, olive, safflower
PA	Palmitoleic acid	Macadamia, palm kernel, coconut

Major Saturated Fatty Acids

Acronym	Fatty Acid Name	Major Dietary Sources
Lauric	Lauric acid	Coconut, dairy, nuts
Myristic	Myristic acid	Coconut, butter
Palmitic	Palmitic acid	Macadamia, palm kernel, coconut, butter, beef, eggs
Stearic	Stearic acid	Macadamia, palm kernel, coconut, eggs

Essential fatty acids

EFA's are fats necessary for adequate health. Eaten in the right proportion, they can also lower inflammation and speed healing. EFA's are long-chain polyunsaturated fatty acids—longer than the linolenic, linoleic and oleic acids. The major EFAs are omega-3s—primarily alpha linolenic acid (ALA), gamma-linoleic acid (GLA), docosahexaenoic acid (DHA) and eicosapentaenoic acid (EPA). EPA and DHA are found in algae, mackerel, salmon, herring, sardines, sablefish (black cod); and omega-6s—primarily linoleic acid, (LA), palmitoleic acid (PA) and arachidonic acid (AA). The term *essential* was originally given with the assumption that these types of fats could not be assembled or produced by the body—they must be taken directly from our food supply.

This assumption, however, is not fully correct. While it is true that we need *some* of these from our diet, our bodies readily convert linoleic acid to arachidonic acid, and ALA to DHA and EPA. Therefore, these fats can be considered essential in some sense, but we do not necessarily have to consume each one of them.

Monounsaturated Fats

Monounsaturated oils are high in omega-9 fatty acids like oleic acid. A monounsaturated fatty acid has one double carbon-hydrogen bonding chain. Oils from seeds, nuts and other plant-based sources have the largest quantities of monounsaturates. Oils that have large proportions of monounsaturates such as olive oil are known to lower inflammation when replacing high saturated fat in diets. Monounsaturates also aid in skin cell health and reduce atopic skin responses.

Monounsaturated fatty acids like oleic acid have been shown in studies to lower heart attack risk, aid blood vessel health, and offer anti-carcinogenic potential. The best sources of omega-9s are olives, sesame seeds, avocados, almonds, peanuts, pecans, pistachio nuts, cashews, hazelnuts, macadamia nuts, several other nuts and their respective oils.

Polyunsaturated Fats

Polyunsaturated fats have at least two double carbon-hydrogen bonds. They come from a variety of plant and marine sources. Omega-3s ALA, DHA and EPA simply have longer chains with more double carbon-hydrogen bonds. ALA, DHA and EPA are known to lower inflammation and increase artery-wall health. These *long-chain* omega-3 polyunsaturates are also considered critical for intestinal health.

The omega-6 fatty acids are the most available form of fat in the plant kingdom. Linoleic acid is the primary omega-6 fatty acid and it is found in most grains and seeds.

Saturated Fats

Saturated fats have multiple fatty acids without double bonds (the hydrogens "saturate" the carbons). They are found among animal fats, and tropical oils such as coconut and palm. Milk products such as butter and whole milk contain saturated fats, along with a special type of healthy linoleic fatty acid called CLA or *conjugated linoleic acid.*

The saturated fats from coconuts and palm differ from animal saturates in that they have shorter chains. This actually gives them—unlike animal saturates—an antimicrobial quality.

Trans Fats

Trans fats are oils that either have been overheated or have undergone hydrogenation. Hydrogenation is produced by heating while bubbling hydrogen ions through the oil. This adds hydrogen and repositions some of the bonds. The "trans" refers to the positioning of part of the molecule in reverse—as opposed to "cis" positioning. The cis positioning is the bonding orientation the body's cell membranes work best with. Trans fats have been known to be a cause for increased radical species in the system; damaging artery walls; contributing to inflammation, heart disease, high LDL levels, liver damage, diabetes, and other metabolic dysfunction (Mozaffarian *et al.* 2009). Trans fat overconsumption slows the conversion of LA to GLA.

It should be noted that CLA is also a trans-fat, but this is a trans fat the body works well with—it is considered a healthy fat.

Arachidonic Acid

The science and research on arachidonic acid was discussed on pages 111-112 and elsewhere. AA is an essential fatty acid, and research has shown that it is essential for infants while they are building their intestinal barriers. However, as we discussed, AA is pro-inflammatory, and too much of it as we age increases the burden on our immune systems, and tends to push our bodies towards hypersensitivity.

As we discussed, AA content is highest among animal meats, fish, fried foods and heavily-processed foods. Plant-based foods contain little or no AA.

The Anti-inflammatory Omega-3s

Research has illustrated that DHA obtained from fish oils and DHA from algae have significant therapeutic and anti-inflammatory effects. The research is so well-known that we hardly need to quote it here.

ALA is the primary omega-3 fatty acid the body can most easily assimilate. Once assimilated, the healthy body will convert ALA to omega-3s, primarily DHA, at a rate of about 7-15%, depending upon the health of the liver. One study of six women performed at England's University of Southampton (Burdge *et al.* 2002) showed a conversion rate of 36% from ALA to DHA and other omega-3s. A follow-up study of men at Southampton showed ALA conversion to the omega-3s occurred at an average of 16%.

DHA readily converts to EPA by the body. EPA degrades quickly if unused in the body. It is easily converted from DHA as needed. Our bodies store DHA and not EPA.

It appears that the anti-inflammatory effects of DHA in particular relates to a modulation of a gene factor called NF-kappaB. The NF-kappaB is involved in signaling among cytokine receptors. With more DHA consumption, the transcription of the NF-kappaB gene sequence is reduced. This seems to reduce inflammatory signaling (Singer *et al.* 2008).

Because much of the early research on the link between fatty acids and inflammatory disease was performed using fish oil, it was assumed that both EPA and DHA fatty acids reduced inflammation. Recent research from the University of Texas' Department of Medicine/Division of Clinical Immunology and Rheumatology (Rahman *et al.* 2008) has clarified it is DHA that is primarily implicated in reducing inflammation. DHA was shown to inhibit RANKL-induced pro-inflammatory cytokines, and a number of inflammation steps, while EPA did not.

The process of converting ALA to DHA and other omega-3s requires an enzyme produced in the liver called delta-6 desaturase. Some people—especially those who have a poor diet, are immune-suppressed, or burdened with toxicity such as cigarette smoke—may not produce this enzyme very well. As a result, they may not convert as much ALA to DHA and EPA.

For those with low levels of DHA—or for those with problems converting ALA and DHA—DHA microalgae can be supplemented. These algae produce significant amounts of DHA. They are the foundation for the DHA molecule all the way up the food chain, including fish. This is how fish get their DHA, in other words. Three algae species— *Crypthecodinium cohnii*, *Nitzschia laevis* and *Schizochytrium spp.*—are now in commercial production and available in oil and capsule form.

Microalgae-derived DHA is preferable to fish or fish oils. Fish and fish oils typically contain saturated fats and may also—depending upon their origin—contain toxins such as mercury and PCBs (though to their credit, many producers also carefully distill their fish oil). However, we should note that salmon contain a considerable amount of arachidonic acid as well (Chilton 2006). And finally, algae-derived DHA does not strain fish populations.

One study (Arterburn *et al.* 2007) measured pro-inflammatory arachidonic acid levels within the body before and after supplementation with algal DHA. It was found that arachidonic acid levels decreased by 20% following just one dose of 100 milligrams of algal DHA.

In a study by researchers from The Netherlands' Wageningen University Toxicology Research Center (van Beelen *et al.* 2007), all three species of commercially produced algal oil showed equivalency with fish oil in their inhibition of cancer cell growth. Another study (Lloyd-Still *et al.* 2007) of twenty cystic fibrosis patients concluded that 50 milligrams of algal DHA was readily absorbed, maintained DHA bioavailability immediately, and increased circulating DHA levels by four to five times.

In a randomized open-label study (Arterburn *et al.* 2008), researchers gave 32 healthy men and women either algal DHA oil or cooked salmon for two weeks. After the two weeks, plasma levels of circulating DHA were bioequivalent.

We should include that ALA, the plant-based omega-3 oil, also produces anti-inflammatory activity. In studies at Wake Forest University (Chilton *et al.* 2008), for example, flaxseed oil produced anti-inflammatory effects, along with borage oil and echium oil (both also containing GLA).

Gamma Linoleic Acid

As mentioned earlier, a wealth of studies have confirmed that GLA reduces or inhibits the inflammatory response. Leukotrienes produced by arachidonic acid stimulate inflammation, while leukotrienes produced by GLA block the conversion of polyunsaturated fatty acids to arachidonic acid. This means that GLA reduces the inflammatory response.

A healthy body will convert linoleic acid into GLA readily, utilizing the same delta-6 desaturase enzyme used for ALA to DHA conversion.

From GLA, the body produces *dihomo-gamma linoleic acid,* which cycles through the body as an eicosinoid. GLA aids in skin health, and downregulates the inflammatory and hypersensitivity allergic response.

In addition to conversion from LA, GLA can be also obtained from the oils of borage seeds, evening primrose seed, hemp seed, and from spirulina. Excellent food sources of LA include chia seeds, seed, hemp-seed, grapeseed, pumpkin seeds, sunflower seeds, safflower seeds, soybeans, olives, pine nuts, pistachio nuts, peanuts, almonds, cashews, chestnuts, and their respective oils.

The conversion of LA to GLA (and ALA to DHA) is reduced by trans-fat consumption, smoking, pollution, stress, infections, and various chemicals that affect the liver.

The Healthy Fat Balance

In a meta-study by researchers from the University of Crete's School of Medicine (Margioris 2009), numerous studies showed that long-chain polyunsaturated omega-3s tend to be anti-inflammatory while omega-6 oils tend to be pro-inflammatory.

This, however, simplifies the equation too much. Most of the research on fats has also shown that most omega-6s are healthy oils. Balance is the key. Let's look at the research:

In a study by researchers from the University of Guelph in Ontario (Tulk and Robinson 2009), eight middle-aged men with metabolic disorder were tested for the inflammatory effects resulting from changing their fat content proportion between omega-3 and omega-6. The men were divided into two groups, one eating a high saturated fat diet with a proportion of 20:1 between omega-6 and omega-3, and the other eating a diet of 2:1 (high omega-3 diet). Both groups were tested before and after the diet change. Testing after the diet change showed that the high omega-3 diet did not change the inflammatory marker tests.

The proportion between omega-6s and omega-3s is thus recommended to be about one or two to one (1-2:1). The current Western American diet has been estimated to be about twenty to thirty to one (20-30:1) for the proportion between omega-6 and omega-3. This imbalance (of too much omega-6 and too little omega-3) has been associated with a number of inflammatory diseases, including arthritis, heart disease, ulcerative colitis, Crohn's disease, and others. When fat consumption is out of balance, the body's metabolism will trend towards inflammation. This is because omega-6 oils convert more easily to arachidonic acid than do omega-3s. AA seems to push the body toward the processes of inflammation (Simopoulos 1999).

We also know that reducing dietary saturated fats and increasing omega-6 polyunsaturated fats reduces inflammation, cardiovascular disease, high cholesterol and diabetes (Ros and Mataix 2008).

The relationships were cleared up in a study performed at Sydney's Heart Research Institute (Nicholls et al. 2008). Here fourteen adults consumed meals either rich in saturated fats or omega-6 polyunsaturated fats.

They were tested following each meal for various inflammation and cholesterol markers. The results showed that the high saturated fat meal increased inflammatory activities and decreased the liver's production of HDL cholesterol; whereas HDL levels and the liver's anti-inflammatory capacity were increased after the omega-6 meals.

What this tells us is that the omega-3/omega-6 story is complicated by the saturated fat content of the diet and subsequent liver function. High saturated fat diets increase (bad) LDL content and reduce the anti-inflammatory and antioxidant capacities of the liver. Diets lower in saturated fat and higher in omega-6 and omega-3 fats encourage antioxidant and anti-inflammatory activity.

We also know that diets high in monounsaturated fats—such as the Mediterranean Diet—are also associated with significant anti-inflammatory effects. Mediterranean diets contain higher levels of monounsaturated fats like oleic acids (omega-9) as well as higher proportions of fruits and vegetables, and lower proportions of saturated fats (Basu *et al.* 2006).

High saturated fat diets are also associated with increased obesity, and a number of studies have shown that obesity is directly related to inflammatory diseases—including allergies as we've discussed. High saturated fat diets and diets high in trans fatty acids have also been clearly shown to accompany higher levels of inflammation and inflammatory factors such as IL-6 and CRP (Basu *et al.* 2006).

Noting the research showing the relationships between the different fatty acids and inflammation, and the condition of the liver (which can be burdened by too much saturated fat), scientists have logically arrived at a model for dietary fat consumption for a person who is either dealing with or wants to prevent inflammation-oriented diseases such as food sensitivities:

Omega-3	25%-30% of dietary fats
Omega-6+Omega-9	40%-50% of dietary fats
Saturated	5%-10% of dietary fats
GLA	10%-20% of dietary fats
Trans-Fats	0% of dietary fats

Fermented Foods

We've discussed in depth that probiotics and enzymes can prevent and even help resolve food sensitivities. Here is another angle on that research: Eating fermented versions of foods that we are sensitive to.

The rationale is that probiotics will change the structure of foods as they ferment the food. In many cases they produce enzymes that digest and break down macromolecular versions of the sugars and proteins that we might be sensitive to. They will present to the digestive tract a different, often more digestible form of the nutrient along with numerous enzymes that aid in further digestion and assimilation.

Fermented foods also deliver to the digestive tract colonies of probiotics that can colonize and continue to help break down those food macromolecules that often cause sensitivities. While fermented foods may only present temporary residents, they will typically endure for a couple of weeks, and during that time provide numerous benefits. During that two weeks, we can eat another meal of the fermented food to help replenish those colonies.

Illustrating this, researchers from the Department of Food Science and Human Nutrition at the University of Illinois (Frias *et al.* 2008) studied the sensitivity response (or, as the researchers termed it, "*immunoreactivity*") of soybeans in the cracked bean form and in the flour state before and after fermentation with probiotics. They fermented some of the cracked beans and flour with *Aspergillus oryzae*, *Rhizopus oryzae*, *Lactobacillus plantarum*, and *Bacillus subtilis*. These are fermenting bacteria are commonly used to make various probiotic cultured foods such as tempeh and sauerkraut.

The researchers used ELISA tests and the Western blot test to quantify IgE immunoglobulin response with human plasma. They found that all of the fermentation processes dramatically decreased the immunoreactivity of the soybeans and flours. Soy flour fermented with *L. plantarum* exhibited the highest reduction, with a 96-99% lower immunoreactivity levels. *R. oryzae* and *A. oryzae* reduced immunoreactivity by 66% and 68% respectively. *B. subtilis* produced from 81% to 86% reduction in immunoreactivity to the soy.

In addition, a positive side effect of the fermentation was the improvement of the protein quality of the soy products. After fermentation with *R. oryzae*, for example, levels of the amino acids alanine and threonine were increased, making the soy products more nutritious!

The bottom line is that this research illustrates what healthy colonies of probiotics can do within the intestinal tract. Probiotics process foods. During their processing, they reduce the immune system's sensitivity to the foods. This is a subtle process related to the probiotics' activity. Now why would probiotics increase the tolerance for otherwise-sensitive foods? Think about it. Let's say that you are living in a house that is too cold. Would you let the cold continue until you freeze to death? No. You would work hard to get the house warm enough so you could continue to survive and maybe even live in comfort. It is a survival issue. In the same way, symbiotic bacteria that are living within our intestines want to remain alive and comfortable, and make their stay as hospitable as possible. In order to do that, they help process nutrients in such a way that works best for our bodies. This keeps us healthy, which also keeps them healthy.

Here is a sampling of some of the world's favorite probiotic foods:

Traditional Yogurt

Traditional yogurt is produced using *L. bulgaricus* and *S. thermophilus*. Commercial preparations sometimes include L. acidophilus, but the use of *L. acidophilus* in yogurt will rarely result in the final product containing *L. acidophilus*. This is because *L. bulgaricus* is a hardy organism, and it will easily overtake *L. acidophilus* within a culture. Note also that in commercial yogurt preparations that are pasteurized after culturing, there are few or no living probiotics remaining after pasteurization. Some manufacturers culture the milk after pasteurization. This will result in a healthy probiotic culture.

Traditional Kefir

Kefir is a traditional drink originally developed in the Caucasus region of what is now considered Southern Russia, Georgia, Armenia and Azerbaijan. Kefir uses fermented milk mixed with kefir grains that resemble little chunks of cauliflower. Kefir typically contains *L. bulgaricus* and *S. thermophilus*. Cow's milk is most used, but sheep's milk, goat's milk or deer milk can also be used.

Traditional Buttermilk

Buttermilk is a soured beverage that was originally curdled from cream. Traditional buttermilk utilized the acids that probiotic bacteria produce for curdling. Today, forced curdling is done using commercially available acidic products such as lemon juice or vinegar. This however, does not result in the probiotic cultures of traditional buttermilk, unless of course, raw probiotic milk is utilized as a base.

This also goes for butter and cottage cheese. Both were probiotic foods until modern dairies decided that there was no value in the probiotics that naturally occur from grass-fed cows.

Traditional Kimchi

Kimchi is a fermented cabbage with a wonderful history from Korea. Kimchi was considered a ceremonial food served to emperors and ambassadors. It was also highly regarded as a healing and tonic food. There are a variety of different recipes of kimchi, depending upon the region and occasion. *Lactobacillus kimchii* is the typical probiotic colonizer, but others have also been used.

Traditional Miso

Miso is an ancient fermented food from Japan. A well-made miso will contain over 160 strains of aerobic probiotic bacteria. This is because the ingredients are perfect prebiotics for these probiotics. Miso is produced by fermenting beans and grains. Soybeans are often used, but other types of beans are also used. *Aspergillus oryzae* or koji is typically used as a fermenting base. When other beans other than soy are used, they will produce different varieties of miso. Shiromiso is white miso, kuromiso is black miso, and akamiso is red miso. They are each made with different beans. There are also various other miso recipies, many of which are highly guarded by their makers.

Traditional Shoyu

Shoyu is a traditional form of soy sauce made by blending a mixture of cooked soybeans and wheat, again with koji, or *Aspergillus oryzae*. The combination is fermented for an extended time. The aging process for shoyu is dependent upon the storage temperature and cooking methods used, and is also regarded as a secret by many producers.

Traditional Tempeh

Tempeh is an aged and fermented soybean food. It is extremely healthy and contains a combination of probiotics and naturally metabolized soy. Tempeh is made by first soaking dehulled soybeans for 10-12 hours. The beans are then cooked for 20 minutes and strained. The dry, cooked beans are then mixed with a tempeh starter containing *Rhyzopus oryzae*, *Rhizopus oligosporus* or both. The flattened and aged cake will be full with white mycelium (fungal roots) when it is ready. This tasty food can then be eaten raw, baked, or toasted.

Traditional Kombucha Tea

Traditional kombucha tea is an ancient beverage from the orient. Its use dates back many centuries; and was used by China and Taiwanese emperors, as well as Russian, and Eastern Europe peoples, where its reputation grew.

Recent research has revealed that kombucha was originally derived from kefir grains developed for fermentation. The kefir was exported to

China, where the grains were added to tea with sugar rather than milk. The result was a combination of probiotic bacteria and yeasts that can include (depending upon the evolution of the mother culture) *Acetobacter xylinum*, *Acetobacter xylinoides*, *Glucobacter bluconicum*, *Acetobacter aceti*, *Saccharomycodes Ludwigii*, *Schizosaccharomyces pombe*, and *Picha fermentans*—and possibly some other species.

The fermenting of these organisms renders a beverage that is full of nutrients and enzymes as well as healthy probiotics. While the probiotic count may not be as high as yogurt or kefir, the range of probiotics will be wider.

Traditional Lassi

Lassi is a traditional beverage once enjoyed by kings and governors in ancient India. Lassi is still very popular in India. It is quite simple to make, as it is made with yogurt, fruit and spices. Quite simply, it is a blend of diluted yogurt with fruit pulp—often mango is used in the traditional lassi. A little salt, turmeric and sweetener give it a sweet-n-salty taste. Other spices are also sometimes used. Sugar is often added in today's versions, but honey and/or fruit would be preferable, health-wise.

Traditional Sauerkraut

Sauerkraut is a traditional German fermented food. It is made quite simply, by blending shredded cabbage and pickling salt with *Lactobacillus plantarum* and *L. brevis* fermentation cultures.

More information on probiotic foods, supplements and the science of probiotics may be found in the author's two books on probiotics: *Probiotics–Protection Against Infection* (2009), and *Oral Probiotics* (2010).

Pasteurization

French chemist Louis Pasteur developed pasteurization in the 1860s to disprove the notion of spontaneous generation—a theory that some put forth to explain how life arose from chemicals. Pasteurization is by far the process that commercial food manufacturers use the most to reduce bacteria in foods and beverages. Most, but certainly not all bacteria colonies are removed with this process.

Today, pasteurization is used for practically every commercially packaged food that has significant water or moisture content. This includes practically every shelf-stable canned food, sauce and mix in jars. Today even vegetables, nuts, fruit, pre-packaged dinners, entrees, and refrigerated juices are also commonly pasteurized.

Pasteurization is the treatment of a food to the point where a large percentage of the bacteria are eliminated. There are five basic types of pasteurization: Holder or steam pasteurization, high temperature or flash pasteurization, ultra high pasteurization, irradiation pasteurization, and gas pasteurization. These methods heat a food to a very high temperature, shoot radiation into the food, or spray the food with gas, respectively.

Holder, vat, tunnel or steam pasteurization requires bringing the food or liquid to 140-145 degrees Fahrenheit for a period of about thirty minutes. For many foods, this takes place by heating the product after being packaged. Cans, for example, will be heated in an airtight, jacketed chamber. This might follow additional kettle cooking and "hot-filling."

Steam or tunnel pasteurization is used for many sauces and juices, especially those packaged in glass. Before this stage the product may still be heated and hot-packed. Following filling, the jar or container is sealed and placed on a conveyor belt, which carries it through a heated tunnel. The tunnel bakes the product while hot water is sprayed onto the package. This creates a blanket of hot steam in the tunnel, heating the package and its contents to the desired temperature. Following the hot steam, a cooling section of the tunnel sprays colder water on it to cool the product down.

Flash or high pasteurization (also called HTST for "high temperature, short time") is done primarily on liquids or slurry products. HTST will take the liquid to 160-165 degrees for 15 seconds. For some liquids, the temperature and time is different. Regular milk (non-UHT), for example, is typically pasteurized by heating to 120 degrees for about 20 seconds. HTST is typically done by running the product through a series of pipes and heat exchanger plates that boost its temperature quickly. Following this, the product is filled into the container. Some processors will still run it through another heating tunnel after packing to prevent contamination in the package. Note that the term "flash pasteurized" has been used in marketing to imply a system somehow less damaging than high temp pasteurization.

Ultra pasteurization (UP) will heat the liquid higher, sometimes over 200 degrees F, for a few seconds. Time and temperature can range, depending upon the product and the desired outcome. The intense heat of ultra pasteurization typically doubles the food's shelf life compared to regular pasteurization.

Then there is ultra high temperature pasteurization, or UHT. UHT will usually heat the food or liquid to about 280 degrees F, but only for a period from a half-second to two or three seconds. This is done mostly for liquids, which are run through a number of extreme heat exchanging chambers before being packaged—usually in an 'aseptic' vacuum package.

UHT will typically allow a product to be put on the dry shelf for an extended period. This process is also sometimes incorrectly referred to as sterilization.

Irradiation pasteurization is a growing method of reducing microorganisms from produce and other products. Because it does not raise the temperature of the product as high as other methods, it is also sometimes marketed as "cold pasteurization." Imported produce is now commonly irradiated as shipments arrive by air or by sea. Increasingly, large U.S. food producers irradiate their raw products because the appearance and flavor of the product is often better preserved. The most common method uses cobalt-60 radiation. X-rays and gamma radiation are also used. Irradiation is not allowed in organic produce. Worker health in irradiation plants has also been a concern.

Gas pasteurization is used for a limited number of foods. Almonds and other nuts, for example are sometimes pasteurized by gassing them with either propylene oxide or hot steam. Organic nut production, of course, does not allow propylene oxide.

For milk and other liquids, UHT and HTST also accompany homogenization. Homogenization blends and mixes the product significantly, which can alter molecular polarity and structure.

Commercial foods that have higher acidity (usually with a pH of less than 4.6) and/or intense sugar content may be able to skip pasteurization. Commercial manufacturers usually have to pass a state pH test before they can package a liquid product without pasteurization. Most acidic juices like orange, apple, carrot and berry used to be commercially available fresh. After an apple juice "outbreak" of *E. coli* in the 1990s, many regulators began requiring HTST for mass-distributed refrigerated fruit juices. Raw milk has been readily available commercially for thousands of years until recent years. Before government regulators have increasingly banned or restricted commercial distribution of raw packaged foods, raw milk was a wonderfully natural, probiotic beverage.

A few foods that are commercially unpasteurized include some balsamic vinegars, kombucha tea, hummus, honey, maple syrup, and a variety of probiotic-fermented foods. We might ask why fermented and probiotic foods can escape pasteurization? Because they've been naturally acidified by probiotic bacteria to a degree that discourages growth of pathogenic microbes. As we've discussed, probiotics consume sugars and carbohydrates, and secrete healthy acids, which also repel pathogenic organisms.

Pasteurization, on the other hand, does not by any means kill all the microbes present. It can significantly reduce it, yes. At best, pasteurization systems will lower *plate count* levels down by about 99%. This means, for example, if there are one trillion bacteria colony-forming units in the food in the beginning, there might still be 10 billion CFU left after pasteurization. For HST pasteurization, the removal rate is higher, about 99.9% removal. This means for a one trillion CFU initial population, there might be a billion CFU population left after heat treatment.

Now we might ask; how many colony-forming units would it take of a bacteria species to make us sick? A billion is plenty, as long as there is food in the form of sugars and carbohydrates, and a reasonable growth temperature.

Consequences of Pasteurization

Most nutrients are heat-sensitive. Vitamin C, fat-soluble vitamins A, E and B vitamins are reduced during pasteurization. Many proteins and glycoproteins are denatured during pasteurization. Important plant nutrients such as anthocyanins and polyphenols are also reduced during pasteurization, along with various enzymes. Proteins are denatured or broken down when heated for long. While this can aid in amino acid absorption, it can also form unrecognized peptide combinations. In milk, for example, nutritious whey protein, or lactabumin, will denature into various peptide combinations, some of which are not readily absorbed.

A 2008 study on strawberry puree from the University of Applied Sciences in Switzerland showed a 37% reduction in vitamin C and a significant loss in antioxidant potency after pasteurization. A 1998 study from Brazil's Universidade Estadual de Maringa determined that Barbados cherries lost about 14% of their vitamin C content after pasteurization. During heat treatment, vitamin C will also convert to dehydroascorbic acid together with a loss of bioflavonoids.

A 2008 study at Spain's Cardenal Herrera University determined that glutathione peroxidase—an important antioxidant contained in milk—was significantly reduced by pasteurization. In 2006, the University also released a study showing that lysine content was significantly decreased by milk pasteurization. A 2005 study at the Universidade Federal do Rio Grande determined that pasteurizing milk reduced vitamin A (retinol) content from an average of 55 micrograms to an average of 37 micrograms. A study at North Carolina State University in 2003 determined that HTST pasteurization significantly reduced conjugated linoleic acid (CLA) content—an important fatty acid in milk shown to reduce cancer and encourage good fat metabolism.

A 2006 study on bayberries at the Southern Yangtze University determined that plant antioxidants such as anthocyanins and polyphenolics were reduced from 12-32% following UHT pasteurization. Polyphenols are the primary nutrients in fruits and vegetables that render anticarcino-genic and antioxidant effects.

One of the most important loss from pasteurization is its enzyme content. Diary and plant foods contain a variety of enzymes that aid in the assimilation or catalyzing of nutrients and antioxidants. These include xanthenes, lysozymes, lipases, oxidases, amylases, lactoferrins and many others. The body uses food enzymes in various ways. Some enzymes, such as papain from papaya and bromelain from pineapples, dissolve artery plaque and reduce inflammation. While the body makes many of its own enzymes, it also absorbs some food enzymes or uses their components to make new ones.

Pasteurization also typically leaves the food or beverage with a resid-ual caramelized flavor due to the conversation of the enzymes, flavonoids and sugars to other compounds. In milk, for example, there is a substan-tial conversion from lactose to lactulose after UHT pasteurization. Lactu-lose can cause intestinal cramping, nausea and vomiting.

In the case of pasteurized juices, pasteurization can leave a highly acidic constituency, which can irritate our mucous membranes and intes-tines—especially in the case of already-acidic fruits.

As for irradiation, there is little research on the resulting nutrient con-tent outside of a few microwave studies (which showed decreased nutrient content and the formation of undesirable metabolites). Thus there is some evidence that irradiation may denature some protein and nutrients.

Whole foods in nature's packages are significantly different from pas-teurized processed foods. Fresh whole foods produced by plants contain various antioxidants and enzymes that reduce the ability of microorgan-isms to grow. The Creator also provided whole foods with peels and shells that protect nutrients and keep most microorganisms out. Micro-organisms may invade the outer shell or peel somewhat, but the peel's pH, dryness and density—together with the pH of the inner fruit—work as barriers to most microorganisms.

For this reason, most fruits and nuts can be easily stored for days and weeks without having significant microbiological risk. Once the peel or shell is removed, the inner fruit, juice or nut must be eaten quickly to prevent contamination, depending upon the fruit's sugar content.

Whole natural foods also contain polysaccharides and oligosaccha-rides that combine nutrients and sugar within large molecules. These complex molecules are often difficult for pathogenic bacteria to break them down for food. Once processing takes place, however, the sugars are broken down into more simplified form, allowing microbial growth. Why? Because simple sugars provide convenient food and energy sources to growing bacteria and fungi colonies. This means processed food feeds pathogenic organisms and makes available to the intestines those byproducts that may stimulate an immune response.

As for milk and milk products, raw milk will contain a number of probiotics that mother cow produces to keep the milk balanced and wholesome. Just as they balance our body's microbiotic content, the probiotics in milk will typically prevent microorganism overgrowth and infection. Let's discuss this a bit further:

Raw vs. Pasteurized Milk

Remember the study by researchers at Switzerland's University of Basel (Waser *et al.* 2007). The researchers studied of 14,893 children between the ages of five and 13 from five different European countries, including 2,823 children from farms and 4,606 children attending a Steiner School (known for its farm-based living and instruction). The researchers found that drinking farm milk was associated with decreased incidence of allergies and asthma. In other words, the raw milk was found to be the largest single determinant of this reduced allergy and asthma incidence among farm children. Why?

Raw milk from the cow contains a host of bacteria. In a healthy, mostly grass-fed cow, these bacteria are primarily probiotics. This is because a grass diet provides prebiotics that promote the cow's own probiotic colonies. Should the cow be fed primarily dried grass and dried grains, probiotic counts will be reduced, and replaced by pathogenic bacteria. As a result, most non-grass fed herds must be given lots of antibiotics to help keep their bacteria counts low. Probiotics, on the other hand, naturally keep bacteria counts down.

As a result, the non-grass fed cow's milk will have higher pathogenic bacteria counts than grass-fed cows. This means that the milk itself will also have high counts. When the non-grass-fed cow's milk is pasteurized, the heat kills most of these bacteria. The result is a milk containing dead pathogenic bacteria parts. These are primarily proteins and peptides, which get mixed with the milk and are eventually consumed with the milk.

In other words, pasteurization may kill the living pathogenic bacteria, but it does not get rid of the bacteria proteins. This might be compared to cooking an insect: If an insect landed in our soup we could surely cook it until it died. But the soup would still contain the insect parts.

Now the immune system of most people, and especially infants with their hypersensitive immune system, is trained to attack and discard pathogenic bacteria. And how does the body identify pathogenic bacteria? From their proteins.

In the case of pasteurized commercial milk, the immune system can still identify heat-killed microorganism body parts and proteins and launch an immune response against these proteins. This was shown in research from the University of Minnesota two decades ago (Takahashi *et al.* 1992).

It is not surprising that weak immune systems readily reject pasteurized cow's milk. In comparison, raw milk has far fewer microorganism content in general, most of which are probiotic in content. This was confirmed by tests done by a local California organic milk farm, who tested their raw milk against standardized tests from conventional milk farms.

In addition, pasteurization breaks apart or denatures many of the proteins and sugar molecules. This was illustrated by researchers from Japan's Nagasaki International University (Nodake *et al.* 2010), who found that when beta-lactoglobulin was conjugated with dextran-glycylglycine, its allergenicity decreased. This occurred by shielding epitope reception on cell membranes. A dextran is a very long chain of glucose molecules—a polysaccharide. In this case, the polysaccharide is joined with the amino acid, glycine.

This is not surprising. Natural whole cow's milk contains special polysaccharides called oligosaccharides. They are largely indigestible polysaccharides that feed our intestinal bacteria. Because of this trait, these indigestible sugars are called prebiotics.

Whole milk contains a number of these oligosaccharides, including oligogalactose, oligolactose, galacto-oligosaccharides (GOS) and transgalactooligosaccharides (TOS). These polysaccharides provide a number of benefits. Not only are they some of the more preferred food for probiotics: they also reduce the ability of pathogenic bacteria like *E. coli* to adhere to intestinal cells.

These oligosaccharides also provide bonds that reduce the incidence of beta-lactoglobulin, through the combination of being food for probiotics and the availability of the buffering effect of long-chain polysaccharides on radical molecules.

This reduction of beta-lactoglobulin has been directly observed in humans and animals after supplementation with probiotics (Taylor *et al.* 2006; Adel-Patient *et al.* 2005; Prioult *et al.* 2003).

Galacto-oligosaccharides are produced by conversion from enzymes in healthy cows and mothers.

Homogenization

The homogenization process is an emulsion of the fatty and watery parts of milk. It blends the butter fat that normally floats to the top, with the liquid portion of the milk. Traditionally, people simply shook the milk to blend the fat and liquid. Homogenization pushes the milk though a filter screen, which reduces the fat molecule size. This unbinding of fat molecules can slightly change the taste of the milk, and expose the fats to possible oxidation.

But does homogenization increase milk's allergenicity or intolerance factors?

Researchers from Finland's University of Helsinki (Paajanen *et al.* 2003) gave 45 people with lactose intolerance homogenized and/or non-homogenized milk for five days. Their study was randomized, double-blinded, and crossed-over. They found differences in symptoms during the five days among homogenized and non-homogenized milk drinkers. About half of the patients better tolerated the non-homogenized milk. But the other half better tolerated the homogenized milk. The researchers concluded that homogenization does not make a difference among lactose-intolerance drinkers.

The limitations of this study were that there may have been differences between the digestive health and precise sensitivities between the two groups. Though all had lactose-intolerance, those who tolerated the non-homogenized milk could have also had sensitivities to the denatured fatty acids, while the other group might have been tolerant to the reduction in fatty acids size typical of homogenized milk.

The bottom line is that the jury is still out on homogenization. What is for certain is that the fats in homogenized milk are different from the fats in raw milk.

The Benefits of Raw Whole Milk

While some children are sensitized to milk, milk should not be ignored as a healthy food for infants in most cases. Cow's milk contains many of the nutrients found in mother's milk. These include a host of vitamins, proteins, nucleotides, minerals, probiotics, immunoglobulins and healthy fatty acids. Raw milk also helps support the intestinal barrier.

Researchers from the University of Malawi College of Medicine (Brewster *et al.* 1997)—in Southeastern Africa—tested intestinal permeability and disease progression among 533 kwashiorkori-ridden children. Kwashiorkori is a protein- assimilation disease often seen among children in poor countries, and is typically accompanied by increased intestinal permeability.

The researchers compared a local mix of maize-soya-egg to the standard milk diet given in kwashiorkor treatment. Intestinal permeability significantly improved among the milk diet group. Fatalities among the milk group were 14% versus 21% among the maize group. The maize group also experienced more infections and gained less weight compared to the milk group.

Raw whole milk is a substantial food for children, and pregnant or lactating mothers, assuming that:

> The milk comes from cows that have been primarily grass-fed. When cows eat grass, they nourish their natural probiotic colonies. They also have stronger immune systems with which to battle pathogenic microorganisms. This means that the milk that comes out will have more probiotics and fewer pathogens. When cows are grass-fed they also receive more sunlight, which increases the health of their own immune systems. Just as in the case of a healthy mother, when cows' immune systems are stronger, they will produce more nourishing milk, which is healthier for the milk consumer.

> The cows receive no synthetic or genetically modified growth hormones. Growth hormones injected into cows have been shown to produce higher levels of IGF-1 in the milk and human body after drinking milk from growth hormones-injected cows. The American Public Health Association stated in a 2009 Policy Release regarding the use of growth hormones in dairy cows, after a review of the evidence, that, *"elevated IGF-1 levels in human blood are associated with higher rates of colon, breast, and prostate cancers."* Indeed, researchers from the University of Cincinnati's College of Medicine (Biro *et al.* 2010) studied 1,239 girls from 6-8 years old. They found that girls in this age group are reaching puberty at double the rate they did just ten years ago.

> The cows receive little or no antibiotics. These antibiotics will travel through the milk into the body. Here they can weaken the immune system and set up a greater susceptibility of antibiotic-resistant microorganisms.

> The milk (from grass-fed cows) is not pasteurized. Pasteurization kills all the beneficial microorganisms cows provide that promote healthy probiotics in the gut.

At least within the United States, the consumer should check to be sure that the dairy is registered with the state and undergoes continuous microorganism control. This means the state tests the milk periodically. Also the dairy should test every batch of milk and should be able to supply their customers with test results. These should show coliform counts less than 10 bacteria per mL of milk (also the same as pasteurized milk).

For those readers whose states ban the sale of raw milk; organic milk, yogurt and kefir are probably the best alternatives. Organic milk from a smaller dairy will typically come from predominantly grass-fed cows. They will also not receive hormones or antibiotics (organic cows can receive antibiotics if they are sick, but must then be separated from the milking herd for a significant period of time).

Note that lactose-intolerant persons should do fine with fresh raw milk from an organic dairy. This is not a guarantee, but the owner of one of the largest raw milk dairies in California has informed the author that many of his raw milk customers are lactose-intolerant.

How does this work? The probiotics in the cow have large colonies of lactobacilli. These species love to break down lactose and they produce lactase. They also consume a number of the polysaccharides in raw milk.

If pasteurized milk is the only option, it can be mixed with yogurt or kefir to increase its probiotic benefit and digestion. This will supply the microorganisms that can help break down the lactose and proteins in the milk to better prepare it for digestion.

Note that as for this and any other information, the reader should consult their health provider before making any significant changes to their diet. Any experimentation with raw milk or any other severely sensitized food should be done in the supervision of a health expert prepared to deal with severe allergic responses.

Why the big disclaimer again? This is because while this information is based upon science, food sensitivities can still be tricky and unique. It always pays to be cautious, moderate and careful.

The A1 Milk Hypothesis

As long as we are on the topic of milk, we should probably help clear up the controversy revolving around A1 and A2 milk.

During the late 1990s, some researchers published studies that apparently indicated that a molecule called beta-CM-7, which results from the breakdown of milk in the colon, could cause autism, juvenile diabetes, allergies, schizophrenia, Parkinson's disease and heart disease among those who drank a type of milk dubbed "A1 milk" (McLachlan 2001, Elliott *et al.* 1999, Laugesen and Elliott 2003) .

The molecular culprit under investigation was beta-casomorphin-7 (beta-CM-7), which was apparently found in higher quantities in some milks than others: And seemingly from some cows more than others. As the theory goes, countries that so happened to have more A1 cows and A1 milk also suffer from higher rates of those diseases mentioned above.

These researchers also happened to be armed with the alternative: conveniently referred to "A2 milk."

As the theory goes, A1 milk was the result of a seeming mutation that occurred sometime between 5,000 and 10,000 years ago, apparently at the point when cows were being domesticated in Europe. This produced what is now called the A1 breed of cow and cow's milk. A2 cows, according to the hypothesis, have not undergone this mutation.

Apparently, A2 cows include some of the Guernsey and the Jersey cows. Most Asian and African cows are supposedly also A2 cows according to tests apparently conducted by the A2 Corporation, who happens to own the patent on the testing. In addition, goats, yaks and sheep theoretically produce primarily A2 milk: Again, according to the A2 Corporation tests. Holsteins, for example, and most other commercial breeds of cows in the U.S., apparently produce primarily A1 milk.

The A1 versus A2 milk controversy has raged over the past few years. Apparently, it is the beta-casein protein that is the cause of concern. Beta casein contains 229 amino acids, of which proline apparently lies at the 67th position in A2 cows. Meanwhile, A1 cows theoretically produce beta casein with a histidine-converted amino acid at this position.

The hypothesis claims that the proline amino acid within the A2 beta casein will strongly bond to this protein called beta-CM-7. This supposedly prevents its release, where as in the case of the histidine beta casein from the A1 cows, the beta-CM-7 will be released within the gut when the A1 milk is consumed.

All of this said, there is good reason to believe that the A2 milk hypothesis is unfounded. For example, the New Zealand Food Safety Authority commissioned a study in 2004 to investigate the claims. The review, led by Professor Boyd Swinburn from Melbourne Australia's Deakin University, concluded little evidence that A1 milk produced an increased risk of disease.

In addition, in 2009 the European Food Safety Authority (EFSA) reviewed the evidence on A1 and A2 milk, and they also could not establish a relationship between A1 milk proteins and increased disease.

The very interesting thing about all this is that it is not all about the science. There are corporate interests with profit motives involved. More specifically, as mentioned, the A2 Corporation holds a patent on the testing for beta-CM-7. It also holds a strangle-hold on the conversion of A1 herds to A2 herds, through the artificial insemination of an A2A2 bull, sold by, you guessed it, the A2 Corporation.

A critical question that this brings up is how can independent researchers verify the hypotheses that certain cows are A1 and others are A2 if the test cannot be conducted (with objectivity) outside of the A2 Corporation's patent? This seeming conflict of the patent (along with other issues about the A2 milk research) was highlighted in a critical review published by the *European Journal of Clinical Nutrition* (Truswell) in 2005, which also criticized the data and science of the hypothesis.

To further research this issue, the author spoke to a CEO of a large dairy who had previously inquired directly to the A2 Corporation in order to have his herd of cows tested for the A1 or A2 genes. He was told that the test is currently unavailable.

It should also be understood that autism, diabetes, neurological diseases and heart disease are traceable to a number of associations. There are many, even multiple associations possible among these diseases, from diet to genetics, to air pollution, to nutrients, to toxins, and to sunlight.

In fact, much of the A2 research grounds itself on epidemiological research associating previously unrelated elements of these disease rates and the assumption of the genetic makeup of most milk herds among those countries.

Curiously, these same countries that supposedly have higher levels of A2 milk are also known for other associations, including a higher consumption of animal products in general, higher levels of toxins, colder weather and less sunshine.

New Zealand's University of Otago biochemistry researcher Dr. T.R. Merriman (2009) has pointed out that these "A1 countries" are specifically associated with geographical latitude. He illustrated that a number of studies have associated those countries further away from the equator as having greater incidence of type-1 diabetes. Dr. Merriman also documented that significant research illustrates that type-1 diabetes is associated with lower levels of vitamin D (a product of sunshine). This data, as Dr. Merriman puts it, *"convincingly implicate vitamin D deficiency in T1D [type-1 diabetes]."*

In addition, a number of studies have now linked schizophrenia, Parkinson's disease and other neurological conditions with vitamin D deficiency. In a recent review done by French neurological researchers (Annweiler *et al.* 2010), 127 studies confirmed an association between these disorders and vitamin D deficiency. They concluded that, *"Vitamin D has been associated with many neurological functions and its deficiency with dysfunction."*

In another recent study, researchers (Amato *et al.* 2010) found that both schizophrenia and Parkinson's, along with others, were associated with *"Latitude-Related Genes (LRGs)."* They commented: *"We found a strong enrichment of LRGs in the set of genes associated to schizophrenia."* They also concluded that, *"several diseases show latitudinal clinals such as hypertension, cancer, dismetabolic conditions, schizophrenia, Parkinson's disease and many more."*

As far as heart disease goes, various studies have also linked vitamin D exposure to heart disease. A study from researchers at Utah's Intermountain Medical Center (Anderson *et al.* 2010) found, after reviewing 41,504 relevant patient records, that, *"The vitamin D levels were also highly associated with coronary artery disease, myocardial infarction, heart failure, and stroke..."*

In addition, an extensive review by Dr. Colin Campbell (2006) found that countries with increased incidence of heart disease were also associated with an increase of animal-based diets among those countries.

In other words, A1-A2 research has not been corroborated by any official government study or review, nor is it substantiated by direct clinical research. The A1-A2 evidence is circumstantial, unverifiable and based upon broad epidemiological research that associates populations supposedly having A1 milk with many other associations common to them, including their diet, geographical location and the availability of sunshine. In other words, there are many other possible causes for the diseases that A1 milk is purported to cause.

Healthy Cooking

While raw whole foods are often more wholesome to the body, some foods must be cooked to make them digestible. Some have put forth that cooking a food that causes an allergic reaction may reduce its allergenicity. This is not true for all allergens. In some cases, a particular allergen might be reduced or somehow broken down to a component that the body is not sensitive to. This may be more likely for food intolerances, but is dependent upon the specific sensitivity.

For example, German researchers (Worm *et al.* 2009) found that heat-treating and processing of hazelnuts reduces their allergenicity among hazelnut allergic people.

It may also depend upon the person and their tolerance as well. Researchers at Switzerland's University Hospital (Ballmer-Weber *et al.* 2002) gave patients with celery allergies raw celery, cooked celery (at 110 degrees for 15 minutes) and celery spice. Six out of 11 patients tested were sensitive to the minimally cooked celery. Five of five patients were sensitive to celery spice. The researchers also tried extended cooking of celery to see if that would change its sensitivity. In most cases, it didn't.

So the element of cooking is highly unique to the person, and dependent upon the food and the sensitivity. As we become more tolerant to foods previously sensitive to, we can test whether we are more tolerant to their cooked or raw versions. This can be tested using the protocols and safety nets discussed earlier. Once a level of tolerance is determined, the food can be slowly and gradually added back to the diet in the form the body is more tolerant to.

What is more important to consider is how much cooking and processing we are doing to our foods. How much cooking is necessary? Yes, cooking some foods often increases their digestibility. This is particularly important with grain-based foods and beans. Cooking these foods will help break down their fibers and complex carbohydrates into more digestible forms.

Also, many vegetables are better cooked, or even better, steamed. Steaming vegetables with a covered pot will preserve more nutrients, while softening some of fibers that hold nutrients. Foods such as beets, asparagus, broccoli, rhubarb, squash and many others are delicious and nutritious after being steamed or lightly boiled in clean water.

Other plant foods are best eaten raw. These include lettuce, cucumbers, avocado and many others. Because the nutrients in these foods are not so tightly bound within the cell walls of the plants, they can be destroyed by the heat and/or easily separated from the food during cooking.

A healthy diet strikes a balance between raw and cooked foods. A perfect way to accomplish this at dinner time is with a salad that includes seeds; cooked grains and/or beans; and a nice sauce. Breakfast and lunch can include fresh fruit; nuts; and fermented dairy with slightly cooked grains such as oats and barley. Snacks can go raw or otherwise. Raw, boiled or lightly roasted nuts and seeds also make especially healthy and slow-digesting snacks with essential fatty acid content.

Adding Anti-inflammatory Spices to Our Meals

We can also spice our cooked foods with excellent and flavorful anti-inflammatory herbs. We discussed a number of herbs earlier that research has shown will reduce inflammation and strengthen the immune system earlier. As a reminder, these include:

> Ginger (*Zingiber officinalis*)
> Cayenne (*Capiscium frutescens* or *Capiscium annum*)
> Turmeric (*Curcuma longa*)
> Basil (*Osimum basilicum*)
> Rosemary (*Rosmarinus officinalis*)
> Oregano (*Origanum vulgare*)
> Reishi mushroom (*Ganoderma spp.*)
> Garlic (*Allium sativum*)
> Onions (*Allium cepa L.*)

It should be noted that there is a great difference between a spice dose and a therapeutic dose. A therapeutic dose of one or more of these spices will typically be larger than a spice dose. The sign of a therapeutic dose of these spices within a dish is when the spice can be readily tasted. That is, the pungent flavor of the spice stands out in the food. If the amount of spice simply flavors the food a little, then it will probably not be enough to stimulate any immune response. If the spice can be specifically tasted (for example, *"that dish tastes garlicy"* or *"tastes peppery"*) then the spice will likely be enough to stimulate a therapeutic response.

That said, if multiple spices are used, the dose of each spice can be smaller. After all, the meal should also taste good. This, however, is why traditional Chinese and Indian food is so spicy. The recipes come from therapeutic traditions.

Another element of the therapeutic dose is consistency. It is not enough to have one or more of these spices once a week with a particular dish. The spice(s) should be added to at least one meal every day.

In addition, care must be taken to protect therapeutic spices from degradation. This can occur when spices are left in the light or sun for an extended period, or when spices are left open to oxygen. Often spices are left in kitchen racks that are exposed to the lights of the kitchen and window, or left in unsealed containers or shakers. Oxygen and light degrade the biochemical constituents that give these spices their therapeutic properties.

This latter point is likely one of the main reasons our culinary spices are not considered therapeutic. Leaving the spice exposed can take place during processing, packaging and shipping; as well as in the kitchen. Therefore, we should consider purchasing our therapeutic spices from a bulk herb store, or from suppliers or brands that respect their therapeutic nature.

By far the best way to consume or add these foods to our diet is in their fresh form. Many of these herbs can be grown in our garden or purchased from a local farmers' market or grocery store in their fresh form. The fresh form will contain a maximum of active constituents. This is because their beneficial constituents are naturally sealed within the plant's cell walls.

Note also that these anti-inflammatory herbal spices (and most of the other natural products contained in this chapter) will typically not stimulate a therapeutic response immediately. Depending upon the status of the immune system, it may take weeks or months before the daily dosing of these natural elements is seen in the form of modulating the immune response.

The Natural Rotary Diet

The *"Rotary Diversified Diet"* was first proposed by Dr. Herbter Rinkel in 1934. The diet was intended to prevent food sensitivities and work with foods that a person had become sensitive to. This isn't to say that traditional medicines around the world have not also treated with rotational diets—they have.

Dr. Rinkel's diet used a system of rotational cycles where different foods and food groups were alternated in a very disciplined manner. The principle used is that if a particular food or food group is too frequently eaten, the body may become intolerant to it. While the research absolutely proving this is sparse, Dr. Rinkel and many other physicians of his day, past and present, have observed this sometimes increasing tolerance among their patients. This however, does remind us of SOTI therapy.

The rotary system recognized that similar foods that either cross-reacted, or had similar protein types (such as wheat and barley), could also cause similar sensitivities. Thus food groups were also separated by rotations in the diet. Food groupings are discussed in detail in Chapter Three.

The rotary diet proposed that a particular food should not be eaten again for at least four to seven days later. If it is eaten sooner, it could promote sensitivity, according to the theory. If eaten any further out, it could also cause sensitivity due to the body no longer recognizing it. This later point has been confirmed in peanut allergy SOTI research, as discussed earlier. Foods must be eaten somewhat regularly to remain recognizable, in other words.

Dr. Rinkel's rotary diet also included slowly introducing foods that the body was previously sensitive to. He proposed that these sensitive foods are gradually introduced into the cycle in small increments: like SOTI.

The rotary diet proposed by Dr. Rinkel and modified by others is quite difficult for most people to maintain because of the discipline required. Quite simply, most people have certain foods that are more available seasonally, and there are foods we simply like to eat more frequently than others.

Also we should add that the author is aware of no hard evidence that consistently eating a certain food will result in a sensitivity to that food. On the contrary, we can look to the Asian continent and their food staples, which include rice and other particular foods that are regionally domestic to their diets. Among many Chinese and Indian nationals, for example—who have had one of the lowest disease rates worldwide—every meal through the day is often similar. These indigenous populations did not have enough wealth to be rotating their diet daily, let alone by the meal. There might be seasonal rotation due to the availability of certain crops, however. But following a particular harvest, that food might still be eaten at every meal.

Furthermore, among these traditional populations, food allergy rates have been some of the lowest in the world.

We would propose that should a person utilize the research supplied in this text, they will see that there are certain types of diets and lifestyles that are known to discourage food sensitivities. These embrace a variety of different foods and food groups that may be *naturally* rotated.

By *naturally rotated,* we mean that if a person focuses on eating primarily seasonal, mostly-locally grown foods, then there will be a natural rotation to the diet. It is also no coincidence that the body works better on slower-digesting foods such as grains and oils during the winter, and faster-digesting foods such as fruits and vegetables during the summer months.

This doesn't mean that we avoid fruits and vegetables during the winter, however. But it may mean that we are eating more grains and oils during the winter than we do during the summer. And it is no coincidence there are more fruits and vegetables available locally during the summer. Often it is too hot in the summer to eat a heavy meal, while salads and fruits with smaller amounts of dairy and grains are digested quite easily during hot weather.

Genetically, our bodies have been tuning to these seasonal foods for thousands of years. We can embrace nature's seasonal rotations while we embrace our energy levels and digestive levels.

Inside of this seasonal rotation, we can also eat a varied diet that is naturally rotated. This will often suit our tastes and our body's nutritional needs as well. One dinner can feature root-oriented foods such as yams, sweet potatoes or potatoes, while the next dinner can feature grains. The next dinner can feature a nut-based, or a bean-based dish.

Other meals can be rotated in the same way. Breakfasts can rotate between a variety of combinations of grains, dairy, fruits and nuts. Beans, vegetables, nuts, dairy and fruits can be rotated at lunch as well, according to our dietary liking, the foods' local availability and seasonal availability.

The rotary diet would still be extremely useful for working in foods we have been sensitive to. We can slowly and gradually work in small amounts of a particular food as documented in the SOTI section. The first rotation might include an amount as small as a tiny spec of the food. Assuming little or no reaction, the amount would be gradually increased as documented in the research, depending upon our level of sensitivity and the supervision of our health professional.

After a period of consistent gradual increase, the food can be added to a weekly rotation of the food, and the quantity of the food could be increased monthly until achieving the desired (moderate) dose.

The exact protocol would be highly unique, depending upon the food, the level of sensitivity, and the goal. If the goal is to be able to eat the food regularly, then this process must continue with increasing doses. If the goal is to tolerate a small amount of the food in the case of accidental ingestion, then the same small amount can be consumed periodically to continue the tolerance.

Again, for anyone with a severe allergy response, this process should be supervised by a trained health professional.

Probiotic Supplementation Strategies

The supplementation of probiotics to discourage food sensitivities must be done with the science in mind. This is vital, because not every species, every strain and every dose has been shown to be useful for food sensitivities. Rather, research has shown that specific species and strains, used in specific doses alongside prebiotic-rich diets are most beneficial, as we've illustrated in this book.

First we should know which species aid in food sensitivities. After reviewing hundreds of clinical studies, some quoted in this book and many more discussed in the author's *Probiotics–Protection Against Infection* (2009), we summarize here the probiotics that have been shown useful for food sensitivities. Under each species, the specific effects found in the research to contribute to its being beneficial for preventing and helping to resolve food sensitivities is listed (refer to the author's probiotics text mentioned above for reference specifics):

Lactobacillus acidophilus

Lactobacillus acidophilus is by far the most familiar probiotic to most of us, and is also by far the most-studied probiotic species to date. They are one of the main residents of the human gut, although supplemented strains may still be transient. In addition to helping digest lactose, probably the most important benefit of *L. acidophilus* is their ability to inhibit the growth of pathogenic intestinal microorganisms such as *Candida albicans*, *Escherichia coli*, *Helicobacter pylori*, *Salmonella*, *Shigella* and *Staphylococcus* species.

The research has shown that under certain conditions *L. acidophilus:*
➢ Help digest milk
➢ Reduce stress-induced GI problems
➢ Inhibit *E. coli*
➢ Reduce infection from rotavirus

➢ Reduce necrotizing enterocolitis
➢ Reduce intestinal permeability
➢ Control *H. pylori*
➢ Modulate PGE2 and IgA
➢ Reduce dyspepsia
➢ Modulate IgG
➢ Relieve and inhibit IBS and colitis
➢ Inhibit and control *Clostridium* spp.
➢ Inhibit *Bacteroides* spp.
➢ Inhibit *Candida* spp. Overgrowths
➢ Reduce allergic response
➢ Decrease allergic symptoms
➢ Inhibit upper respiratory infections

Lactobacillus helveticus

L. helveticus was made popular by cheese-makers from Switzerland. The Latin word *Helvetia* refers to Switzerland. *L. helveticus* is used to make Swiss cheese and other varietals, as it produces lactic acid but not other probiotic metabolites that can often make cheese taste bitter or sour.

The research has shown that under certain conditions *L. helveticus:*

➢ Normalize gut colonization similar to breast-fed infants among formula-fed infants

Lactobacillus salivarius

L. salivarius are residents of most humans. They are found in the mouth, small intestines, colon, and vagina. They are hardy bacteria that can live in both oxygen and oxygen-free environments. *L. salivarius* is one of the few bacteria species that can also thrive in salty environments. *L. salivarius* produce prolific amounts of lactic acid, which makes them hardy defenders of the teeth and gums. They also produce a number of antibiotics, and are speedy colonizers.

The research has shown that under certain conditions *L. salivarius:*

➢ Inhibit mutans streptococci in the mouth
➢ Reduce dental carries
➢ Reduce gingivitis and periodontal disease
➢ Reduce mastitis
➢ Reduce risk of strep throat caused by *S. pyogenes*
➢ Reduce ulcerative colitis and IBS
➢ Inhibit *E. coli*
➢ Inhibit *Salmonella* spp.
➢ Inhibit *Candida albicans*

Lactobacillus casei

L. *casei* are transient bacteria within the human body, but are residents of cow intestines. Thus they are readily found in naturally raw milk and colostrum. L. *casei* have been reported to reduce allergy symptoms and increase immune response. This is accomplished by their regulating the immune system's CHS, CD8 and T-cell responsiveness—an effect seen among immunosuppressed patients. L. *casei* are also competitive bacteria that will overtake other probiotics in a combined supplement. So it is best to supplement L. *casei* individually.

The research has shown that under certain conditions L. *casei*:

➢ Inhibit pathogenic microbial infections
➢ Reduce occurrence, risk and symptoms of IBS
➢ Inhibit severe systemic inflammatory response syndrome
➢ Inhibit respiratory tract infections
➢ Inhibit bronchitis
➢ Maintain remission of diverticular disease
➢ Inhibit *H. pylori* (and ulcers)
➢ Reduce allergy symptoms
➢ Inhibit *Pseudomonas aeruginosa*
➢ Decrease milk intolerance
➢ Increase CD3+ and CD4+
➢ Increase phagocytic activity
➢ Support liver function
➢ Decrease proinflammatory cytokine TNF-alpha
➢ Strengthen the immune system
➢ Inhibit and reduce diarrhea episodes
➢ Stimulate cytokine interleukin-1beta (IL-1b)
➢ Stimulate interferon-gamma
➢ Inhibit *Clostridium difficile*
➢ Reduce asthma symptoms
➢ Reduce constipation
➢ Decrease beta-glucuronidase
➢ Stimulate natural killer cell activity (NK-cells)
➢ Increase IgA levels
➢ Increase lymphocytes
➢ Decrease IL-6 (pro-inflammatory)
➢ Increase IL-12 (stimulates NK-cells)
➢ Reduce lower respiratory infections
➢ Inhibit *Candida* overgrowth
➢ Inhibit vaginosis
➢ Prevent colorectal tumor growth
➢ Restore NK-cell activity in smokers
➢ Stimulate the immune system among the elderly
➢ Increase CD56 lymphocytes
➢ Decrease rotavirus infections

➢ Decrease colds and influenza
➢ Reduce risk of bladder cancer
➢ Increase (good) HDL-cholesterol
➢ Decrease triglycerides
➢ Decrease blood pressure
➢ Inhibit viral infections
➢ Inhibit malignant pleural effusions secondary to lung cancer
➢ Reduce cervix tumors when used in combination radiation therapy
➢ Inhibit tumor growth of carcinomatous peritonitis/stomach cancer
➢ Break down nutrients for bioavailability

Lactobacillus rhamnosus

Much of the research on this species has been done on a particular strain, *L. rhamnosus* GG. *L. rhamnosus* GG have been shown in numerous studies to significantly stimulate the immune system and inhibit allergic inflammatory response as noted earlier. This is not to say, however, that non-GG strains will not perform similarly. In fact, studies with *L. rhamnosus* GR-1, *L. rhamnosus* 573/L, and *L. rhamnosus* LC705 strains have also showed positive results. The GG strain is trademarked by the Valio Ltd. Company in Finland and patented in 1985 by two scientists, Dr. Sherwood Gorbach and Dr. Barry Goldin, who also led most of the exhaustive research on this strain.

The research has shown that under certain conditions *L. rhamnosus:*
➢ Inhibit a number of pathogenic microbial infections
➢ Improve glucose control
➢ Reduce risk of respiratory infections
➢ Decrease beta-glucosidase
➢ Reduce eczema
➢ Reduce colds and flu
➢ Strengthen the immune system
➢ Increase IgA levels in mucosal membrane
➢ Increase IgA levels in mothers breast milk
➢ Inhibit *Pseudomonas aeruginosa* infections in respiratory tract
➢ Inhibit *Clostridium difficile*
➢ Inhibit enterobacteria
➢ Reduce IBS symptoms
➢ Decrease IL-12, IL-2+ and CD69+ T-cells in IBS
➢ Reduce constipation
➢ Reduce the risk of colon cancer
➢ Modulate skin IgE sensitization
➢ Inhibit *H. pylori* (ulcer-causing)
➢ Reduce atopic dermatitis in children
➢ Increase Hib IgG levels in allergy-prone infants

➤ Reduce colic
➤ Stimulate IgM, IgA and IgG levels (modulates IgE)
➤ Stabilize intestinal barrier function (decreased permeability)
➤ Increase INF-gamma
➤ Modulate IL-4
➤ Help prevent atopic eczema
➤ Reduce *Streptococcus mutans*
➤ Stimulate tumor killing activity among NK-cells
➤ Stimulate IL-10 (anti-inflammatory)
➤ Reduce inflammation

Lactobacillus reuteri

L. reuteri is a species found residing permanently in humans. As a result, most supplemented strains attach fairly well, though temporarily, and stimulate colony growth for resident *L. reuteri* strains. *L. reuteri* will colonize in the stomach, duodenum and ileum regions. *L. reuteri* will also significantly modulate the immune response of the gastrointestinal mucosal membranes. This means that *L. reuteri* are useful for many of the same digestive ailments that *L. acidophilus* are also effective for. *L. reuteri* also have several other effects, including the restoration of our oral cavity bacteria. They also produce a significant amount of antibiotics.

The research has shown that under certain conditions *L. reuteri:*

➤ Inhibit gingivitis
➤ Reduce pro-inflammatory cytokines
➤ Stimulate growth and feeding among preterm infants
➤ Inhibit and suppress *H. pylori*
➤ Decrease dyspepsia
➤ Reduce nausea
➤ Reduce flatulence
➤ Reduce diarrhea (rotavirus and non-rotavirus)
➤ Reduce TGF-beta2 in breast-feeding mothers (reducing eczema)
➤ Reduce salivary *mutans streptococcus*
➤ Strengthen the immune system
➤ Reduce plaque on teeth
➤ Decrease symptoms of IBS
➤ Increase (inflammatory) CD4+ and CD25 T-cells (in IBS)
➤ Decrease (inflammatory) TNF-alpha (in IBS)
➤ Decrease (inflammatory) IL-12 (in IBS)
➤ Reduce eczema-specific IgEs in infants
➤ Reduce infant colic
➤ Reduce colds and influenza
➤ Stabilize intestinal barrier function (intestinal permeability)
➤ Decrease atopic dermatitis

Lactobacillus plantarum

L. plantarum has been part of the human diet for thousands of years. They are used in numerous fermented foods, including sauerkraut, gherkins, olive brines, sourdough bread, Nigerian ogi and fufu, kocha from Ethiopia, sour mifen noodles from China, Korean kim chi and other traditional foods. *L. plantarum* are also found in dairy and cow dung.

L. plantarum is a hardy strain. The bacteria have been shown to survive all the way through the intestinal tract. Temperature for optimal growth is 86-95 degrees F. *L. plantarum* are not permanent residents, however. When supplemented, they vigorously attack pathogenic bacteria, and create an environment hospitable for incubated resident strains to expand before departing. *L. plantarum* also produce lysine, and a number of antibiotics including lactolin. They also strengthen the mucosal membrane and reduce intestinal permeability.

The research has shown that under certain conditions, *L. plantarum:*

➢ Strengthen the immune system
➢ Help restore healthy liver enzymes (alcohol-induced liver injury)
➢ Reduce frequency and severity of respiratory diseases
➢ Reduce intestinal permeability
➢ Inhibit various intestinal pathobiotics (incl. *Clostridium difficile*)
➢ Reduce Th2 (inflammatory) levels and increase Th1/Th2 ratio
➢ Reduce inflammatory responses
➢ Reduce symptoms of multiple traumas among injured patients
➢ Reduce fungal infections
➢ Reduce IBS symptoms
➢ Reduce pancreatic sepsis (infection)
➢ Reduce (inflammatory) interleukin-6 (IL-6) levels
➢ Decrease flatulence

Lactobacillus bulgaricus

We owe the *bulgaricus* name to Ilya Mechnikov, who named it after the Bulgarians—who used the bacteria to make the fermented milks that produced the original kefirs apparently related to their extreme longevity. In the 1960s and 1970s Russian researchers, notably Dr. Ivan Bogdanov and others, began focused research on *L. bulgaricus*. Early studies indicated antitumor effects. As the research progressed into Russian clinical research and commercialization, it became obvious that even heat-killed *L. bulgaricus* cell fragments have immune system stimulating benefits.

L. bulgaricus bacteria are transients that assist in *bifidobacteria* colony growth. They significantly stimulate the immune system and have antitumor effects. They also produce antibiotic and antiviral substances such as bulgarican and others. *L. bulgaricus* bacteria have also been reported to have anti-herpes properties. *L. bulgaricus* require more heat to colonize than many probiotics—at 104-109 degrees F.

The research has shown that under certain conditions *L. bulgaricus:*

➤ Reduce intestinal permeability
➤ Decrease IBS symptoms
➤ Help manage HIV symptoms
➤ Stimulate TNF-alpha
➤ Stimulate IL-1beta
➤ Decrease diarrhea (rotavirus and non-rotavirus)
➤ Decrease nausea
➤ Increase phagocytic activity
➤ Increase leukocyte levels
➤ Increase immune response
➤ Increase CD8+ levels
➤ Lower CD4+/CD8+ ratio (reducing inflammation)
➤ Increase IFN-gamma
➤ Lower total cholesterol
➤ Lower LDL levels
➤ Lower triglycerides
➤ Inhibit viruses
➤ Reduce salivary mutans in the mouth
➤ Increase absorption of dairy (lactose)
➤ Increase white blood cell counts after chemotherapy
➤ Increase IgA (immunity) to rotavirus
➤ Reduce intestinal bacteria

Bifidobacterium bifidum

These are normal residents in the human intestines, and by far the largest residents in terms of colonies. Their greatest populations occur in the colon, but also inhabit the lower small intestines. Breast milk typically contains large populations of *B. bifidum* along with other bifidobacteria. *B. bifidum* are highly competitive with yeasts such as *Candida albicans*. As a result, their populations may be decimated by large yeast overgrowths. This will also result in a number of endotoxins, including ammonia, being leached out of the colon into the bloodstream. As a result, *B. bifidum* populations are extremely important to the health of the liver, as has been illustrated in the research. They produce an array of antibiotics such as bifidin and various antimicrobial biochemicals such as formic acid. *B. bifidus* populations can also be severely damaged by the use of pharmaceutical antibiotics.

The research has shown that under certain conditions _B. bifidum:_

➢ Increase cell regeneration in alcohol-induced liver injury
➢ Stimulate immunity in very low birth weight infants
➢ Increase TGF-beta (anti-inflammatory) levels
➢ Reduce allergies
➢ Reduce _H. pylori_ colonization
➢ Increase CD8+ T-cells as needed
➢ Establish infant microflora
➢ Inhibit _E. coli_
➢ Reduce intestinal bacteria infections
➢ Reduce acute diarrhea (rotavirus and non-rotavirus)

Bifidobacterium infantis

B. infantis are also normal residents of the human intestines—primarily among children. As implicated in the name, infants colonize a significant number of _B. infantis_ in their early years. They will also colonize in the vagina, leading to the newborn's first exposure to protective probiotic bacteria. For this reason, it is important that pregnant mothers consider probiotic supplementation with _B. infantis_. _B. infantis_ are largely anaerobic, and thrive within the darkest regions, where they can produce profuse quantities of acetic acid, lactic acid and formic acid to acidify the intestinal tract.

The research has shown that under certain conditions, _B. infantis:_

➢ Reduce acute diarrhea (rotavirus and non-rotavirus)
➢ Reduce or eliminate symptoms of IBS
➢ Reduce death among very low birth weight infants
➢ Increase immunity among very low birth weight infants
➢ Establish infant microflora
➢ Normalize Th1/Th2 ratio
➢ Reduce inflammatory allergic responses
➢ Normalize IL-10/IL-12 ratio
➢ Improve immune system efficiency

Bifidobacterium longum

B. longum are also normal inhabitants of the human digestive tract. They predominate the colon but also live in the small intestines. They are one of our top four bifidobacteria inhabitants. Like _B. infantis_, they produce acetic, lactic and formic acid. Like other bifidobacteria, they resist the growth of pathogenic bacteria, and thus reduce the production of harmful nitrites and ammonia. _B. longum_ also produce B vitamins. Healthy breast milk contains significant _B. longum_.

The research has shown that under certain conditions _B. longum:_

➤ Reduce death among very low birth weight infants
➤ Reduce sickness among very low birth weight infants
➤ Reduce acute diarrhea (rotavirus and non-rotavirus)
➤ Reduce vomiting
➤ Reduce nausea
➤ Reduce ulcerative colitis
➤ Reduce or alleviate symptoms of IBS
➤ Stabilize intestinal barrier function (decreased permeability)
➤ Inhibit _H. pylori_
➤ Increase TGF-beta1 (anti-inflammatory) levels
➤ Decrease (inflammatory) TNF-alpha
➤ Decrease (inflammatory) IL-10 cytokines
➤ Reduce lactose-intolerance symptoms
➤ Reduce diarrhea
➤ Increase helper T-cells type2 (Th2)
➤ Increase (anti-inflammatory) IL-6
➤ Reduce (inflammatory) Th1
➤ Reduce pro-inflammatory IL-12 and interferon
➤ Stimulate healing of liver in cirrhosis
➤ Reduce constipation
➤ Reduce hypersensitivity
➤ Reduce IBS symptoms
➤ Inhibit intestinal pathogenic bacteria
➤ Decrease prostate cancer risk
➤ Decrease itching, nasal blockage and rhinitis in allergies
➤ Reduce (inflammatory) NF-kappaB
➤ Reduce (inflammatory) IL-8 levels
➤ Reduce progression of chronic liver disease
➤ Increase absorption of dairy nutrients

Bifidobacterium animalis/B. lactis

B. animalis was previously thought to be distinct from _B. lactis_, but today they are considered the same species with _B. lactis_ being a subspecies of _B. animalis_. _B. lactis_ has also been described as _Streptococcus lactis_. They are transient bacteria typically present in raw milk. They are also used as starters for traditional cheeses, cottage cheeses and buttermilks. They are also found among certain plants.

The research has shown that under certain conditions _B. animalis:_

➤ Reduce constipation
➤ Improve digestive comfort
➤ Decrease total cholesterol
➤ Increase blood glucose control
➤ Reduce respiratory diseases (severity and frequency)

➢ Strengthen the immune system
➢ Reduce salivary mutans in mouth
➢ Increase body weight among preterm infants
➢ Reduce (inflammatory) CRP levels
➢ Reduce (inflammatory) TNF-alpha levels
➢ Reduce acute diarrhea (rotavirus and non-rotavirus)
➢ Reduce (inflammatory) IL-10 levels
➢ Reduce (inflammatory) TGF-beta1 levels
➢ Reduce inflammatory responses
➢ Reduce (inflammatory) CDE4+CD54(+) cytokines
➢ Stimulate improvement in atopic dermatitis patients
➢ Reduce IBS symptoms
➢ Reduce diarrhea
➢ Normalize bowel movements
➢ Decrease intestinal permeability
➢ Reduce blood levels of interferon-gamma
➢ Stimulate IgA among milk-allergy infants
➢ Improve atopic dermatitis symptoms and sensitivity
➢ Inhibit *H. pylori*
➢ Reduce allergic inflammation
➢ Increase T-cell activity as needed
➢ Increase immunity among the elderly
➢ Increase absorption of dairy

Bifidobacterium breve

B. breve are also normal inhabitants of the human digestive tract—living mostly within the colon. They produce prolific acids, and also B vitamins. Like the other bifidobacteria, they also reduce ammonia-producing bacteria in the colon, aiding the health of the liver. Latin *brevis* means short.

The research has shown that under certain conditions *B. breve*:

➢ Reduce severe systemic inflammatory response syndrome
➢ Increase resistance to respiratory infection
➢ Reduce (inflammatory) TNF-alpha
➢ Reduce (inflammatory) IL-10
➢ Reduce (inflammatory) TGF-beta1
➢ Reduce IBS symptoms
➢ Decrease (pro-colon cancer) beta-glucoronidase
➢ Inhibit *H. pylori*
➢ Increase antipoliovirus vaccination effectiveness
➢ Reduce acute diarrhea (rotavirus and non-rotavirus)
➢ Reduce allergy symptoms
➢ Increase growth weights among very low birth weight infants

Streptococcus thermophilus

Streptococcus thermophilus are common participants in yogurt making. They are also used in cheese making, and are even sometimes found in pasteurized milk. They will colonize at higher temperatures, from 104-113 degrees F. This is significant because this bacterium readily produces lactase, which breaks down lactose. (This is the only streptococci known to do this.) Like many other supplemented probiotics, *S. thermophilus* are temporary microorganisms in the human body. Their colonies will typically inhabit the system for a week or two before exiting (unless consistently consumed). During that time, however, they will help set up a healthy environment to support resident colony growth. Like other probiotics, *S. thermophilus* also produce a number of different antibiotic substances, including acids that deter the growth of pathogenic bacteria.

The research has shown that under certain conditions *S. thermophilus:*

➤ Reduce acute diarrhea (rotavirus and non-rotavirus)
➤ Reduce intestinal permeability
➤ Inhibit *H. pylori*
➤ Help manage AIDS symptoms
➤ Increase lymphocytes among low-WBC patients
➤ Increase (anti-inflammatory) IL-1beta
➤ Decrease (inflammatory) IL-10
➤ Increase tumor necrosis factor-alpha (TNF-a)
➤ Increase absorption of dairy
➤ Decrease symptoms of IBS
➤ Inhibit *Clostridium difficile*
➤ Increase immune function among the elderly
➤ Restore infant microflora similar to breast-fed infants
➤ Increase (anti-inflammatory) CD8+
➤ Increase (anti-inflammatory) IFN-gamma
➤ Reduce acute gastroenteritis (diarrhea)
➤ Reduce baby colic
➤ Reduce symptoms of atopic dermatitis
➤ Reduce nasal cavity infections
➤ Increase HDL-cholesterol
➤ Increase growth in preterm infants
➤ Reduce intestinal bacteria
➤ Reduce upper respiratory tract infections from *Staphylococcus aureus*, *Streptococcus pneumoniae*, beta-hemolytic streptococci, and *Haemophilus influenzae*
➤ Reduce salivary mutans streptococci in the mouth
➤ Reduce flare-ups of chronic pouchitis
➤ Reduce LDL-cholesterol in overweight subjects
➤ Reduce ulcerative colitis

Saccharomyces boulardii

S. boulardii are yeasts (fungi). They render a variety of preventative and therapeutic benefits to the body. Yet should this or another yeast colony grow too large, they can quickly become a burden to the body due to their dietary needs (primarily refined sugars) and waste products. *S. boulardii* are known to enhance IgA—which, as we've discussed, will typically reduce IgE atopic sensitivities. This is likely why this probiotic helps clear skin disorders. *S. boulardii* also help control diarrhea, and have been shown to be helpful in Crohn's disease and irritable bowel issues. *S. boulardii* have also been shown to be useful in combating cholera bacteria (*Vibrio cholerae*).

The research has shown that under certain conditions *S. boulardii*:

➤ Decrease infectious *Entameba histolytica* (intestinal)
➤ Inhibit *H. pylori*
➤ Decrease intestinal permeability
➤ Decrease diarrhea infections
➤ Stimulate T-cells as needed
➤ Decrease C-reactive protein
➤ Decrease beta-glucoronidase enzyme (associated with colon cancer)
➤ Inhibit *E. coli*
➤ Reduce ulcerative colitis
➤ Reduce symptoms of Crohn's disease
➤ Reduce *Clostridium difficile*

Probiotic Supplement Considerations

The main consideration in probiotic supplementation is consuming live organisms. These are typically labeled as "CFU" which stands for *colony forming units*. In other words, live probiotics will produce new colonies once inside the intestines. Dead ones will not. So the key is keeping the probiotics alive while in the capsule and supplement bottle, until we are ready to consume them. Here are a few considerations about probiotic supplements:

Capsules

Vegetable capsules contain less moisture than gelatin or enteric-coated capsules. Even a little moisture in the capsule can increase the possibility of waking up the probiotics while in the bottle. Once woken up, they will starve and die. Enteric coating can minimally protect the probiotics within the stomach, assuming they have survived in the bottle. Some manufactures use oils to help protect the probiotics in the stomach. In all cases, encapsulated freeze-dried probiotics should be refrigerated (no matter what the label says) at all times during shipping, at the store, and at home. Dark containers also better protect the probiotics from light exposure, which can kill them.

Powders

Powders of freeze-dried probiotics are subject to deterioration due to increased exposure to oxygen and light. Powders should be refrigerated in dark containers and sealed tightly to be kept viable. They should also be consumed with liquids or food, preferably dairy or fermented dairy. If used as to insert into the vagina, a douche mixture with water and a little yogurt is preferable.

Caplets/Tablets

Some tablet/caplets have special coatings that provide viability through to the intestines without refrigeration. If not, those tablets would likely be in the same category as encapsulated products, in terms of requiring refrigeration.

Shells or Beads

These can provide longer shelf viability without refrigeration and better survive the stomach. However, because of the size of the shell, these typically come with less CFU quantity, increasing the cost of a therapeutic dose. Another drawback may be that the intestines must dissolve this thick shell. An easy test is to examine the stool to be sure that the beads or shells aren't coming out the other end whole.

Lozenges

These are new and exciting ways to supplement with probiotics. A correctly formulated chewable or lozenge can inoculate the mouth, nose and throat with beneficial bacteria to compete with and fight off pathogenic bacteria as they enter or reside in our nose, throat, mouth and even lungs. However, the probiotics in a lozenge will not likely survive the stomach acids and penetrate the intestines.

Still, lozenges are an excellent way to protect against new infections and prevent sore throats when we are traveling or working in enclosed spaces. The bacteria in a lozenge or chewable ease out as we are sucking or chewing, leaving probiotics dispersed throughout our gums and throat, rendering increased immunity. This type of supplement should still be kept sealed, airtight and cool. Refer to the author's book *Oral Probiotics* (2010) for detailed information regarding species and strategies for oral probiotic lozenges.

Liquid Supplements

There are several probiotic supplements in small liquid form. One brand has a long tradition and a hardy, well-researched strain. A liquid probiotic should be in a light-sealed, refrigerated container. It should also contain some dairy or other probiotic-friendly culture, giving the probiotics some food while they are waiting for delivery.

Probiotic Hydrotherapy

This method of supplementation is probably the best way to implant live colonies of probiotics into the lower colon. Colon hydrotherapy (or colonic) is one of the healthiest things we can do for preventative and therapeutic health. Colon hydrotherapy is performed by a certified colon hydrotherapist who uses specialized (and sanitary) equipment to flush out the colon. This colon flushing usually takes about 30 minutes. Once the process is complete, the hydrotherapist can "insert" a blend of probiotics into the tube and "pump" the probiotics directly into our colon. Colon hydrotherapy is a wonderful treatment recommended for most anyone, especially those with disorders related to autoimmunity, allergies and food sensitivities.

Colonic treatments are relatively inexpensive, especially for their benefit. Two to three colonics a year is often recommended for ultimate colon health. Those with sensitive or irritable bowels should consult with their health professional before submitting to a colonic, however.

Probiotic Dosage

A good dosage for intestinal probiotics for prevention and maintenance can be ten to fifteen billion CFU (*colony forming units*) per day. Total intake during an illness or therapeutic period, however, will often double or triple that dosage. Much of the research shown in this text utilized 20 billion to 40 billion CFU per day, about a third of that dose for children and a quarter of that dose for infants. (*B. infantis* is often the supplement of choice for babies.)

Supplemental oral probiotic dosages can be far less (100 million to two billion), especially when the formula contains the hardy *L. reuteri*.

People who must take antibiotics for life-threatening reasons can alternate doses of probiotics between their antibiotic dosing. The probiotic dose can be at least two hours before or after the antibiotic dose. (Always consult with the prescribing doctor first.)

Remember that these dosages depend upon delivery to the intestines. Therefore, a product that passes into the stomach with little protection would likely not deliver well to the intestines. Such a supplement would likely require higher dosage to achieve the desired effects.

Hydration

One might think that hydration is completely unrelated to food sensitivities. This is absolutely false.

The intestinal mucosal membrane is primarily water. In a dehydrated state, this mucosal membrane thins. It is for this reason that research on water drinking has found that many ulcerated conditions can be cured simply by drinking adequate water (Batmanghelidj 1997).

The immune system is also irrevocably aligned with the body's water availability. The immune system utilizes water to produce lymph fluid. Lymph fluid circulates immune cells throughout the body so that they can target specific intruders. The lymph is also used to escort toxins out of the body.

Water in general is needed to speed the removal of toxins, from every organ and tissue system.

Water also increases the availability of oxygen to cells. Water balances the level of free radicals. Water flushes and replenishes the digestive tract. Thus, water is necessary for the proper digestion of food. The gastric cells and intestinal wall cells require water for proper functioning.

Water is also intimately involved in the release of histamine. Research has revealed that increased levels of histamine are released during periods of dehydration, in order to help provide water balance within the bloodstream, tissues, kidneys and other organs (Batmanghelidj 1987; Batmanghelidj 1990).

A rule of thumb accepted by many experts, and consistent with government studies, would be to drink one-half ounce of water per pound of body weight per day.

Drinking just any water is not advised. Care must be taken to drink water that is pure yet naturally mineralized. Research has confirmed that distilled water and soft water are not advisable. Please refer to the author's book, *Pure Water* (2010) for the specific research that concludes which types of water and filtration methods are the healthiest.

Exercise

Nutrition researchers from The Netherlands' Wageningen University (Chin *et al.* 2000) found that as elderly people became more frail, their immune systems weakened and they became more sensitive to certain foods. The researchers studied 112 elderly subjects with an average age of 79 years old. The research compared the effects of vitamin supplementation and exercise with food sensitivities. They found that vitamin supplementation did not slow the rate of sensitivity to foods, but exercise did slow the rate of food sensitivity among the elderly men and women.

We are not surprised about the vitamin supplementation. While even antioxidant vitamins such as C and E have been shown to strengthen the body's immune system, isolated vitamins do not have the cofactors and buffers needed for a balanced effect. This is also why studies on isolated vitamins such as E have been inconclusive. Nature produces several forms of vitamin E, which includes alpha-, beta-, gamma- and delta-tocopherols. When these are isolated they do not have the same effects as when they are naturally presented in foods. Also, we might add that elderly persons often do not absorb isolated nutrients very well. Food-based nutrition is the best strategy, although sometimes isolated nutrients become necessary in order to avoid a deficiency.

As far as exercise goes, this is one of the most assured ways of strengthening the immune system and thus increasing tolerance. When we exercise, we contract muscles. Muscle contraction is what circulates (or pumps) lymph around the body through the lymph vessels. This is because the lymphatic system does not have a heart like the circulatory system has. The lymphatic system relies on muscle contraction for circulation.

Lymph circulation is critical because while immune cells are also circulated through the blood, much of our immune cells, cytokines and immunoglobulins are circulated through the lymph. Lymph also carries out of the body those broken-down toxins and cell parts after the immune system has done its job. And recent research has revealed that parts of the lymphatic system also houses and incubates probiotics in ducts such as the vermiform appendix (Randal, *et al.* 2007).

And of course exercise also circulates oxygen, nutrients and immune cells throughout the body using the bloodstream. The bloodstream also carries out of the body those detoxification byproducts as well. Exercise also stimulates the thymus gland, and speeds up healing of the intestinal cell walls. In all, exercise is one of the best and cheapest therapies available to boost immunity and tolerance.

Environmental Strategies

As we discussed in Chapter Four, a number of studies over the past decade have found that children living in rural areas were less likely to have allergies, especially asthma and food sensitivities. For years, doctors and researchers have been supposing that this effect was coming from the increased exposures to the various allergens. In other words, the theory has been that the immune system becomes more tolerant when it is exposed to increased levels of potential toxins.

Remember the research from Switzerland's University of Basel (Waser *et al.* 2007). The study of 14,893 children, including 2,823 children from farms and 4,606 Steiner children, found that farm living and farm milk in particular, resulted in lower incidence of allergies. While we can attribute much of the effect to the natural probiotics in farm milk, rural living and the increased plant-food diets of the Steiner children also indicate lifestyles that decrease allergy rates among children.

Remember also the other studies quoted earlier that showed that food sensitivities were higher in industrialized countries and among those living in urban areas.

The hypothesis that the more exposure to toxins, the more tolerant the immune system becomes has now come under scrutiny. The problem with this theory is that if this was the case, those living in cities should become more tolerant to smog and other pollutants, and thus should have even lower levels of asthma than those living in rural regions where smog exposure is reduced.

A number of studies have shown the opposite. For example, a study done by the Arizona Health Care Cost Containment System (Smith *et al.* 2010) found that urban residents had a 55% greater likelihood of asthma than rural residents. The study followed 3,013 persons.

The real issue here is that the immune system of a human has evolved over millions of years with nature. The healthy immune system is genetically set up to ultimately recognize nature's toxins and deal with them appropriately through IgA responses and liver detoxification systems. Occasionally, the natural immune system also launches a hyper-inflammatory response to an invasion of viruses and/or bacteria. These are dealt with appropriately; and the immune system memorizes the invader. This memory serves to protect the body from a reinvasion, typically without the need for hyper-inflammation.

However, our increasingly synthetic environments are corrupting the immune system, producing hypersensitivity. They are overloading the immune system with a variety of chemical toxins that the immune system and its probiotic helpers have never encountered at these levels.

This barrage is producing an immune system fallout. Normal processes of mucosal membrane barriers and intestinal wall barriers are being destroyed. This in turn damages the body's ability to properly break down nutrients, leaving the intestinal wall exposed to macromolecules new to the immune system.

The destruction of the mucosal membranes of the mouth and digestive tract also weakens the body's IgA response. Out of desperation, the immune system responds with hypersensitivity, sometimes even to elements that were consumed for decades.

Urban industrialized areas expose people to environments with an increased amount of these synthetic toxins. It is for this reason that undeveloped countries and urban areas have less food sensitivity.

Reversing Increased Intestinal Permeability

As we've discussed extensively in this text, the scientific evidence points to the fact that many food sensitivities are caused by or worsened by the weakening and breakdown of the intestinal mucosal membrane and intestinal barrier. Once the barrier has broken down, toxins and food macromolecules can come into contact with intestinal tissues and the bloodstream. As this takes place, the immune system launches an attack and "marks" the offenders as dangerous foreigners.

Assuming a weakened immune system, if one of these "marks" included an innocent and otherwise nutritious food molecule that simply did not get properly broken down in the digestive tract, then that food macromolecule—many times a protein—can stimulate a systemic immune system response.

Once marked, IgE immunoglobulins are programmed to look for those food proteins on an ongoing basis. Every exposure will cause IgE to lock on and stimulate the systemic immune response. This mechanism has been described over and over in the research, and has been verified through peer-reviewed clinical studies as we've shown in this text.

Now the question is how to rebuild the mucosal membrane and the intestinal barrier.

Throughout this book we have discussed a variety of toxins (including those listed on pages 141-142) that can weaken the immune system. Most of these toxins are also implicated in the weakening of the mucosal membrane and intestinal barrier. Is this a coincidence?

The fact is, the intestinal barrier is *part* of the body's immune system. It is the body's most important first and/or second line of defense against invading microorganisms and toxins. This barrier also prevents larger, undigested food molecules from penetrating the body's tissues and invoking a hypersensitive response.

We have also thoroughly investigated not only the causes of the breakdown of the mucosal membrane and intestinal barrier, but also laid out a variety of strategies to reverse increased intestinal permeability. These have ranged from dietary strategies to herbs, probiotics, water and exercise. While some of these may not directly heal the barrier, most will at least strengthen the immune system to help detoxify the body of some of the elements that weaken the mucosal membrane and brush barrier.

Decreasing the body's toxic load combined with a healthy, predominantly plant-based diet will also help our gastric and intestinal cells regenerate a healthy mucosal membrane. This will help reduce the toxic burden upon the cells of the intestinal wall, which will in turn help the intestines regenerate a healthy brush barrier.

As we illustrated in the section on s-methylmethionine, many plants—especially leafy green vegetables—produce substances that will directly stimulate the rebuilding of the mucosal membrane within the stomach and intestines. In the case of s-methylmethionine, research has confirmed its ability to heal ulcers, colitis and gastritis. To this we added plant-based foods that stimulate enzyme activity and provide other nutrients used to produce a healthy mucosal membrane.

We also showed that probiotics help reverse intestinal permeability.

We must remember that the cells within the intestines have some of the fastest turnover rates of all the body's cells. Most of these cells will divide and be replaced by new cells within a week. While this doesn't necessarily mean we can heal the intestinal brush barrier within that short a period of time, it does mean that gradually, over several generations of new, healthier intestinal cells, the brush barrier can gradually be rebuilt.

Keeping Track: The Food Diary

The biggest pitfall in any food sensitivity is ignorance. Nearly every epidemiological study performed on food sensitivities underscores a similar problem: That many people assume they are allergic or intolerant to some food or food group without adequate confirmation. For this reason, professional consultation and testing along the lines discussed in the first chapter are required to confirm the sensitivity and whether it is a food allergy or an intolerance.

Even professional diagnosis can be difficult (and costly) to establish without careful tracking and self-assessment. It is one thing to have a negative reaction after we ate something. But it is quite another to have a severe response after we eat but not be clear on what food(s) caused that severe response. In this case, knowledge can literally save our lives.

The key is the food diary. A food diary simply allows for jotting down what foods are eaten at each meal and what (if any) responses followed. If there is any negative response later, that is also written into the food diary, along with the time and the severity. A sample diary format is given on the following page:

Food Diary

Meal Date/ Time	Foods Eaten	Reaction Time	Reaction Description	Reaction Severity (1-10)

Over some time, this diary should pinpoint those foods we might be sensitive to. The diary will also be an invaluable tool for any diagnostician to use. They will help us in a historical context, as we begin to adjust our diet, strengthen our immune system and explore oral tolerance strategies.

Conclusion: Putting it All Together

One of the possible solutions that we completely left out of this discussion was the *avoidance diet*. This is quite simply avoiding the offending food. This is actually probably the most clinically-applied treatment to food sensitivities in North America. And it has provided great success among those who have embraced it. We can also say that the majority of food sensitivity sufferers in Western countries have been told by their health professionals that there is no other option: We have a food sensitivity and that's that. While we might accidentally outgrow it someday, we are pretty much stuck with it. *So live with it,* we are told.

Yet we find that this very advice, which includes the fact that a person may outgrow a food sensitivity, says something extremely important: *We can outgrow our food sensitivities.* This says, basically, that it is *possible.* And not only is it possible, but a very large segment of the population that contracts a food sensitivity will outgrow it.

The point that Western physicians seem to be missing is that since the body *can* outgrow it, there must be a *mechanism* for outgrowing an allergy. After all, the body is not a lottery system, where some people just so happen to get lucky while others are not so lucky. This sort of mind-set would also lead us to the conclusion that it wouldn't matter if we dropped an atomic bomb on a city, because everything is simply luck.

The fact is, those who have outgrown their sensitivities experienced a modulation of their immune system. Their immune system began tolerating something they were previously sensitive to. How does this occur?

We have discussed the mechanics of this at length in this book. By strengthening the immune system, *we increase the ability of the immune system to adapt to and tolerate what is not inherently dangerous.*

By strengthening our immune system, we give our bodies the ability to recognize that a peanut protein is not really life-threatening. We give the immune system the ability to re-adjust its priorities to what is *really* life-threatening.

Furthermore, we have shown how a burdened, weakened immune system can become hypersensitive to those foods that should be getting broken down and supplying the body with nutrients.

All of the nutritional, herbal, probiotic and lifestyle information in this text illustrates *scientifically proven* methods to unburden and strengthen the immune system. These methods are not simply the opinions of the author. These methods are not simply a particular fad diet or innovative therapy. They are peer-reviewed, tried-and-true methods that have been proven to strengthen the immune system and/or specifically help the immune system adapt to those foods that our immune systems might have mistakenly become sensitive to.

This doesn't mean, however, that we will not have to partake in an elimination diet while we work on strengthening our immune system. No part of this text has suggested that a person simply ignore the body's responses and arbitrarily begin to gorge on the food. While eating the offending food might be a reasonable goal, there is a safe approach, as we've discussed.

Remember also that this discussion is for research purposes, and the food-sensitive person should consult with their health professional before making radical changes to their diet, supplementation and/or lifestyle.

There are numerous herbs, formulas, foods and lifestyle changes suggested in this chapter. Some may apply to a particular situation while others won't apply or could even worsen the condition. This of course depends largely upon the type of food sensitivity, ones particular constitution, and the manner of application of the strategy. This is one reason to be in consultation with a health professional who has expertise in these areas, especially for a person with severe reactions.

Another reason is that choosing the right herbal formulation of herbs can be downright complex. The reader may have noticed that there were several Chinese and Ayurvedic formulations discussed in this chapter. In other words, not even a Traditional Chinese Medicine doctor or Ayurvedic doctor will necessarily recommend the same thing to different people. Doctors of Chinese medicine and Ayurvedic medicine will carefully review the constitution of the patient and specify those herbs that apply to the particular constitution of the patient.

One way to utilize this text might be to present the book to ones health professional. Perhaps they already know how to apply many of these strategies. Or perhaps they are unaware of some of them. Or they are unaware of the research showing how efficacious some of these methods are. At the very least, they may be open enough to look through the research and suggest a program that integrates some of these with their current treatment strategy.

This does not mean that a person cannot, assuming they are not anaphylactic, have consulted with a health professional about the nature of their sensitivity and/or have a level of education that permits them to select those herbs and foods that most apply to their constitution. But the reader must understand that this text is not a prescription for any particular situation. It is an educational reference.

The reader must understand that there are so many different types of food sensitivities, from IgE allergies to simple intolerances. There are as many foods that one can be sensitive to as there are foods. And there are a host of different scenarios that can create a food sensitivity. We can almost say that practically every food sensitivity case is as unique as each person. Therefore, to offer any general prescriptive scenario for dealing with this expanse of uniqueness would be seriously short-sighted, and misleading to the reader.

What we have done is offered well-founded and tested techniques that have been peer-reviewed by modern scientists and/or traditional healers over the centuries. We have provided the background and research on techniques that have been effective for more than a few people, and have been clinically applied repeatedly.

The bottom line of this text is that we should not give up on our body's ability to heal itself. We must not assume that our body is a static machine programmed forever to have certain food sensitivities. We should not assume that a food sensitivity is a life sentence.

To the contrary, we can see from the research provided here that the human body is a highly fluid mechanism. The immune systems and its relative tolerances can quite often change. The immune system might be able to easily fight off a rhinovirus exposure immediately with no cold symptoms one day, and yet succumb to a 3-5 day hold-down of sneezing and coughing to the same type of exposure another day. What was the difference? Was the rhinovirus stronger in the latter case? Possibly, but not likely. What is more likely is that the immune system was weaker in the latter case. The immune system had to resort to a more urgent technique to remove the virus infection, due to its weakened state or the level of exposure. The immune system was weaker than the exposure, in other words.

The body is a fluid mechanism. We know that every cell in the body will die and be replaced by a new cell within about every seven years. Intestinal cells, as discussed above, will be replaced within just a few days. Some nerve and stem cells may live a bit longer. But every other cell—within every organ and tissue system in the body—will be replaced within weeks or months. Furthermore, the cells are constantly recycling molecules and nutrients over their life spans. In fact, researchers have determined that the body will have an entirely new molecular constitution at least every five years.

In other words, the molecules within our body are constantly being replaced by new molecules. The old molecules are purged and sent into the environment, and new ones are coming in from our foods, water and environment. This means that, from a molecular basis, within five years we will have a different body: A body replaced by new molecules and cells. This might be compared to looking at a waterfall: The waterfall might look the same, but the water that makes up the waterfall is constantly changing.

Therefore, there is no reason why our bodies cannot undergo change. There is no reason why the body's immune cells cannot become tolerant to something they were previously sensitive to. The research supports this. A majority of children outgrow allergies and food intolerances. Many adults also grow out of food sensitivities. And most of us will become temporarily sensitive to one food or another sometime in our lifetimes.

The message here is quite simple: Consider the body a fluid molecular machine. Is it well-oiled? Is it well-maintained? Are we taking care of it? Are we putting the best molecular fuel in it? Just as in any machine, the better the fuel, the better it runs. The body is no different.

Let's encourage our body to change for the better by feeding it better molecular fuel. The reward will be more than just becoming tolerant to a few foods. The bigger reward will be more resistance to disease, clearer thinking, a better heart, more stamina, and a more-productive life.

References and Bibliography

Abbott M, Hayward S, Ross W, Godefroy SB, Ulberth F, Van Hengel AJ, Roberts J, Akiyama H, Popping B, Yeung JM, Wehling P, Taylor SL, Poms RE, Delahaut P. Validation procedures for quantitative food allergen ELISA methods: community guidance and best practices. *J AOAC Int.* 2010 Mar-Apr;93(2):442-50.

Adel-Patient K, Ah-Leung S, Creminon C, Nouaille S, Chatel JM, Langella P, Wal JM. Oral administration of recombinant Lactococcus lactis expressing bovine beta-lactoglobulin partially prevents mice from sensitization. *Clin Exp Allergy.* 2005 Apr;35(4):539-46.

Aggarwal BB, Harikumar KB. Potential therapeutic effects of curcumin, the anti-inflammatory agent, against neurodegenerative, cardiovascular, pulmonary, metabolic, autoimmune and neoplastic diseases. *Int J Biochem Cell Biol.* 2009 Jan;41(1):40-59.

Aggarwal BB, Sung B. Pharmacological basis for the role of curcumin in chronic diseases: an age-old spice with modern targets. *Trends Pharmacol Sci.* 2009 Feb;30(2):85-94.

Agne PS, Bidat E, Agne PS, Rance F, Paty E. Sesame seed allergy in children. *Eur Ann Allergy Clin Immunol.* 2004 Oct;36(8):300-5.

Agostoni C, Fiocchi A, Riva E, Terracciano L, Sarratud T, Martelli A, Lodi F, D'Auria E, Zuccotti G, Giovannini M. Growth of infants with IgE-mediated cow's milk allergy fed different formulas in the complementary feeding period. *Pediatr Allergy Immunol.* 2007 Nov;18(7):599-606.

Ahmed T, Fuchs GJ. Gastrointestinal allergy to food: a review. *J Diarrhoeal Dis Res.* 1997 Dec;15(4):211-23.

Aho K, Koskenvuo M, Tuominen J, Kaprio J. Occurrence of rheumatoid arthritis in a nationwide series of twins. *J Rheumatol.* 1986 Oct;13(5):899-902.

Airola P. *How to Get Well.* Phoenix, AZ: Health Plus, 1974.

Akkol EK, Güvenç A, Yesilada E. A comparative study on the antinociceptive and anti-inflammatory activities of five Juniperus taxa. *J Ethnopharmacol.* 2009 Jun 6.

Alemán A, Sastre J, Quirce S, de las Heras M, Carnés J, Fernández-Caldas E, Pastor C, Blázquez AB, Vivanco F, Cuesta-Herranz J. Allergy to kiwi: a double-blind, placebo-controlled food challenge study in patients from a birch-free area. *J Allergy Clin Immunol.* 2004 Mar;113(3):543-50.

Alexander DD, Cabana MD. Partially hydrolyzed 100% whey protein infant formula and reduced risk of atopic dermatitis: a meta-analysis. *J Pediatr Gastroenterol Nutr.* 2010 Apr;50(4):422-30.

Alexandrakis M, Letourneau R, Kempuraj D, Kandere-Grzybowska K, Huang M, Christodoulou S, Boucher W, Seretakis D, Theoharides TC. Flavones inhibit Proliferation and increase mediator content in human leukemic mast cells (HMC-1). *Eur J Haematol.* 2003 Dec;71(6):448-54.

Al-Harrasi A, Al-Saidi S. Phytochemical analysis of the essential oil from botanically certified oleogum resin of Boswellia sacra (Omani Luban). *Molecules.* 2008 Sep 16;13(9):2181-9.

Almqvist C, Garden F, Xuan W, Mihrshahi S, Leeder SR, Oddy W, Webb K, Marks GB; CAPS team. Omega-3 and omega-6 fatty acid exposure from early life does not affect atopy and asthma at age 5 years. *J Allergy Clin Immunol.* 2007 Jun;119(6):1438-44.

Al-Mustafa AH, Al-Thunibat OY. Antioxidant activity of some Jordanian medicinal plants used traditionally for treatment of diabetes. *Pak J Biol Sci.* 2008 Feb 1;11(3):351-8.

Altman RD, Marcussen KC. Effects of a ginger extract on knee pain in patients with osteoarthritis. *Arthritis Rheum.* 2001 Nov;44(11):2531-8.

Amato R, Pinelli M, Monticelli A, Miele G, Cocozza S. Schizophrenia and Vitamin D Related Genes Could Have Been Subject to Latitude-driven Adaptation. *BMC Evol Biol.* 2010 Nov 11;10(1):351.

American Conference of Governmental Industrial Hygienists. *Threshold limit values for chemical substances and physical agents in the work environment.* Cincinnati, OH: ACGIH, 1986.

American Dietetic Association; Dietitians of Canada. Position of the American Dietetic Association and Dietitians of Canada: vegetarian diets. *Can J Diet Pract Res.* 2003 Summer;64(2):62-81.

Ammon HP. Boswellic acids in chronic inflammatory diseases. *Planta Med.* 2006 Oct;72(12):1100-16.

Anand P, Thomas SG, Kunnumakkara AB, Sundaram C, Harikumar KB, Sung B, Tharakan ST, Misra K, Priyadarsini IK, Rajasekharan KN, Aggarwal BB. Biological activities of curcumin and its analogues (Congeners) made by man and Mother Nature. *Biochem Pharmacol.* 2008 Dec 1;76(11):1590-611.

Anderson JL, May HT, Horne BD, Bair TL, Hall NL, Carlquist JF, Lappé DL, Muhlestein JB; Intermountain Heart Collaborative (IHC) Study Group. Relation of vitamin D deficiency to cardiovascular risk factors, disease status, and incident events in a general healthcare population. *Am J Cardiol.* 2010 Oct 1;106(7):963-8.

Anderson RC, Anderson JH. Acute toxic effects of fragrance products. *Arch Environ Health.* 1998 Mar-Apr;53(2):138-46.

Andoh T, Zhang Q, Yamamoto T, Tayama M, Hattori M, Tanaka K, Kuraishi Y. Inhibitory Effects of the Methanol Extract of Ganoderma lucidum on Mosquito Allergy-Induced Itch-Associated Responses in Mice. *J Pharmacol Sci.* 2010 Oct 8.

Andre C, Andre F, Colin L, Cavagna S. Measurement of intestinal permeability to mannitol and lactulose as a means of diagnosing food allergy and evaluating therapeutic effectiveness of disodium cromoglycate. Ann Allergy. 1987 Nov;59(5 Pt 2):127-30.

André C, André F, Colin L. Effect of allergen ingestion challenge with and without cromoglycate cover on intestinal permeability in atopic dermatitis, urticaria and other symptoms of food allergy. *Allergy*. 1989;44 Suppl 9:47-51.

André C. Food allergy. Objective diagnosis and test of therapeutic efficacy by measuring intestinal permeability. *Presse Med.* 1986 Jan 25;15(3):105-8.

Andre F, Andre C, Feknous M, Colin L, Cavagna S. Digestive permeability to different-sized molecules and to sodium cromoglycate in food allergy. *Allergy Proc.* 1991 Sep-Oct;12(5):293-8.

Angioni A, Barra A, Russo MT, Coroneo V, Dessi S, Cabras P. Chemical composition of the essential oils of Juniperus from ripe and unripe berries and leaves and their antimicrobial activity. *J Agric Food Chem.* 2003 May 7;51(10):3073-8.

Anim-Nyame N, Sooranna SR, Johnson MR, Gamble J, Steer PJ. Garlic supplementation increases peripheral blood flow: a role for interleukin-6? *J Nutr Biochem.* 2004 Jan;15(1):30-6.

Annweiler C, Schott AM, Berrut G, Chauviré V, Le Gall D, Inzitari M, Beauchet O. Vitamin D and ageing: neurological issues. *Neuropsychobiology.* 2010 Aug;62(3):139-50.

Aoki T, Usuda Y, Miyakoshi M, Tamura K, Herberman RB. Low natural killer syndrome: clinical and immunologic features. *Nat Immun Cell Growth Regul.* 1987;6(3):116-28.

Apáti P, Houghton PJ, Kite G, Steventon GB, Kéry A. In-vitro effect of flavonoids from Solidago canadensis extract on glutathione S-transferase. *J Pharm Pharmacol.* 2006 Feb;58(2):251-6.

APHA (American Public Health Association). Opposition to the Use of Hormone Growth Promoters in Beef and Dairy Cattle Production. Policy Date: 11/10/2009. Policy Number: 20098. http://www.apha.org/advocacy/policy/id=1379. Accessed Nov. 24, 2010.

Araki K, Shinozaki T, Irie Y, Miyazawa Y. Trial of oral administration of Bifidobacterium breve for the prevention of rotavirus infections. *Kansenshogaku Zasshi.* 1999 Apr;73(4):305-10.

Argento A, Tiraferri E, Marzaloni M. Oral anticoagulants and medicinal plants. An emerging interaction. *Ann Ital Med Int.* 2000 Apr-Jun;15(2):139-43.

Arshad SH, Bateman B, Sadeghnejad A, Gant C, Matthews SM. Prevention of allergic disease during childhood by allergen avoidance: the Isle of Wight prevention study. *J Allergy Clin Immunol.* 2007 Feb;119(2):307-13.

Arslan G, Kahrs GE, Lind R, Froyland L, Florvaag E, Berstad A. Patients with subjective food hypersensitivity: the value of analyzing intestinal permeability and inflammation markers in gut lavage fluid. *Digestion.* 2004;70(1):26-35.

Arslanoglu S, Moro GE, Schmitt J, Tandoi L, Rizzardi S, Boehm G. Early dietary intervention with a mixture of prebiotic oligosaccharides reduces the incidence of allergic manifestations and infections during the first two years of life. *J Nutr.* 2008 Jun;138(6):1091-5.

Arterburn LM, Oken HA, Bailey Hall E, Hamersley J, Kuratko CN, Hoffman JP. Algal-oil capsules and cooked salmon: nutritionally equivalent sources of docosahexaenoic acid. *J Am Diet Assoc.* 2008 Jul;108(7):1204-9.

Arterburn LM, Oken HA, Hoffman JP, Bailey-Hall E, Chung G, Rom D, Hamersley J, McCarthy D. Bioequivalence of Docosahexaenoic acid from different algal oils in capsules and in a DHA-fortified food. *Lipids.* 2007 Nov;42(11):1011-24.

Asero R, Antonicelli L, Arena A, Bommarito L, Caruso B, Colombo G, Crivellaro M, De Carli M, Della Torre E, Della Torre F, Heffler E, Lodi Rizzini F, Longo R, Manzotti G, Marcotulli M, Melchiorre A, Minale P, Morandi P, Moreni B, Moschella A, Murzilli F, Nebiolo F, Poppa M, Randazzo S, Rossi G, Senna GE. Causes of food-induced anaphylaxis in Italian adults: a multi-centre study. *Int Arch Allergy Immunol.* 2009;150(3):271-7.

Asero R, Antonicelli L, Arena A, Bommarito L, Caruso B, Crivellaro M, De Carli M, Della Torre E, Della Torre F, Heffler E, Lodi Rizzini F, Longo R, Manzotti G, Marcotulli M, Melchiorre A, Minale P, Morandi P, Moreni B, Moschella A, Murzilli F, Nebiolo F, Poppa M, Randazzo S, Rossi G, Senna GE. EpidemAAITO: features of food allergy in Italian adults attending allergy clinics: a multi-centre study. *Clin Exp Allergy.* 2009 Apr;39(4):547-55.

Asero R, Mistrello G, Roncarolo D, Amato S, Caldironi G, Barocci F, van Ree R. Immunological cross-reactivity between lipid transfer proteins from botanically unrelated plant-derived foods: a clinical study. *Allergy.* 2002 Oct;57(10):900-6.

Ashrafi K, Chang FY, Watts JL, Fraser AG, Kamath RS, Ahringer J, Ruvkun G. Genome-wide RNAi analysis of Caenorhabditis elegans fat regulatory genes. *Nature.* 2003 Jan 16;421(6920):268-72.

Atkinson W, Sheldon TA, Shaath N, Whorwell PJ. Food elimination based on IgG antibodies in irritable bowel syndrome: a randomised controlled trial. *Gut.* 2004 Oct;53(10):1459-64.

Atsumi T, Tonosaki K. Smelling lavender and rosemary increases free radical scavenging activity and decreases cortisol level in saliva. *Psychiatry Res.* 2007 Feb 28;150(1):89-96.

Bachas-Daunert S, Deo SK. Should genetically modified foods be abandoned on the basis of allergenicity? *Anal Bioanal Chem.* 2008 Oct;392(3):341-6.

Badar VA, Thawani VR, Wakode PT, Shrivastava MP, Gharpure KJ, Hingorani LL, Khiyani RM. Efficacy of Tinospora cordifolia in allergic rhinitis. *J Ethnopharmacol.* 2005 Jan 15;96(3):445-9.

Baker DH. Comparative nutrition and metabolism: explication of open questions with emphasis on protein and amino acids. *Proc Natl Acad Sci U S A.* 2005 Dec 13;102(50):17897-902.

Baker SM. *Detoxification and Healing.* Chicago: Contemporary Books, 2004.

Balch P, Balch J. *Prescription for Nutritional Healing.* New York: Avery, 2000.

Ballentine R. *Diet & Nutrition: A holistic approach.* Honesdale, PA: Himalayan Int., 1978.

Ballentine R. *Radical Healing.* New York: Harmony Books, 1999.

Ballmer-Weber BK, Hoffmann A, Wüthrich B, Lüttkopf D, Pompei C, Wangorsch A, Kästner M, Vieths S. Influence of food processing on the allergenicity of celery: DBPCFC with celery spice and cooked celery in patients with celery allergy. *Allergy.* 2002 Mar;57(3):228-35.

Ballmer-Weber BK, Holzhauser T, Scibilia J, Mittag D, Zisa G, Ortolani C, Oesterballe M, Poulsen LK, Vieths S, Bindslev-Jensen C. Clinical characteristics of soybean allergy in Europe: a double-blind, placebo-controlled food challenge study. *J Allergy Clin Immunol.* 2007 Jun;119(6):1489-96.

Ballmer-Weber BK, Vieths S, Lüttkopf D, Heuschmann P, Wüthrich B. Celery allergy confirmed by double-blind, placebo-controlled food challenge: a clinical study in 32 subjects with a history of adverse reactions to celery root. *J Allergy Clin Immunol.* 2000 Aug;106(2):373-8.

Banno N, Akihisa T, Yasukawa K, Tokuda H, Tabata K, Nakamura Y, Nishimura R, Kimura Y, Suzuki T. Anti-inflammatory activities of the triterpene acids from the resin of Boswellia carteri. *J Ethnopharmacol.* 2006 Sep 19;107(2):249-53.

Bant A, Kruszewski J. Increased sensitization prevalence to common inhalant and food allergens in young adult Polish males. *Ann Agric Environ Med.* 2008 Jun;15(1):21-7.

Barau E, Dupont C. Modifications of intestinal permeability during food provocation procedures in pediatric irritable bowel syndrome. *J Pediatr Gastroenterol Nutr.* 1990 Jul;11(1):72-7.

Barnes M, Cullinan P, Athanasaki P, MacNeill S, Hole AM, Harris J, Kalogeraki S, Chatzinikolaou M, Drakonakis N, Bibaki-Liakou V, Newman Taylor AJ, Bibakis I. Crete: does farming explain urban and rural differences in atopy? *Clin Exp Allergy.* 2001 Dec;31(12):1822-8.

Barnetson RS, Drummond H, Ferguson A. Precipitins to dietary proteins in atopic eczema. *Br J Dermatol.* 1983 Dec;109(6):653-5.

Barrager E, Veltmann JR Jr, Schauss AG, Schiller RN. A multicentered, open-label trial on the safety and efficacy of methylsulfonylmethane in the treatment of seasonal allergic rhinitis. *J Altern Complement Med.* 2002 Apr;8(2):167-73.

Basu A, Devaraj S, Jialal I. Dietary factors that promote or retard inflammation. *Arterioscler Thromb Vasc Biol.* 2006 May;26(5):995-1001.

Bateman B, Warner JO, Hutchinson E, Dean T, Rowlandson P, Gant C, Grundy J, Fitzgerald C, Stevenson J. The effects of a double blind, placebo controlled, artificial food colourings and benzoate preservative challenge on hyperactivity in a general population sample of preschool children. *Arch Dis Child.* 2004 Jun;89(6):506-11.

Batista R, Martins I, Jeno P, Ricardo CP, Oliveira MM. A proteomic study to identify soya allergens—the human response to transgenic versus non-transgenic soya samples. *Int Arch Allergy Immunol.* 2007;144(1):29-38.

Batmanghelidj F. Neurotransmitter histamine: an alternative view point, *Science in Medicine Simplified.* Falls Church, VA: Foundation for the Simple in Medicine, 1990.

Batmanghelidj F. Pain: a need for paradigm change. *Anticancer Res.* 1987 Sep-Oct;7(5B):971-89.

Batmanghelidj F. *Your Body's Many Cries for Water.* 2nd Ed. Vienna, VA: Global Health, 1997.

Beasley R, Clayton T, Crane J, von Mutius E, Lai CK, Montefort S, Stewart A; ISAAC Phase Three Study Group. Association between paracetamol use in infancy and childhood, and risk of asthma, rhinoconjunctivitis, and eczema in children aged 6-7 years: analysis from Phase Three of the ISAAC programme. *Lancet.* 2008 Sep. 20;372(9643):1039-48.

Becker KG, Simon RM, Bailey-Wilson JE, Freidlin B, Biddison WE, McFarland HF, Trent JM. Clustering of non-major histocompatibility complex susceptibility candidate loci in human autoimmune diseases. *Proc Natl Acad Sci U S A.* 1998 Aug 18;95(17):9979-84.

Beddoe AF. *Biologic Ionization as Applied to Human Nutrition.* Warsaw: Wendell Whitman, 2002.

Beecher GR. Phytonutrients' role in metabolism: effects on resistance to degenerative processes. *Nutr Rev.* 1999 Sep;57(9 Pt 2):S3-6.

Belcaro G, Cesarone MR, Errichi S, Zulli C, Errichi BM, Vinciguerra G, Ledda A, Di Renzo A, Stuard S, Dugall M, Pellegrini L, Gizzi G, Ippolito E, Ricci A, Cacchio M, Cipollone G, Ruffini I, Fano F, Hosoi

M, Rohdewald P. Variations in C-reactive protein, plasma free radicals and fibrinogen values in patients with osteoarthritis treated with Pycnogenol. *Redox Rep.* 2008;13(6):271-6.

Bell IR, Baldwin CM, Schwartz GE, Illness from low levels of environmental chemicals: relevance to chronic fatigue syndrome and fibromyalgia. *Am J Med.* 1998;105 (suppl 3A).:74-82. S.

Bell SJ, Potter PC. Milk whey-specific immune complexes in allergic and non-allergic subjects. *Allergy.* 1988 Oct;43(7):497-503.

Bellanti JA, Zeligs BJ, Malka-Rais J, Sabra A. Abnormalities of Th1 function in non-IgE food allergy, celiac disease, and ileal lymphonodular hyperplasia: a new relationship? Ann *Allergy Asthma Immunol.* 2003 Jun;90(6 Suppl 3):84-9.

Ben, X.M., Zhou, X.Y., Zhao, W.H., Yu, W.L., Pan, W., Zhang, W.L., Wu, S.M., Van Beusekom, C.M., Schaafsma, A. (2004) Supplementation of milk formula with galactooligosaccharides improves intestinal micro-flora and fermentation in term infants. *Chin Med J.* 117(6):927-931, 2004.

Benard A, Desreumeaux P, Huglo D, Hoorelbeke A, Tonnel AB, Wallaert B. Increased intestinal permeability in bronchial asthma. *J Allergy Clin Immunol.* 1996 Jun;97(6):1173-8.

Bengmark S. Curcumin, an atoxic antioxidant and natural NFkappaB, cyclooxygenase-2, lipooxygenase, and inducible nitric oxide synthase inhibitor: a shield against acute and chronic diseases. *JPEN J Parenter Enteral Nutr.* 2006 Jan-Feb;30(1):45-51.

Bengmark S. Immunonutrition: role of biosurfactants, fiber, and probiotic bacteria. Nutrition. 1998 Jul-Aug;14(7-8):585-94.

Benlounes N, Dupont C, Candalh C, Blaton MA, Darmon N, Desjeux JF, Heyman M. The threshold for immune cell reactivity to milk antigens decreases in cow's milk allergy with intestinal symptoms. *J Allergy Clin Immunol.* 1996 Oct;98(4):781-9.

Ben-Shoshan M, Harrington DW, Soller L, Fragapane J, Joseph L, St Pierre Y, Godefroy SB, Elliot SJ, Clarke AE. A population-based study on peanut, tree nut, fish, shellfish, and sesame allergy prevalence in Canada. *J Allergy Clin Immunol.* 2010 Jun;125(6):1327-35.

Ben-Shoshan M, Kagan R, Primeau MN, Alizadehfar R, Turnbull E, Harada L, Dufresne C, Allen M, Joseph L, St Pierre Y, Clarke A. Establishing the diagnosis of peanut allergy in children never exposed to peanut or with an uncertain history: a cross-Canada study. *Pediatr Allergy Immunol.* 2010 Sep;21(6):920-6.

Bensky D, Gable A, Kaptchuk T (transl.). *Chinese Herbal Medicine Materia Medica.* Seattle: Eastland Press, 1986.

Bentz S, Hausmann M, Piberger H, Kellermeier S, Paul S, Held L, Falk W, Obermeier F, Fried M, Schölmerich J, Rogler G. Clinical relevance of IgG antibodies against food antigens in Crohn's disease: a double-blind cross-over diet intervention study. *Digestion.* 2010;81(4):252-64.

Bergner P. *The Healing Power of Garlic.* Prima Publishing, Rocklin CA 1996.

Berin MC, Yang PC, Ciok L, Waserman S, Perdue MH. Role for IL-4 in macromolecular transport across human intestinal epithelium. Am J Physiol. 1999 May;276(5 Pt 1):C1046-52.

Berkow R., (Ed.) *The Merck Manual of Diagnosis and Therapy.* 16th Edition. Rahway, N.J.: Merck Research Labs, 1992.

Berseth CL, Mitmesser SH, Ziegler EE, Marunycz JD, Vanderhoof J. Tolerance of a standard intact protein formula versus a partially hydrolyzed formula in healthy, term infants. Nutr J. 2009 Jun 19;8:27.

Berteau O and Mulloy B. 2003. Sulfated fucans, fresh perspectives: structures, functions, and biological properties of sulfated fucans and an overview of enzymes active toward this class of polysaccharide. *Glycobiology.* Jun;13(6):29R-40R.

Beyer K, Morrow E, Li XM, Bardina L, Bannon GA, Burks AW, Sampson HA. Effects of cooking methods on peanut allergenicity. *J Allergy Clin Immunol.* 2001;107:1077-81.

Bhandari U, Sharma JN, Zafar R. The protective action of ethanolic ginger (Zingiber officinale) extract in cholesterol fed rabbits. *J Ethnopharmacol.* 1998 Jun;61(2):167-71.

Bielory BP, Perez VL, Bielory L. Treatment of seasonal allergic conjunctivitis with ophthalmic corticosteroids: in search of the perfect ocular corticosteroid in the treatment of allergic conjunctivitis. *Curr Opin Allergy Clin Immunol.* 2010 Oct;10(5):469-77.

Bielory L, Lupoli K. Herbal interventions in asthma and allergy. *J Asthma.* 1999;36:1–65.

Bielory L, Russin J, Zuckerman GB. Clinical efficacy, mechanisms of action, and adverse effects of complementary and alternative medicine therapies for asthma. *Allergy Asthma Proc.* 2004;25:283–91.

Bindslev-Jensen C, Skov PS, Roggen EL, Hvass P, Brinch DS. Investigation on possible allergenicity of 19 different commercial enzymes used in the food industry. *Food Chem Toxicol.* 2006 Nov;44(11):1909-15.

Biro FM, Galvez MP, Greenspan LC, Succop PA, Vangeepuram N, Pinney SM, Teitelbaum S, Windham GC, Kushi LH, Wolff MS. Pubertal assessment method and baseline characteristics in a mixed longitudinal study of girls. *Pediatrics.* 2010 Sep;126(3):e583-90.

Bischoff SC. Food allergy and eosinophilic gastroenteritis and colitis. *Curr Opin Allergy Clin Immunol.* 2010 Jun;10(3):238-45.

Bjarnason I, MacPherson A, Hollander D. Intestinal permeability: an overview. *Gastroenterology.* 1995 May;108(5):1566-81.

REFERENCES AND BIBLIOGRAPHY

Bjornsson E, Janson C, Plaschke P, Norrman E, Sjoberg O (1996) Prevalence of sensitization to food allergies in adult Swedes. *Ann Allergy Asthma Immunol.* 77: 327–332.

Blázquez AB, Mayer L, Berin MC. Thymic Stromal Lymphopoietin Is Required for Gastrointestinal Allergy but Not Oral Tolerance. *Gastroenterology.* 2010 Jun 23.

Boccafogli A, Vicentini L, Camerani A, Cogliati P, D'Ambrosi A, Scolozzi R. Adverse food reactions in patients with grass pollen allergic respiratory disease. *Ann Allergy.* 1994 Oct;73(4):301-8.

Bode C, Bode JC. Effect of alcohol consumption on the gut. *Best Pract Res Clin Gastroenterol.* 2003 Aug;17(4):575-92.

Bodinier M, Legoux MA, Pineau F, Triballeau S, Segain JP, Brossard C, Denery-Papini S. Intestinal translocation capabilities of wheat allergens using the Caco-2 cell line. *J Agric Food Chem.* 2007 May 30;55(11):4576-83.

Boehm, G., Lidestri, M., Casetta, P., Jelinek, J., Negretti, F., Stahl, B., Martini, A. (2002) Supplementation of a bovine milk formula with an oligosaccharide mixture increases counts of faecal bifidobacteria in preterm infants. *Arch Dis Child Fetal Neonatal Ed.* 86: F178-F181

Bolhaar ST, Tiemessen MM, Zuidmeer L, van Leeuwen A, Hoffmann-Sommergruber K, Bruijnzeel-Koomen CA, Taams LS, Knol EF, van Hoffen E, van Ree R, Knulst AC. Efficacy of birch-pollen immunotherapy on cross-reactive food allergy confirmed by skin tests and double-blind food challenges. *Clin Exp Allergy.* 2004 May;34(5):761-9.

Bolleddula J, Goldfarb J, Wang R, Sampson H, Li XM. Synergistic Modulation Of Eotaxin And Il-4 Secretion By Constituents Of An Anti-asthma Herbal Formula (ASHMI) In Vitro. *J Allergy Clin Immunol.* 2007;119:S172.

Bongartz D, Hesse A. Selective extraction of quercetrin in vegetable drugs and urine by off-line coupling of boronic acid affinity chromatography and high-performance liquid chromatography. *J Chromatogr B Biomed Appl.* 1995 Nov 17;673(2):223-30.

Bongaerts GP, Severijnen RS. Preventive and curative effects of probiotics in atopic patients. *Med Hypotheses.* 2005;64(6):1089-92.

Borchers AT, Hackman RM, Keen CL, Stern JS, Gershwin ME. Complementary medicine: a review of immunomodulatory effects of Chinese herbal medicines. *Am J Clin Nutr.* 1997 Dec;66(6):1303-12.

Borchert VE, Czyborra P, Fetscher C, Goepel M, Michel MC. Extracts from Rhois aromatica and Solidaginis virgaurea inhibit rat and human bladder contraction. *Naunyn Schmiedebergs Arch Pharmacol.* 2004 Mar;369(3):281-6.

Böttcher MF, Jenmalm MC, Voor T, Julge K, Holt PG, Björkstén B. Cytokine responses to allergens during the first 2 years of life in Estonian and Swedish children. *Clin Exp Allergy.* 2006 May;36(5):619-28.

Bouchez-Mahiout I, Pecquet C, Kerre S, Snégaroff J, Raison-Peyron N, Laurière M. High molecular weight entities in industrial wheat protein hydrolysates are immunoreactive with IgE from allergic patients. *J Agric Food Chem.* 2010 Apr 14;58(7):4207-15.

Boverhof DR, Gollapudi BB, Hotchkiss JA, Osterloh-Quiroz M, Woolhiser MR. A draining lymph node assay (DLNA) for assessing the sensitizing potential of proteins. *Toxicol Lett.* 2010 Mar 15;193(2):144-51.

Boyce JA, Assa'ad A, Burks AW, Jones SM, Sampson HA, Wood RA, Plaut M, Cooper SF, Fenton MJ. Guidelines for the Diagnosis and Management of Food Allergy in the United State. *Natl Instit of Health.* 2010 Dec. NIH Publ No. 11-7700.

Bradette-Hébert ME, Legault J, Lavoie S, Pichette A. A new labdane diterpene from the flowers of Solidago canadensis. *Chem Pharm Bull.* 2008 Jan;56(1):82-4.

Brandtzaeg P. Food allergy: separating the science from the mythology. *Nat Rev Gastroenterol Hepatol.* 2010 Jul;7(7):380-400.

Breuer K, Heratizadeh A, Wulf A, Baumann U, Constien A, Tetau D, Kapp A, Werfel T. Late eczematous reactions to food in children with atopic dermatitis. *Clin Exp Allergy.* 2004 May;34(5):817-24.

Brewster DR, Manary MJ, Menzies IS, Henry RL, O'Loughlin EV. Comparison of milk and maize based diets in kwashiorkor. *Arch Dis Child.* 1997 Mar;76(3):242-8.

Brighenti F, Valtueña S, Pellegrini N, Ardigò D, Del Rio D, Salvatore S, Piatti P, Serafini M, Zavaroni I. Total antioxidant capacity of the diet is inversely and independently related to plasma concentration of high-sensitivity C-reactive protein in adult Italian subjects. *Br J Nutr.* 2005 May;93(5):619-25.

Brody J. *Jane Brody's Nutrition Book.* New York: WW Norton, 1981.

Brostoff J, Gamlin L, Brostoff J. *Food Allergies and Food Intolerance: The Complete Guide to Their Identification and Treatment.* Rochester, VT: Healing Arts, 2000.

Brownstein D. *Salt: Your Way to Health.* West Bloomfield, MI: Medical Alternatives, 2006.

Brown-Whitehorn TF, Spergel JM. The link between allergies and eosinophilic esophagitis: implications for management strategies. *Expert Rev Clin Immunol.* 2010 Jan;6(1):101-9.

Bublin M, Pfister M, Radauer C, Oberhuber C, Bulley S, Dewitt AM, Lidholm J, Reese G, Vieths S, Breiteneder H, Hoffmann-Sommergruber K, Ballmer-Weber BK. Component-resolved diagnosis of kiwifruit allergy with purified natural and recombinant kiwifruit allergens. *J Allergy Clin Immunol.* 2010 Mar;125(3):687-94, 694.e1.

Buchanan AD, Green TD, Jones SM, Scurlock AM, Christie L, Althage KA, Steele PH, Pons L, Helm RM, Lee LA, Burks AW. Egg oral immunotherapy in nonanaphylactic children with egg allergy. *J Allergy Clin Immunol.* 2007 Jan;119(1):199-205.

Bucher X, Pichler WJ, Dahinden CA, Helbling A. Effect of tree pollen specific, subcutaneous immunotherapy on the oral allergy syndrome to apple and hazelnut. *Allergy.* 2004 Dec;59(12):1272-6.

Budzianowski J. Coumarins, caffeoyltartaric acids and their artifactual methyl esters from Taraxacum officinale leaves. *Planta Med.* 1997 Jun;63(3):288.

Bueno L. Protease activated receptor 2: a new target for IBS treatment. *Eur Rev Med Pharmacol Sci.* 2008 Aug;12 Suppl 1:95-102.

Bundy R, Walker AF, Middleton RW, Booth J. Turmeric extract may improve irritable bowel syndrome symptomology in otherwise healthy adults: a pilot study. *J Altern Complement Med.* 2004 Dec;10(6):1015-8.

Burdge GC, Jones AE, Wootton SA. Eicosapentaenoic and docosapentaenoic acids are the principal products of alpha-linolenic acid metabolism in young men. *B J Nutr.* 2002 Oct;88(4):355-63.

Buret AG. How stress induces intestinal hypersensitivity. *Am J Pathol.* 2006 Jan;168(1):3-5.

Burits M, Asres K, Bucar F. The antioxidant activity of the essential oils of Artemisia afra, Artemisia abyssinica and Juniperus procera. *Phytother Res.* 2001 Mar;15(2):103-8.

Burks AW, James JM, Hiegel A, Wilson G, Wheeler JG, Jones SM, Zuerlein N. Atopic dermatitis and food hypersensitivity reactions. *J Pediatr.* 1998;132(1):132-6.

Burks W, Jones SM, Berseth CL, Harris C, Sampson HA, Scalabrin DM. Hypoallergenicity and effects on growth and tolerance of a new amino acid-based formula with docosahexaenoic acid and arachidonic acid. *J Pediatr.* 2008 Aug;153(2):266-71.

Burney PG, Luczynska C, Chinn S, Jarvis D (1994) The European Community Respiratory Health Survey. *Eur Respir J.* 7: 954–960.

Busse PJ, Wen MC, Huang CK, Srivastava K, Zhang TF, Schofield B, Sampson HA, Li XM. Therapeutic effects of the Chinese herbal formula, MSSM-03d, on persistent airway hyperreactivity and airway remodeling. *J Allergy Clin Immunol.* 2004;113:S220.

Butani L, Afshinnik A, Johnson J, Javaheri D, Peck S, German JB, Perez RV. Amelioration of tacrolimus-induced nephrotoxicity in rats using juniper oil. *Transplantation.* 2003 Jul 27;76(2):306-11.

Butkus SN, Mahan LK. Food allergies: immunological reactions to food. *J Am Diet Assoc.* 1986 May;86(5):601-8.

Byrne AM, Malka-Rais J, Burks AW, Fleischer DM. How do we know when peanut and tree nut allergy have resolved, and how do we keep it resolved? *Clin Exp Allergy.* 2010 Sep;40(9):1303-11.

Cabanillas B, Pedrosa MM, Rodríguez J, González A, Muzquiz M, Cuadrado C, Crespo JF, Burbano C. Effects of enzymatic hydrolysis on lentil allergenicity. *Mol Nutr Food Res.* 2010 Mar 19.

Caffarelli C, Coscia A, Baldi F, Borghi A, Capra L, Cazzato S, Migliozzi L, Pecorari L, Valenti A, Cavagni G. Characterization of irritable bowel syndrome and constipation in children with allergic diseases. *Eur J Pediatr.* 2007 Dec;166(12):1245-52.

Caffarelli C, Petroccione T. False-negative food challenges in children with suspected food allergy. *Lancet.* 2001 Dec 1;358(9296):1871-2.

Cahn J, Borzeix MG. Administration of procyanidolic oligomers in rats. Observed effects on changes in the permeability of the blood-brain barrier. *Sem Hop.* 1983 Jul 7;59(27-28):2031-4.

Calder PC. Dietary modification of inflammation with lipids. *Proc Nutr Soc.* 2002 Aug;61(3):345-58.

Calvani M, Giorgio V, Miceli Sopo S. Specific oral tolerance induction for food. A systematic review. *Eur Ann Allergy Clin Immunol.* 2010 Feb;42(1):11-9.

Caminiti L, Passalacqua G, Barberi S, Vita D, Barberio G, De Luca R, Pajno GB. A new protocol for specific oral tolerance induction in children with IgE-mediated cow's milk allergy. *Allergy Asthma Proc.* 2009 Jul-Aug;30(4):443-8.

Campbell TC, Campbell TM. *The China Study.* Dallas, TX: Benbella Books, 2006.

Canani RB, Ruotolo S, Auricchio L, Caldore M, Porcaro F, Manguso F, Terrin G, Troncone R. Diagnostic accuracy of the atopy patch test in children with food allergy-related gastrointestinal symptoms. *Allergy.* 2007 Jul;62(7):738-43.

Canonica GW, Passalacqua G. Noninjection routes for immunotherapy. *J Allergy Clin Immunol.* 2003 Mar;111(3):437-48; quiz 449.

Cantani A, Micera M. Natural history of cow's milk allergy. An eight-year follow-up study in 115 atopic children. *Eur Rev Med Pharmacol Sci.* 2004 Jul-Aug;8(4):153-64.

Cantani A, Micera M. The prick by prick test is safe and reliable in 58 children with atopic dermatitis and food allergy. *Eur Rev Med Pharmacol Sci.* 2006 May-Jun;10(3):115-20.

REFERENCES AND BIBLIOGRAPHY

Cao G, Alessio HM, Cutler RG. Oxygen-radical absorbance capacity assay for antioxidants. *Free Radic Biol Med.* 1993 Mar;14(3):303-11.

Cao G, Shukitt-Hale B, Bickford PC, Joseph JA, McEwen J, Prior RL. Hyperoxia-induced changes in antioxidant capacity and the effect of dietary antioxidants. *J Appl Physiol.* 1999 Jun;86(6):1817-22.

Caramia G. The essential fatty acids omega-6 and omega-3: from their discovery to their use in therapy. *Minerva Pediatr.* 2008 Apr;60(2):219-33.

Carroccio A, Cavataio F, Montalto G, D'Amico D, Alabrese L, Iacono G. Intolerance to hydrolysed cow's milk proteins in infants: clinical characteristics and dietary treatment. *Clin Exp Allergy.* 2000 Nov;30(11):1597-603.

Carroll D. *The Complete Book of Natural Medicines.* New York: Summit, 1980.

Caruso M, Frasca G, Di Giuseppe PL, Pennisi A, Tringali G, Bonina FP. Effects of a new nutraceutical ingredient on allergen-induced sulphidoleukotrienes production and CD63 expression in allergic subjects. *Int Immunopharmacol.* 2008 Dec 20;8(13-14):1781-6.

Cataldo F, Accomando S, Fragapane ML, Montaperto D; SIGENP and GLNBI Working Groups on Food Intolerances. Are food intolerances and allergies increasing in immigrant children coming from developing countries? *Pediatr Allergy Immunol.* 2006 Aug;17(5):364-9.

Cats A, Kuipers EJ, Bosschaert MA, Pot RG, Vandenbroucke-Grauls CM, Kusters JG. Effect of frequent consumption of a Lactobacillus casei-containing milk drink in Helicobacter pylori-colonized subjects. *Aliment Pharmacol Ther.* 2003 Feb;17(3):429-35.

Cavaleiro C, Pinto E, Gonçalves MJ, Salgueiro L. Antifungal activity of Juniperus essential oils against dermatophyte, Aspergillus and Candida strains. *J Appl Microbiol.* 2006 Jun;100(6):1333-8.

Celakovská J, Vaněčková J, Ettlerová K, Ettler K, Bukac J. The role of atopy patch test in diagnosis of food allergy in atopic eczema/dermatitis syndrom in patients over 14 years of age. *Acta Medica (Hradec Kralove).* 2010;53(2):101-8.

Celikel S, Karakaya G, Yurtsever N, Sorkun K, Kalyoncu AF. Bee and bee products allergy in Turkish beekeepers: determination of risk factors for systemic reactions. *Allergol Immunopathol (Madr).* 2006 Sep-Oct;34(5):180-4.

Cereijido M, Contreras RG, Flores-Benítez D, Flores-Maldonado C, Larre I, Ruiz A, Shoshani L. New diseases derived or associated with the tight junction. *Arch Med Res.* 2007 Jul;38(5):465-78.

Chafen JJ, Newberry SJ, Riedl MA, Bravata DM, Maglione M, Suttorp MJ, Sundaram V, Paige NM, Towfigh A, Hulley BJ, Shekelle PG. Diagnosing and managing common food allergies: a systematic review. *JAMA.* 2010 May 12;303(18):1848-56.

Chahine BG, Bahna SL. The role of the gut mucosal immunity in the development of tolerance versus development of allergy to food. *Curr Opin Allergy Clin Immunol.* 2010 Aug;10(4):394-9.

Chaitow L, Trenev N. *ProBiotics.* New York: Thorsons, 1990.

Chaitow L. *Conquer Pain the Natural Way.* San Francisco: Chronicle Books, 2002.

Chakürski I, Matev M, Koïchev A, Angelova I, Stefanov G. Treatment of chronic colitis with an herbal combination of Taraxacum officinale, Hipericum perforatum, Melissa officinaliss, Calendula officinalis and Foeniculum vulgare. *Vutr Boles.* 1981;20(6):51-4.

Chan CK, Kuo ML, Shen JJ, See LC, Chang HH, Huang JL. Ding Chuan Tang, a Chinese herb decoction, could improve airway hyper-responsiveness in stabilized asthmatic children: a randomized, double-blind clinical trial. *Pediatr Allergy Immunol.* 2006;17:316–22.

Chandra RK. Prospective studies of the effect of breast feeding on incidence of infection and allergy. *Acta Paediatr Scand.* 1979 Sep;68(5):691-4.

Chaney M, Ross M. *Nutrition.* New York: Houghton Mifflin, 1971.

Chang CI, Chen WC, Shao YY, Yeh GR, Yang NS, Chiang W, Kuo YH. A new labdane-type diterpene from the bark of Juniperus chinensis Linn. *Nat Prod Res.* 2008;22(13):1158-62.

Chang TT, Huang CC, Hsu CH. Clinical evaluation of the Chinese herbal medicine formula STA-1 in the treatment of allergic asthma. *Phytother Res.* 2006;20:342–7.

Chang TT, Huang CC, Hsu CH. Inhibition of mite-induced immunoglobulin E synthesis, airway inflammation, and hyperreactivity by herbal medicine STA-1. *Immunopharmacol Immunotoxicol.* 2006;28:683–95.

Chapat L, Chemin K, Dubois B, Bourdet-Sicard R, Kaiserlian D. Lactobacillus casei reduces CD8+ T cell-mediated skin inflammation. *Eur J Immunol.* 2004 Sep;34(9):2520-8.

Characterization and quantitation of Antioxidant Constituents of Sweet Pepper (Capsicum annuum - Cayenne). *J Agric Food Chem.* 2004 Jun 16;52(12):3861-9.

Charles K. Food allergies are becoming more common. *N.Y. Daily News.* 2008. May 20.

Chatzi L, Apostolaki G, Bibakis I, Skypala I, Bibaki-Liakou V, Tzanakis N, Kogevinas M, Cullinan P. Protective effect of fruits, vegetables and the Mediterranean diet on asthma and allergies among children in Crete. *Thorax.* 2007 Aug;62(8):677-83.

Chao A, Thun MJ, Connell CJ, McCullough ML, Jacobs EJ, Flanders WD, Rodriguez C, Sinha R, Calle EE. Meat consumption and risk of colorectal cancer. *JAMA.* 2005 Jan 12;293(2):172-82.

Chatzi L, Torrent M, Romieu I, Garcia-Esteban R, Ferrer C, Vioque J, Kogevinas M, Sunyer J. Mediterranean diet in pregnancy is protective for wheeze and atopy in childhood. *Thorax.* 2008 Jun;63(6):507-13.

Chavali SR, Weeks CE, Zhong WW, Forse RA. Increased production of TNF-alpha and decreased levels of dienoic eicosanoids, IL-6 and IL-10 in mice fed menhaden oil and juniper oil diets in response to an intraperitoneal lethal dose of LPS. *Prostaglandins Leukot Essent Fatty Acids.* 1998 Aug;59(2):89-93.

Chehade M, Aceves SS. Food allergy and eosinophilic esophagitis. *Curr Opin Allergy Clin Immunol.* 2010 Jun;10(3):231-7.

Chen HJ, Shih CK, Hsu HY, Chiang W. Mast cell-dependent allergic responses are inhibited by ethanolic extract of adlay (Coix lachryma-jobi L. var. ma-yuen Stapf) testa. *J Agric Food Chem.* 2010 Feb 24;58(4):2596-601.

Cheney G, Waxler SH, Miller IJ. Vitamin U therapy of peptic ulcer; experience at San Quentin Prison. *Calif Med.* 1956 Jan;84(1):39-42.

Chevrier MR, Ryan AE, Lee DY, Zhongze M, Wu-Yan Z, Via CS. Boswellia carterii extract inhibits TH1 cytokines and promotes TH2 cytokines in vitro. *Clin Diagn Lab Immunol.* 2005 May;12(5):575-80.

Chilton FH, Rudel LL, Parks JS, Arm JP, Seeds MC. Mechanisms by which botanical lipids affect inflammatory disorders. *Am J Clin Nutr.* 2008 Feb;87(2):498S-503S.

Chilton FH, Tucker L. *Win the War Within.* New York: Rodale, 2006.

Chin A Paw MJ, de Jong N, Pallast EG, Kloek GC, Schouten EG, Kok FJ. Immunity in frail elderly: a randomized controlled trial of exercise and enriched foods. *Med Sci Sports Exerc.* 2000 Dec;32(12):2005-11.

Choi SY, Sohn JH, Lee YW, Lee EK, Hong CS, Park JW. Characterization of buckwheat 19-kD allergen and its application for diagnosing clinical reactivity. *Int Arch Allergy Immunol.* 2007;144(4):267-74.

Choi SZ, Choi SU, Lee KR. Phytochemical constituents of the aerial parts from Solidago virga-aurea var. gigantea. *Arch Pharm Res.* 2004 Feb;27(2):164-8.

Chopra RN, Nayar SL, Chopra IC, eds. *Glossary of Indian Medicinal plants.* New Delhi: CSIR, 1956.

Christopher J. *School of Natural Healing.* Springville UT: Christopher Publ, 1976.

Chrubasik S, Pollak S. Pain management with herbal antirheumatic drugs. *Wien Med Wochenschr.* 2002;152(7-8):198-203.

Chu YF, Liu RH. Cranberries inhibit LDL oxidation and induce LDL receptor expression in hepatocytes. *Life Sci.* 2005;77(15):1892-1901. 27.

Chung SY, Butts CL, Maleki SJ, Champagne ET (2003) Linking peanut allergenicity to the processes of maturation, curing, and roasting. *J Agric Food Chem.* 51: 4273–4277.

Cingi C, Demirbas D, Songu M. Allergic rhinitis caused by food allergies. *Eur Arch Otorhinolaryngol.* 2010 Sep;267(9):1327-35.

Clark AT, Islam S, King Y, Deighton J, Anagnostou K, Ewan PW. Successful oral tolerance induction in severe peanut allergy. *Allergy.* 2009 Aug;64(8):1218-20.

Clark AT, Mangat JS, Tay SS, King Y, Monk CJ, White PA, Ewan PW. Facial thermography is a sensitive and specific method for assessing food challenge outcome. *Allergy.* 2007 Jul;62(7):744-9.

Cobo Sanz JM, Mateos JA, Muñoz Conejo A. Effect of Lactobacillus casei on the incidence of infectious conditions in children. *Nutr Hosp.* 2006 Jul-Aug;21(4):547-51.

Codispoti CD, Levin L, LeMasters GK, Ryan P, Reponen T, Villareal M, Burkle J, Stanforth S, Lockey JE, Khurana Hershey GK, Bernstein DI. Breast-feeding, aeroallergen sensitization, and environmental exposures during infancy are determinants of childhood allergic rhinitis. *J Allergy Clin Immunol.* 2010 May;125(5):1054-1060.e1.

Cohen A, Goldberg M, Levy B, Leshno M, Katz Y. Sesame food allergy and sensitization in children: the natural history and long-term follow-up. *Pediatr Allergy Immunol.* 2007 May;18(3):217-23.

Conquer JA, Holub BJ. Dietary docosahexaenoic acid as a source of eicosapentaenoic acid in vegetarians and omnivores. *Lipids.* 1997 Mar;32(3):341-5.

Coombs RR, McLaughlan P. Allergenicity of food proteins and its possible modification. *Ann Allergy.* 1984 Dec;53(6 Pt 2):592-6.

Cooper GS, Miller FW, Germolec DR: Occupational exposures and autoimmune diseases. *Int Immunopharm* 2002, 2:303-313.

Cooper K. *The Aerobics Program for Total Well-Being.* New York: Evans, 1980.

Corbe C, Boissin JP, Siou A. Light vision and chorioretinal circulation. Study of the effect of procyanidolic oligomers (Endotelon). *J Fr Ophtalmol.* 1988;11(5):453-60.

Couzy F, Kastenmayer P, Vigo M, Clough J, Munoz-Box R, Barclay DV. Calcium bioavailability from a calcium- and sulfate-rich mineral water, compared with milk, in young adult women. *Am J Clin Nutr.* 1995 Dec;62(6):1239-44.

Crescente M, Jessen G, Momi S, Höltje HD, Gresele P, Cerletti C, de Gaetano G. Interactions of gallic acid, resveratrol, quercetin and aspirin at the platelet cyclooxygenase-1 level. Functional and modelling studies. *Thromb Haemost.* 2009 Aug;102(2):336-46.

Cuesta-Herranz J, Barber D, Blanco C, Cistero-Bahíma A, Crespo JF, Fernández-Rivas M, Fernández-Sánchez J, Florido JF, Ibáñez MD, Rodríguez R, Salcedo G, Garcia BE, Lombardero M, Quiralte J, Rodriguez J, Sánchez-Monge R, Vereda A, Villalba M, Alonso Díaz de Durana MD, Basagaña M, Carrillo T, Fernández-Nieto M, Tabar AI. Differences among Pollen-Allergic Patients with and without Plant Food Allergy. Int Arch Allergy Immunol. 2010 Apr 23;153(2):182-192.

Cummings M. Human Heredity: Principles and Issues. St. Paul, MN: West, 1988.

D'Auria E, Sala M, Lodi F, Radaelli G, Riva E, Giovannini M. Nutritional value of a rice-hydrolysate formula in infants with cows' milk protein allergy: a randomized pilot study. J Int Med Res. 2003 May-Jun;31(3):215-22.

Davies G. Timetables of Medicine. New York: Black Dog & Leventhal, 2000.

Davin JC, Forget P, Mahieu PR. Increased intestinal permeability to (51 Cr) EDTA is correlated with IgA immune complex-plasma levels in children with IgA-associated nephropathies. Acta Paediatr Scand. 1988 Jan;77(1):118-24.

de Boissieu D, Dupont C, Badoual J. Allergy to nondairy proteins in mother's milk as assessed by intestinal permeability tests. Allergy. 1994 Dec;49(10):882-4.

de Boissieu D, Matarazzo P, Rocchiccioli F, Dupont C. Multiple food allergy: a possible diagnosis in breast-fed infants. Acta Paediatr. 1997 Oct;86(10):1042-6.

De Knop KJ, Hagendorens MM, Bridts CH, Stevens WJ, Ebo DG. Macadamia nut allergy: 2 case reports and a review of the literature. Acta Clin Belg. 2010 Mar-Apr;65(2):129-32.

De Lucca AJ, Bland JM, Vigo CB, Cushion M, Selitrennikoff CP, Peter J, Walsh TJ. CAY-I, a fungicidal saponin from Capsicum sp. fruit. Med Mycol. 2002 Apr;40(2):131-7.

de Martino M, Novembre E, Galli L, de Marco A, Botarelli P, Marano E, Vierucci A. Allergy to different fish species in cod-allergic children: in vivo and in vitro studies. J Allergy Clin Immunol. 1990;86:909-914.

DeMeo MT, Mutlu EA, Keshavarzian A, Tobin MC. Intestinal permeation and gastrointestinal disease. J Clin Gastroenterol. 2002 Apr;34(4):385-96.

De Smet PA. Herbal remedies. N Engl J Med. 2002;347:2046–2056.

Dean C. Death by Modern Medicine. Belleville, ON: Matrix Verite-Media, 2005.

del Giudice MM, Leonardi S, Maiello N, Brunese FP. Food allergy and probiotics in childhood. J Clin Gastroenterol. 2010 Sep;44 Suppl 1:S22-5.

Dengate S, Ruben A. Controlled trial of cumulative behavioural effects of a common bread preservative. J Paediatr Child Health. 2002 Aug;38(4):373-6.

Derebery MJ, Berliner KI. Allergy and its relation to Meniere's disease. Otolaryngol Clin North Am. 2010 Oct;43(5):1047-58.

Desjeux JF, Heyman M. Milk proteins, cytokines and intestinal epithelial functions in children. Acta Paediatr Jpn. 1994 Oct;36(5):592-6.

DesRoches A, Infante-Rivard C, Paradis L, Paradis J, Haddad E. Peanut allergy: is maternal transmission of antigens during pregnancy and breastfeeding a risk factor? J Investig Allergol Clin Immunol. 2010;20(4):289-94.

Deutsche Gesellschaft für Ernährung. Drink distilled water? Med. Mo. Pharm. 1993;16:146.

Devaraj TL. Speaking of Ayurvedic Remedies for Common Diseases. New Delhi: Sterling, 1985.

Diesner SC, Untersmayr E, Pietschmann P, Jensen-Jarolim E. Food Allergy: Only a Pediatric Disease? Gerontology. 2010 Jan 29.

Diğrak M, Ilçim A, Hakki Alma M. Antimicrobial activities of several parts of Pinus brutia, Juniperus oxycedrus, Abies cilicia, Cedrus libani and Pinus nigra. Phytother Res. 1999 Nov;13(7):584-7.

Din FV, Theodoratou E, Farrington SM, Tenesa A, Barnetson RA, Cetnarskyj R, Stark L, Porteous ME, Campbell H, Dunlop MG. Effect of aspirin and NSAIDs on risk and survival from colorectal cancer. Gut. 2010 Dec;59(12):1670-9.

Diop L, Guillou S, Durand H. Probiotic food supplement reduces stress-induced gastrointestinal symptoms in volunteers: a double-blind, placebo-controlled, randomized trial. Nutr Res. 2008 Jan;28(1):1-5.

Dona A, Arvanitoyannis IS. Health risks of genetically modified foods. Crit Rev Food Sci Nutr. 2009 Feb;49(2):164-75.

Donato F, Monarca S, Premi S., and Gelatti, U. Drinking water hardness and chronic degenerative diseases. Part III. Tumors, urolithiasis, fetal malformations, deterioration of the cognitive function in the aged and atopic eczema. Ann. Ig. 2003;15:57-70.

Dooley, M.A. and Hogan S.L. Environmental epidemiology and risk factors for autoimmune disease. Curr Opin Rheum. 2003;15(2):99-103.

D'Orazio N, Ficoneri C, Riccioni G, Conti P, Theoharides TC, Bollea MR. Conjugated linoleic acid: a functional food? Int J Immunopathol Pharmacol. 2003 Sep-Dec;16(3):215-20.

Dotolo Institute. The Study of Colon Hydrotherapy. Pinellas Park, FL: Dotolo, 2003.

Drouault-Holowacz S, Bieuvelet S, Burckel A, Cazaubiel M, Dray X, Marteau P. A double blind randomized controlled trial of a probiotic combination in 100 patients with irritable bowel syndrome. *Gastroenterol Clin Biol.* 2008 Feb;32(2):147-52.

Ducrotté P. Irritable bowel syndrome: from the gut to the brain-gut. *Gastroenterol Clin Biol.* 2009 Aug-Sep;33(8-9):703-12.

Duke J. *The Green Pharmacy.* New York: St. Martins, 1997.

Dunstan JA, Hale J, Breckler L, Lehmann H, Weston S, Richmond P, Prescott SL. Atopic dermatitis in young children is associated with impaired interleukin-10 and interferon-gamma responses to allergens, vaccines and colonizing skin and gut bacteria. *Clin Exp Allergy.* 2005 Oct;35(10):1309-17.

Dunstan JA, Roper J, Mitoulas L, Hartmann PE, Simmer K, Prescott SL. The effect of supplementation with fish oil during pregnancy on breast milk immunoglobulin A, soluble CD14, cytokine levels and fatty acid composition. *Clin Exp Allergy.* 2004 Aug;34(8):1237-42.

Dupont C, Barau E, Molkhou P, Raynaud F, Barbet JP, Dehennin L. Food-induced alterations of intestinal permeability in children with cow's milk-sensitive enteropathy and atopic dermatitis. *J Pediatr Gastroenterol Nutr.* 1989 May;8(4):459-65.

Dupont C, Barau E, Molkhou P. Intestinal permeability disorders in children. *Allerg Immunol (Paris).* 1991 Mar;23(3):95-103.

Dupont C, Barau E. Diagnosis of food allergy in children. *Ann Pediatr (Paris).* 1992 Jan;39(1):5-12.

Dupont C, Soulaines P, Lapillonne A, Donne N, Kalach N, Benhamou P. Atopy patch test for early diagnosis of cow's milk allergy in preterm infants. *J Pediatr Gastroenterol Nutr.* 2010 Apr;50(4):463-4.

Dupuy P, Cassé M, André F, Dhivert-Donnadieu H, Pinton J, Hernandez-Pion C. Low-salt water reduces intestinal permeability in atopic patients. *Dermatology.* 1999;198(2):153-5.

Duran-Tauleria E, Vignati G, Guedan MJ, Petersson CJ. The utility of specific immunoglobulin E measurements in primary care. *Allergy.* 2004 Aug;59 Suppl 78:35-41.

D'Urbano LE, Pellegrino K, Artesani MC, Donnanno S, Luciano R, Riccardi C, Tozzi AE, Ravà L, De Benedetti F, Cavagni G. Performance of a component-based allergen-microarray in the diagnosis of cow's milk and hen's egg allergy. *Clin Exp Allergy.* 2010 Jul 13.

Duwiejua M, Zeitlin IJ, Waterman PG, Chapman J, Mhango GJ, Provan GJ. Anti-inflammatory activity of resins from some species of the plant family Burseraceae. *Planta Med.* 1993 Feb;59(1):12-6.

Dykewicz MS, Lemmon JK, Keaney DL. Comparison of the Multi-Test II and Skintestor Omni allergy skin test devices. *Ann Allergy Asthma Immunol.* 2007 Jun;98(6):559-62.

Eastham EJ, Walker WA. Effect of cow's milk on the gastrointestinal tract: a persistent dilemma for the pediatrician. *Pediatrics.* 1977 Oct;60(4):477-81.

Eaton KK, Howard M, Howard JM. Gut permeability measured by polyethylene glycol absorption in abnormal gut fermentation as compared with food intolerance. *J R Soc Med.* 1995 Feb;88(2):63-6.

Ebers GC, Kukay K, Bulman DE, Sadovnick AD, Rice G, Anderson C, Armstrong H, Cousin K, Bell RB, Hader W, Paty DW, Hashimoto S, Oger J, Duquette P, Warren S, Gray T, O'Connor P, Nath A, Auty A, Metz L, Francis G, Paulseth JE, Murray TJ, Pryse-Phillips W, Nelson R, Freedman M, Brunet D, Bouchard JP, Hinds D, Risch N. A full genome search in multiple sclerosis. *Nat Genet.* 1996 Aug;13(4):472-6.

ECRHS (2002) The European Community Respiratory Health Survey II. *Eur Respir J.* 20: 1071–1079.

Ege MJ, Herzum I, Büchele G, Krauss-Etschmann S, Lauener RP, Roponen M, Hyvärinen A, Vuitton DA, Riedler J, Brunekreef B, Dalphin JC, Braun-Fahrländer C, Pekkanen J, Renz H, von Mutius E; Protection Against Allergy Study in Rural Environments (PASTURE) Study group. Prenatal exposure to a farm environment modifies atopic sensitization at birth. *J Allergy Clin Immunol.* 2008 Aug;122(2):407-12, 412.e1-4.

Eggermont E. Cow's milk protein allergy. *Tijdschr Kindergeneeskd.* 1981 Feb;49(1):16-20.

Ehling S, Hengel M, and Shibamoto T. Formation of acrylamide from lipids. *Adv Exp Med Biol* 2005, 561:223-233.

Ehren J, Morón B, Martin E, Bethune MT, Gray GM, Khosla C. A food-grade enzyme preparation with modest gluten detoxification properties. *PLoS One.* 2009 Jul 21;4(7):e6313.

el-Ghazaly M, Khayyal MT, Okpanyi SN, Arens-Corell M. Study of the anti-inflammatory activity of Populus tremula, Solidago virgaurea and Fraxinus excelsior. *Arzneimittelforschung.* 1992 Mar;42(3):333-6.

El-Ghorab A, Shaaban HA, El-Massry KF, Shibamoto T. Chemical composition of volatile extract and biological activities of volatile and less-volatile extracts of juniper berry (Juniperus drupacea L.) fruit. *J Agric Food Chem.* 2008 Jul 9;56(13):5021-5.

El-Khouly F, Lewis SA, Pons L, Burks AW, Hourihane JO. IgG and IgE avidity characteristics of peanut allergic individuals. *Pediatr Allergy Immunol.* 2007 Nov;18(7):607-13.

Ellingwood F. *American Materia Medica, Therapeutics and Pharmacognosy.* Portland: Eclectic Medical Publ., 1983.

REFERENCES AND BIBLIOGRAPHY

Elliott RB, Harris DP, Hill JP, Bibby NJ, Wasmuth HE. Type I (insulin-dependent) diabetes mellitus and cow milk: casein variant consumption. *Diabetologia*. 1999 Mar;42(3):292-6. Erratum in: Diabetologia 1999 Aug;42(8):1032.

Elwood PC. Epidemiology and trace elements. *Clin Endocrinol Metab*. 1985 Aug;14(3):617-28.

Engel, M.F., Dimethyl sulfoxide in the treatment of scleroderma. *South Med J*. 1972;65:71.

Engler RJ. Alternative and complementary medicine: a source of improved therapies for asthma? A challenge for redefining the specialty? J Allergy Clin Immunol. 2000;106:627–9.

Environmental Working Group. *Human Toxome Project*. 2007. http://www.ewg.org/sites/ humantoxome/. Accessed: 2007 Sep.

EPA. *A Brief Guide to Mold, Moisture and Your Home*. Environmental Protection Agency, Office of Air and Radiation/Indoor Environments Division. EPA 2002;402-K-02-003.

Ernst E. Frankincense: systematic review. *BMJ*. 2008 Dec 17;337:a2813.

Erwin EA, James HR, Gutekunst HM, Russo JM, Kelleher KJ, Platts-Mills TA. Serum IgE measurement and detection of food allergy in pediatric patients with eosinophilic esophagitis. *Ann Allergy Asthma Immunol*. 2010 Jun;104(6):496-502.

EuroPrevall. *WP 1.1 Birth Cohort Update*. 1st Quarter 2006. Berlin, Germany: Charité University Medical Centre.

Eutamene H, Lamine F, Chabo C, Theodorou V, Rochat F, Bergonzelli GE, Corthésy-Theulaz I, Fioramonti J, Bueno L. Synergy between Lactobacillus paracasei and its bacterial products to counteract stress-induced gut permeability and sensitivity increase in rats. *J Nutr*. 2007 Aug;137(8):1901-7.

Evans P, Forte D, Jacobs C, Fredhoi C, Aitchison E, Hucklebridge F, Clow A. Cortisol secretory activity in older people in relation to positive and negative well-being. *Psychoneuroendocrinology*. 2007 Aug 7

Everhart JE. *Digestive Diseases in the United States*. Darby, PA: Diane Pub, 1994.

Exl BM, Deland U, Secretin MC, Preysch U, Wall M, Shmerling DH. Improved general health status in an unselected infant population following an allergen reduced dietary intervention programme. The ZUFF-study-programme. Part I: Study design and 6-month nutritional behaviour. *Eur J Nutr*. 2000 Jun;39(3):89-102.

FAAN. *Public Comment on 2005 Food Safety Survey: Docket No. 2004N-0516 (2005 FSS)*. Fairfax, VA: Food Allergy & Anaphylaxis Network.

Faeste CK, Christians U, Egaas E, Jonscher KR. Characterization of potential allergens in fenugreek (Trigonella foenum-graecum) using patient sera and MS-based proteomic analysis. *J Proteomics*. 2010 May 7;73(7):1321-33.

Faeste CK, Jonscher KR, Sit L, Klawitter J, Løvberg KE, Moen LH. Differentiating cross-reacting allergens in the immunological analysis of celery (Apium graveolens) by mass spectrometry. *J AOAC Int*. 2010 Mar-Apr;93(2):451-61.

Fajac I, Frossard N. Neuropeptides of the nasal innervation and allergic rhinitis. *Rev Mal Respir*. 1994;11(4):357-67.

Fälth-Magnusson K, Kjellman NI, Magnusson KE, Sundqvist T. Intestinal permeability in healthy and allergic children before and after sodium-cromoglycate treatment assessed with different-sized poly-ethyleneglycols (PEG 400 and PEG 1000). *Clin Allergy*. 1984 May;14(3):277-86.

Fälth-Magnusson K, Kjellman NI, Odelram H, Sundqvist T, Magnusson KE. Gastrointestinal permeability in children with cow's milk allergy: effect of milk challenge and sodium cromoglycate as assessed with polyethyleneglycols (PEG 400 and PEG 1000). *Clin Allergy*. 1986 Nov;16(6):543-51.

Fan AY, Lao L, Zhang RX, Zhou AN, Wang LB, Moudgil KD, Lee DY, Ma ZZ, Zhang WY, Berman BM. Effects of an acetone extract of Boswellia carterii Birdw. (Burseraceae) gum resin on adjuvant-induced arthritis in lewis rats. *J Ethnopharmacol*. 2005 Oct 3;101(1-3):104-9.

Fanaro S, Marten B, Bagna R, Vigi V, Fabris C, Peña-Quintana, Argüelles F, Scholz-Ahrens KE, Sawatzki G, Zelenka R, Schrezenmeir J, de Vrese M and Bertino E. Galacto-oligosaccharides are bifidogenic and safe at weaning: A double-blind Randomized Multicenter study. *J Pediatr Gastroent Nutr*. 2009 48; 82-88

Fang SP, Tanaka T, Tago F, Okamoto T, Kojima S. Immunomodulatory effects of gyokuheifusan on INF-gamma/IL-4 (Th1/Th2) balance in ovalbumin (OVA)-induced asthma model mice. *Biol Pharm Bull*. 2005;28:829–33.

Fanigliulo L, Comparato G, Aragona G, Cavallaro L, Iori V, Maino M, Cavestro GM, Soliani P, Sianesi M, Franzè A, Di Mario F. Role of gut microflora and probiotic effects in the irritable bowel syndrome. *Acta Biomed*. 2006 Aug;77(2):85-9.

FAO/WHO Expert Committee. *Fats and Oils in Human Nutrition*. Food and Nutrition Paper. 1994;(57).

Fasano A, Berti I, Gerarduzzi T, Not T, Colletti RB, Drago S, Elitsur Y, Green PH, Guandalini S, Hill ID, Pietzak M, Ventura A, Thorpe M, Kryszak D, Fornaroli F, Wasserman SS, Murray JA, Horvath K. Prevalence of celiac disease in at-risk and not-at-risk groups in the United States: a large multicenter study. *Arch Intern Med*. 2003 Feb 10;163(3):286-92.

Fawell J, Nieuwenhuijsen MJ. Contaminants in drinking water. *Br Med Bull*. 2003;68:199-208.

Felley CP, Corthésy-Theulaz I, Rivero JL, Sipponen P, Kaufmann M, Bauerfeind P, Wiesel PH, Brassart D, Pfeifer A, Blum AL, Michetti P. Favourable effect of an acidified milk (LC-1) on Helicobacter pylori gastritis in man. *Eur J Gastroenterol Hepatol.* 2001 Jan;13(1):25-9.

Fernández-Rivas M, Garrido Fernández S, Nadal JA, Díaz de Durana MD, García BE, González-Mancebo E, Martín S, Barber D, Rico P, Tabar AI. Randomized double-blind, placebo-controlled trial of sublingual immunotherapy with a Pru p 3 quantified peach extract. *Allergy.* 2009 Jun;64(6):876-83.

Fernández-Rivas M, González-Mancebo E, Rodríguez-Pérez R, Benito C, Sánchez-Monge R, Salcedo G, Alonso MD, Rosado A, Tejedor MA, Vila C, Casas ML. Clinically relevant peach allergy is related to peach lipid transfer protein, Pru p 3, in the Spanish population. *J Allergy Clin Immunol.* 2003 Oct;112(4):789-95.

Ferrier L, Berard F, Debrauwer L, Chabo C, Langella P, Bueno L, Fioramonti J. Impairment of the intestinal barrier by ethanol involves enteric microflora and mast cell activation in rodents. *Am J Pathol.* 2006 Apr;168(4):1148-54.

Filipowicz N, Kamiński M, Kurlenda J, Asztemborska M, Ochocka JR. Antibacterial and antifungal activity of juniper berry oil and its selected components. *Phytother Res.* 2003 Mar;17(3):227-31.

Finkelman FD, Boyce JA, Vercelli D, Rothenberg ME. Key advances in mechanisms of asthma, allergy, and immunology in 2009. *J Allergy Clin Immunol.* 2010 Feb;125(2):312-8.

Fiocchi A, Restani P, Bernardo L, Martelli A, Ballabio C, D'Auria E, Riva E. Tolerance of heat-treated kiwi by children with kiwifruit allergy. *Pediatr Allergy Immunol.* 2004 Oct;15(5):454-8.

Fiocchi A, Travaini M, D'Auria E, Banderali G, Bernardo L, Riva E. Tolerance to a rice hydrolysate formula in children allergic to cow's milk and soy. *Clin Exp Allergy.* 2003 Nov;33(11):1576-80.

Fiocchi, A; Restani, P; Riva, E; Qualizza, R; Bruni, P; Restelli, AR; Galli, CL. Meat allergy: I. Specific IgE to BSA and OSA in atopic, beef sensitive children. *J Am Coll Nutr.* 1995 14: 239-244.

Flammarion S, Santos C, Guimber D, Jouannic L, Thumerelle C, Gottrand F, Deschildre A. Diet and nutritional status of children with food allergies. *Pediatr Allergy Immunol.* 2010 Jun 14.

Flandrin, J, Montanari M. (eds.). *Food: A Culinary History from Antiquity to the Present.* New York: Penguin Books, 1999.

Fleischer DM, Conover-Walker MK, Christie L, Burks AW, Wood RA. Peanut allergy: recurrence and its management. *J Allergy Clin Immunol.* 2004 Nov;114(5):1195-201.

Flinterman AE, Pasmans SG, den Hartog Jager CF, Hoekstra MO, Bruijnzeel-Koomen CA, Knol EF, van Hoffen E. T cell responses to major peanut allergens in children with and without peanut allergy. *Clin Exp Allergy.* 2010 Apr;40(4):590-7.

Flinterman AE, van Hoffen E, den Hartog Jager CF, Koppelman S, Pasmans SG, Hoekstra MO, Bruijnzeel-Koomen CA, Knulst AC, Knol EF. Children with peanut allergy recognize predominantly Ara h2 and Ara h6, which remains stable over time. *Clin Exp Allergy.* 2007 Aug;37(8):1221-8.

Food allergy continues to increase. *Child Health Alert.* 2010 Jan;28:2.

Forbes EE, Groschwitz K, Abonia JP, Brandt EB, Cohen E, Blanchard C, Ahrens R, Seidu L, McKenzie A, Strait R, Finkelman FD, Foster PS, Matthaei KI, Rothenberg ME, Hogan SP. IL-9- and mast cell-mediated intestinal permeability predisposes to oral antigen hypersensitivity. *J Exp Med.* 2008 Apr 14;205(4):897-913.

Forestier C, Guelon D, Cluytens V, Gillart T, Sirot J, De Champs C. Oral probiotic and prevention of Pseudomonas aeruginosa infections: a randomized, double-blind, placebo-controlled pilot study in intensive care unit patients. *Crit Care.* 2008;12(3):R69.

Forget P, Sodoyez-Goffaux F, Zappitelli A. Permeability of the small intestine to 51Cr EDTA in children with acute gastroenteritis or eczema. *J Pediatr Gastroenterol Nutr.* 1985 Jun;4(3):393-6.

Forget-Dubois N, Boivin M, Dionne G, Pierce T, Tremblay RE, Pérusse D. A longitudinal twin study of the genetic and environmental etiology of maternal hostile-reactive behavior during infancy and toddlerhood. *Infant Behav Dev.* 2007

Foster S, Hobbs C. *Medicinal Plants and Herbs.* Boston: Houghton Mifflin, 2002.

Fox RD, *Algoculture.* Doctorate Disseration, 1983 Jul.

Francavilla R, Lionetti E, Castellaneta SP, Magistà AM, Maurogiovanni G, Bucci N, De Canio A, Indrio F, Cavallo L, Ierardi E, Miniello VL. Inhibition of Helicobacter pylori infection in humans by Lactobacillus reuteri ATCC 55730 and effect on eradication therapy: a pilot study. *Helicobacter.* 2008 Apr;13(2):127-34.

Frawley D, Lad V. *The Yoga of Herbs.* Sante Fe: Lotus Press, 1986.

Fremont S, Moneret-Vautrin DA, Franck P, Morisset M, Croizier A, Codreanu F, Kanny G. Prospective study of sensitization and food allergy to flaxseed in 1317 subjects. *Eur Ann Allergy Clin Immunol.* 2010 Jun;42(3):103-11.

Frias J, Song YS, Martínez-Villaluenga C, González de Mejia E, Vidal-Valverde C. Immunoreactivity and amino acid content of fermented soybean products. *J Agric Food Chem.* 2008 Jan 9;56(1):99-105.

Fu G, Zhong Y, Li C, Li Y, Lin X, Liao B, Tsang EW, Wu K, Huang S. Epigenetic regulation of peanut allergen gene Ara h 3 in developing embryos. *Planta.* 2010 Apr;231(5):1049-60.

Fujimori S, Gudis K, Mitsui K, Seo T, Yonezawa M, Tanaka S, Tatsuguchi A, Sakamoto C. A randomized controlled trial on the efficacy of synbiotic versus probiotic or prebiotic treatment to improve the quality of life in patients with ulcerative colitis. *Nutrition.* 2009 May;25(5):520-5.

Furrie E, Macfarlane S, Kennedy A, Cummings JH, Walsh SV, O'neil DA, Macfarlane GT. Synbiotic therapy (Bifidobacterium longum/Synergy 1) initiates resolution of inflammation in patients with active ulcerative colitis: a randomised controlled pilot trial. *Gut.* 2005 Feb;54(2):242-9.

Furuhjelm C, Warstedt K, Larsson J, Fredriksson M, Böttcher MF, Fälth-Magnusson K, Duchén K. Fish oil supplementation in pregnancy and lactation may decrease the risk of infant allergy. *Acta Paediatr.* 2009 Sep;98(9):1461-7.

Gagnier JJ, DeMelo J, Boon H, Rochon P, Bombardier C. Quality of reporting of randomized controlled trials of herbal medicine interventions. *Am J Med.* 2006;119:1–11.

Galli E, Ciucci A, Cersosimo S, Pagnini C, Avitabile S, Mancino G, Delle Fave G, Corleto VD. Eczema and food allergy in an Italian pediatric cohort: no association with TLR-2 and TLR-4 polymorphisms. *Int J Immunopathol Pharmacol.* 2010 Apr-Jun;23(2):671-5.

Gamboa PM, Cáceres O, Antepara I, Sánchez-Monge R, Ahrazem O, Salcedo G, Barber D, Lombardero M, Sanz ML. Two different profiles of peach allergy in the north of Spain. *Allergy.* 2007 Apr;62(4):408-14.

Gao X, Wang W, Wei S, Li W. Review of pharmacological effects of Glycyrrhiza radix and its bioactive compounds. *Zhongguo Zhong Yao Za Zhi.* 2009 Nov;34(21):2695-700.

Garcia Gomez LJ, Sanchez-Muniz FJ. Review: cardiovascular effect of garlic (Allium sativum). *Arch Latinoam Nutr.* 2000 Sep;50(3):219-29.

Gardner ML. Gastrointestinal absorption of intact proteins. Annu Rev Nutr. 1988;8:329-50.

Gareau MG, Jury J, Yang PC, MacQueen G, Perdue MH. Neonatal maternal separation causes colonic dysfunction in rat pups including impaired host resistance. *Pediatr Res.* 2006 Jan;59(1):83-8.

Garzi A, Messina M, Frati F, Carfagna L, Zagordo L, Belcastro M, Parmiani S, Sensi L, Marcucci F. An extensively hydrolysed cow's milk formula improves clinical symptoms of gastroesophageal reflux and reduces the gastric emptying time in infants. *Allergol Immunopathol (Madr).* 2002 Jan-Feb;30(1):36-41.

Gastrointestinal permeability in food-allergic children. *Nutr Rev.* 1985 Aug;43(8):233-5.

Gawrońska A, Dziechciarz P, Horvath A, Szajewska H. A randomized double-blind placebo-controlled trial of Lactobacillus GG for abdominal pain disorders in children. *Aliment Pharmacol Ther.* 2007 Jan 15;25(2):177-84.

Geha RS, Beiser A, Ren C, Patterson R, Greenberger PA, Grammer LC, Ditto AM, Harris KE, Shaughnessy MA, Yarnold PR, Corren J, Saxon A. Multicenter, double-blind, placebo-controlled, multiple-challenge evaluation of reported reactions to monosodium glutamate. *J Allergy Clin Immunol.* 2000 Nov;106(5):973-80.

Gerez IF, Shek LP, Chng HH, Lee BW. Diagnostic tests for food allergy. Singapore Med J. 2010 Jan;51(1):4-9.

Ghadioungui P. (transl.) *The Ebers Papyrus.* Academy of Scientific Research. Cairo, 1987.

Ghayur MN, Gilani AH. Ginger lowers blood pressure through blockade of voltage-dependent calcium Channels acting as a cardiotonic pump activator in mice, rabbit and dogs. *J Cardiovasc Pharmacol.* 2005 Jan;45(1):74-80.

Giampietro PG, Kjellman NI, Oldaeus G, Wouters-Wesseling W, Businco L. Hypoallergenicity of an extensively hydrolyzed whey formula. *Pediatr Allergy Immunol.* 2001 Apr;12(2):83-6.

Gibbons E. *Stalking the Healthful Herbs.* New York: David McKay, 1966.

Gibson RA. Docosa-hexaenoic acid (DHA) accumulation is regulated by the polyunsaturated fat content of the diet: Is it synthesis or is it incorporation? *Asia Pac J Clin Nutr.* 2004;13(Suppl):S78.

Gibson, G.R., McCartney, A.L., Rastall, R.A. (2005) Prebiotics and resistance to gastrointestinal infections. *Br J of Nutr.* 93, Suppl. 1, pp31-34.

Gill HS, Rutherfurd KJ, Cross ML, Gopal PK. Enhancement of immunity in the elderly by dietary supplementation with the probiotic Bifidobacterium lactis HN019. *Am J Clin Nutr.* 2001 Dec;74(6):833-9.

Gillman A, Douglass JA. What do asthmatics have to fear from food and additive allergy? *Clin Exp Allergy.* 2010 Sep;40(9):1295-302.

Gionchetti P, Rizzello F, Venturi A, Brigidi P, Matteuzzi D, Bazzocchi G, Poggioli G, Miglioli M, Campieri M. Oral bacteriotherapy as maintenance treatment in patients with chronic pouchitis: a double-blind, placebo-controlled trial. *Gastroenterology.* 2000 Aug;119(2):305-9.

Glück U, Gebbers J. Ingested probiotics reduce nasal colonization with pathogenic bacteria (Staphylococcus aureus, Streptococcus pneumoniae, and b-hemolytic streptococci. *Am J. Clin. Nutr.* 2003;77:517-520.

Gohil K, Packer L. Bioflavonoid-Rich Botanical Extracts Show Antioxidant and Gene Regulatory Activity. *Ann N Y Acad Sci.* 2002:957:70-7.

Goldin BR, Adlercreutz H, Dwyer JT, Swenson L, Warram JH, Gorbach SL. Effect of diet on excretion of estrogens in pre- and postmenopausal women. *Cancer Res.* 1981 Sep;41(9 Pt 2):3771-3.

Goldin BR, Adlercreutz H, Gorbach SL, Warram JH, Dwyer JT, Swenson L, Woods MN. Estrogen excretion patterns and plasma levels in vegetarian and omnivorous women. *N Engl J Med.* 1982 Dec 16;307(25):1542-7.

Goldin BR, Swenson L, Dwyer J, Sexton M, Gorbach SL. Effect of diet and Lactobacillus acidophilus supplements on human fecal bacterial enzymes. *J Natl Cancer Inst.* 1980 Feb;64(2):255-61.

Goldstein JL, Aisenberg J, Zakko SF, Berger MF, Dodge WE. Endoscopic ulcer rates in healthy subjects associated with use of aspirin (81 mg q.d.) alone or coadministered with celecoxib or naproxen: a randomized, 1-week trial. *Dig Dis Sci.* 2008 Mar;53(3):647-56.

Golub E. *The Limits of Medicine.* New York: Times Books, 1994.

Gonipeta B, Parvataneni S, Paruchuri P, Gangur V. Long-term characteristics of hazelnut allergy in an adjuvant-free mouse model. *Int Arch Allergy Immunol.* 2010;152(3):219-25.

Gonlachanvit S. Are rice and spicy diet good for functional gastrointestinal disorders? *J Neurogastroenterol Motil.* 2010 Apr;16(2):131-8.

González Alvarez R, Arruzazabala ML. Current views of the mechanism of action of prophylactic antiallergic drugs. *Allergol Immunopathol (Madr).* 1981 Nov-Dec;9(6):501-8.

González-Pérez A, Aponte Z, Vidaurre CF, Rodríguez LA. Anaphylaxis epidemiology in patients with and patients without asthma: a United Kingdom database review. *J Allergy Clin Immunol.* 2010 May;125(5):1098-1104.e1.

Goossens DA, Jonkers DM, Russel MG, Stobberingh EE, Stockbrügger RW. The effect of a probiotic drink with Lactobacillus plantarum 299v on the bacterial composition in faeces and mucosal biopsies of rectum and ascending colon. *Aliment Pharmacol Ther.* 2006 Jan 15;23(2):255-63.

Gordon BR. Patch testing for allergies. *Curr Opin Otolaryngol Head Neck Surg.* 2010 Jun;18(3):191-4.

Gotteland M, Poliak L, Cruchet S, Brunser O. Effect of regular ingestion of Saccharomyces boulardii plus inulin or Lactobacillus acidophilus LB in children colonized by Helicobacter pylori. *Acta Paediatr.* 2005 Dec;94(12):1747-51.

Grant WB, Holick MF. Benefits and requirements of vitamin D for optimal health: a review. *Altern Med Rev.* 2005 Jun;10(2):94-111.

Grant WB. Solar ultraviolet irradiance and cancer incidence and mortality. *Adv Exp Med Biol.* 2008;624:16-30.

Gray H. *Anatomy, Descriptive and Surgical.* 15th Edition. New York: Random House, 1977.

Gray-Davison F. *Ayurvedic Healing.* New York: Keats, 2002.

Griffith HW. *Healing Herbs: The Essential Guide.* Tucson: Fisher Books, 2000.

Grimshaw KE, King RM, Nordlee JA, Hefle SL, Warner JO, Hourihane JO. Presentation of allergen in different food preparations affects the nature of the allergic reaction—a case series. *Clin Exp Allergy.* 2003 Nov;33(11):1581-5.

Grob M, Reindl J, Vieths S, Wüthrich B, Ballmer-Weber BK. Heterogeneity of banana allergy: characterization of allergens in banana-allergic patients. *Ann Allergy Asthma Immunol.* 2002 Nov;89(5):513-6.

Groschwitz KR, Ahrens R, Osterfeld H, Gurish MF, Han X, Abrink M, Finkelman FD, Pejler G, Hogan SP. Mast cells regulate homeostatic intestinal epithelial migration and barrier function by a chymase/Mcpt4-dependent mechanism. *Proc Natl Acad Sci U S A.* 2009 Dec 29;106(52):22381-6.

Grzanna R, Lindmark L, Frondoza CG. Ginger—an herbal medicinal product with broad anti-inflammatory actions. *J Med Food.* 2005 Summer;8(2):125-32.

Grzybowska-Chlebowczyk U, Woś H, Sieroń AL, Wiecek S, Auguściak-Duma A, Koryciak-Komarska H, Kasznia-Kocot J. Serologic investigations in children with inflammatory bowel disease and food allergy. *Mediators Inflamm.* 2009;2009:512695.

Guandalini S. The influence of gluten: weaning recommendations for healthy children and children at risk for celiac disease. *Nestle Nutr Workshop Ser Pediatr Program.* 2007;60:139-51; discussion 151-5.

Guerin M, Huntley ME, Olaizola M. Haematococcus astaxanthin: applications for human health and nutrition. *Trends Biotechnol.* 2003 May;21(5):210-6.

Gundermann KJ, Müller J. Phytodolor—effects and efficacy of a herbal medicine. *Wien Med Wochenschr.* 2007;157(13-14):343-7.

Gupta R, Sheikh A, Strachan DP, Anderson HR (2006) Time trends in allergic disorders in the UK. *Thorax,* published online. doi: 10.1136/thx.2004.038844.

Guslandi M, Giollo P, Testoni PA. A pilot trial of Saccharomyces boulardii in ulcerative colitis. *Eur J Gastroenterol Hepatol.* 2003 Jun;15(6):697-8.

Gutmanis J. *Hawaiian Herbal Medicine.* Waipahu, HI: Island Heritage, 2001.

Guyonnet D, Woodcock A, Stefani B, Trevisan C, Hall C. Fermented milk containing Bifidobacterium lactis DN-173 010 improved self-reported digestive comfort amongst a general population of adults. A randomized, open-label, controlled, pilot study. *J Dig Dis.* 2009 Feb;10(1):61-70.

Hadjivassiliou M, Davies-Jones GA, Sanders DS, Grünewald RA. Dietary treatment of gluten ataxia. *J Neurol Neurosurg Psychiatry*. 2003 Sep;74(9):1221-4.

Hafström I, Ringertz B, Spångberg A, von Zweigbergk L, Brannemark S, Nylander I, Rönnelid J, Laasonen L, Klareskog L. A vegan diet free of gluten improves the signs and symptoms of rheumatoid arthritis: the effects on arthritis correlate with a reduction in antibodies to food antigens. *Rheumatology (Oxford)*. 2001 Oct;40(10):1175-9.

Haines JL, Ter-Minassian M, Bazyk A, Gusella JF, Kim DJ, Terwedow H, Pericak-Vance MA, Rimmler JB, Haynes CS, Roses AD, Lee A, Shaner B, Menold M, Seboun E, Fitoussi RP, Gartioux C, Reyes C, Ribierre F, Gyapay G, Weissenbach J, Hauser SL, Goodkin DE, Lincoln R, Usuku K, Oksenberg JR, et al. A complete genomic screen for multiple sclerosis underscores a role for the major histocompatability complex. The Multiple Sclerosis Genetics Group. *Nat Genet*. 1996 Aug;13(4):469-71..

Halken S, Hansen KS, Jacobsen HP, Estmann A, Faelling AE, Hansen LG, Kier SR, Lassen K, Lintrup M, Mortensen S, Ibsen KK, Osterballe O, Host A. Comparison of a partially hydrolyzed infant formula with two extensively hydrolyzed formulas for allergy prevention: a prospective, randomized study. *Pediatr Allergy Immunol*. 2000 Aug;11(3):149-61.

Halpern GM, Miller AH. *Medicinal Mushrooms: Ancient Remedies for Modern Ailments*. New York: M. Evans, 2002.

Hamelmann E, Beyer K, Gruber C, Lau S, Matricardi PM, Nickel R, Niggemann B, Wahn U. Primary prevention of allergy: avoiding risk or providing protection? *Clin Exp Allergy*. 2008 Feb;38(2):233-45.

Hamilton RG. Clinical laboratory assessment of immediate-type hypersensitivity. *J Allergy Clin Immunol*. 2010 Feb;125(2 Suppl 2):S284-96.

Hammond BG, Mayhew DA, Kier LD, Mast RW, Sander WJ. Safety assessment of DHA-rich microalgae from Schizochytrium sp. *Regul Toxicol Pharmacol*. 2002 Apr;35(2 Pt 1):255-65.

Han SN, Leka LS, Lichtenstein AH, Ausman LM, Meydani SN. Effect of a therapeutic lifestyle change diet on immune functions of moderately hypercholesterolemic humans. *J Lipid Res*. 2003 Dec;44(12):2304-10.

Hansen KS, Ballmer-Weber BK, Lüttkopf D, Skov PS, Wüthrich B, Bindslev-Jensen C, Vieths S, Poulsen LK. Roasted hazelnuts—allergenic activity evaluated by double-blind, placebo-controlled food challenge. *Allergy*. 2003 Feb;58(2):132-8.

Hansen KS, Ballmer-Weber BK, Sastre J, Lidholm J, Andersson K, Oberhofer H, Lluch-Bernal M, Ostling J, Mattsson L, Schocker F, Vieths S, Poulsen LK. Component-resolved in vitro diagnosis of hazelnut allergy in Europe. *J Allergy Clin Immunol*. 2009 May;123(5):1134-41, 1141.e1-3.

Hansen KS, Khinchi MS, Skov PS, Bindslev-Jensen C, Poulsen LK, Malling HJ. Food allergy to apple and specific immunotherapy with birch pollen. *Mol Nutr Food Res*. 2004 Nov;48(6):441-8.

Hartz C, Lauer I, Del Mar San Miguel Moncin M, Cistero-Bahima A, Foetisch K, Lidholm J, Vieths S, Scheurer S. Comparison of IgE-Binding Capacity, Cross-Reactivity and Biological Potency of Allergenic Non-Specific Lipid Transfer Proteins from Peach, Cherry and Hazelnut. *Int Arch Allergy Immunol*. 2010 Jun 17;153(4):335-346.

Harvald B, Hauge M: Hereditary factors elucidated by twin studies. In *Genetics and the Epidemiology of Chronic Disease*. Edited by Neel JV, Shaw MV, Schull WJ. Washington, DC: Department of Health, Education and Welfare, 1965:64-76.

Hashem MM, Atta AH, Arbid MS, Nada SA, Asaad GF. Immunological studies on Amaranth, Sunset Yellow and Curcumin as food colouring agents in albino rats. *Food Chem Toxicol*. 2010 Jun;48(6):1581-6.

Hata K, Ishikawa K, Hori K, Konishi T. Differentiation-inducing activity of lupeol, a lupane-type triterpene from Chinese dandelion root (Hokouei-kon), on a mouse melanoma cell line. *Biol Pharm Bull*. 2000 Aug;23(8):962-7.

Hattori K, Sasai M, Yamamoto A, Taniuchi S, Kojima T, Kobayashi Y, Iwamoto H, Yaeshima T, Hayasawa H. Intestinal flora of infants with cow milk hypersensitivity fed on casein-hydrolyzed formula supplemented raffinose. *Arerugi*. 2000 Dec;49(12):1146-55.

Hawkes CP, Mulcair S, Hourihane JO. Is hospital based MMR vaccination for children with egg allergy here to stay? *Ir Med J*. 2010 Jan;103(1):17-9.

Heaney RP, Dowell MS. Absorbability of the calcium in a high-calcium mineral water. *Osteoporos Int*. 1994 Nov;4(6):323-4.

Heap GA, van Heel DA. Genetics and pathogenesis of coeliac disease. *Semin Immunol*. May 13 2009.

Helin T, Haahtela S, Haahtela T. No effect of oral treatment with an intestinal bacterial strain, Lactobacillus rhamnosus (ATCC 53103), on birch-pollen allergy: a placebo-controlled double-blind study. *Allergy*. 2002 Mar;57(3):243-6.

Hemmer W, Focke M, Marzban G, Swoboda I, Jarisch R, Laimer M. Identification of Bet v 1-related allergens in fig and other Moraceae fruits. *Clin Exp Allergy*. 2010 Apr;40(4):679-87.

Hendel B, Ferreira P. *Water & Salt: The Essence of Life*. Gaithersburg: Natural Resources, 2003.

Herbert V. Vitamin B12: Plant sources, requirements, and assay. *Am J Clin Nutr.* 1988;48:852-858.

Herman PM, Drost LM. Evaluating the clinical relevance of food sensitivity tests: a single subject experiment. *Altern Med Rev.* 2004 Jun;9(2):198-207.

Heyman M, Grasset E, Ducroc R, Desjeux JF. Antigen absorption by the jejunal epithelium of children with cow's milk allergy. *Pediatr Res.* 1988 Aug;24(2):197-202.

Hiemori M, Eguchi Y, Kimoto M, Yamasita H, Takahashi K, Takahashi K, Tsuji H. Characterization of new 18-kDa IgE-binding proteins in beer. *Biosci Biotechnol Biochem.* 2008 Apr;72(4):1095-8.

Hieta N, Hasan T, Mäkinen-Kiljunen S, Lammintausta K. Sweet lupin—a new food allergen. *Duodecim.* 2010;126(12):1393-9.

Hirose Y, Murosaki S, Yamamoto Y, Yoshikai Y, Tsuru T. Daily intake of heat-killed Lactobacillus plantarum L-137 augments acquired immunity in healthy adults. *J Nutr.* 2006 Dec;136(12):3069-73.

Hobbs C. *Medicinal Mushrooms.* Summertown, TN: Botanica Press, 2003.

Hobbs C. *Stress & Natural Healing.* Loveland, CO: Interweave Press, 1997.

Hoffmann D. *Holistic Herbal.* London: Thorsons, 1983-2002.

Hofmann AM, Scurlock AM, Jones SM, Palmer KP, Lokhnygina Y, Steele PH, Kamilaris J, Burks AW. Safety of a peanut oral immunotherapy protocol in children with peanut allergy. *J Allergy Clin Immunol.* 2009 Aug;124(2):286-91, 291.e1-6.

Holick MF. Sunlight and vitamin D for bone health and prevention of autoimmune diseases, cancers, and cardiovascular disease. *Am J Clin Nutr.* 2004 Dec;80(6 Suppl):1678S-88S.

Holick MF. The vitamin D deficiency pandemic and consequences for nonskeletal health: mechanisms of action. *Mol Aspects Med.* 2008 Dec;29(6):361-8

Holick MF. Vitamin D status: measurement, interpretation, and clinical application. *Ann Epidemiol.* 2009 Feb;19(2):73-8.

Holick MF. Vitamin D: importance in the prevention of cancers, type 1 diabetes, heart disease, and osteoporosis. *Am J Clin Nutr.* 2004 Mar;79(3):362-71.

Holladay, S.D. Prenatal Immunotoxicant Exposure and Postnatal Autoimmune Disease. *Environ Health Perspect.* 1999; 107(suppl 5):687-691.

Hönscheid A, Rink L, Haase H. T-lymphocytes: a target for stimulatory and inhibitory effects of zinc ions. *Endocr Metab Immune Disord Drug Targets.* 2009 Jun;9(2):132-44.

Hooper R, Calvert J, Thompson RL, Deetlefs ME, Burney P. Urban/rural differences in diet and atopy in South Africa. *Allergy.* 2008 Apr;63(4):425-31.

Horrobin DF. Effects of evening primrose oil in rheumatoid arthritis. *Ann Rheum Dis.* 1989 Nov;48(11):965-6.

Hospers IC, de Vries-Vrolijk K, Brand PL. Double-blind, placebo-controlled cow's milk challenge in children with alleged cow's milk allergies, performed in a general hospital: diagnosis rejected in two-thirds of the children. *Ned Tijdschr Geneeskd.* 2006 Jun 10;150(23):1292-7.

Houle CR, Leo HL, Clark NM. A developmental, community, and psychosocial approach to food allergies in children. *Curr Allergy Asthma Rep.* 2010 Sep;10(5):381-6.

Hourihane JO, Grimshaw KE, Lewis SA, Briggs RA, Trewin JB, King RM, Kilburn SA, Warner JO. Does severity of low-dose, double-blind, placebo-controlled food challenges reflect severity of allergic reactions to peanut in the community? *Clin Exp Allergy.* 2005 Sep;35(9):1227-33.

Hsu CH, Lu CM, Chang TT. Efficacy and safety of modified Mai-Men-Dong-Tang for treatment of allergic asthma. *Pediatr Allergy Immunol.* 2005;16:76–81.

Hu C, Kitts DD. Antioxidant, prooxidant, and cytotoxic activities of solvent-fractionated dandelion (Taraxacum officinale) flower extracts in vitro. *J Agric Food Chem.* 2003 Jan 1;51(1):301-10.

Hu C, Kitts DD. Dandelion (Taraxacum officinale) flower extract suppresses both reactive oxygen species and nitric oxide and prevents lipid oxidation in vitro. *Phytomedicine.* 2005 Aug;12(8):588-97.

Hu C, Kitts DD. Luteolin and luteolin-7-O-glucoside from dandelion flower suppress iNOS and COX-2 in RAW264.7 cells. *Mol Cell Biochem.* 2004 Oct;265(1-2):107-13.

Huang D, Ou B, Prior RL. The chemistry behind antioxidant capacity assays. *J Agric Food Chem.* 2005 Mar 23;53(6):1841-56.

Huang M, Wang W, Wei S. Investigation on medicinal plant resources of Glycyrrhiza uralensis in China and chemical assessment of its underground part. *Zhongguo Zhong Yao Za Zhi.* 2010 Apr;35(8):947-52.

Hun L. Bacillus coagulans significantly improved abdominal pain and bloating in patients with IBS. *Postgrad Med.* 2009 Mar;121(2):119-24.

Hunter JO. Do horses suffer from irritable bowel syndrome? *Equine Vet J.* 2009 Dec;41(9):836-40.

Hur YM, Rushton JP. Genetic and environmental contributions to prosocial behaviour in 2- to 9-year-old South Korean twins. *Biol Lett.* 2007 Dec 23;3(6):664-6.

Husby S. Dietary antigens: uptake and humoral immunity in man. *APMIS Suppl.* 1988;1:1-40.

Ibero M, Boné J, Martín B, Martínez J. Evaluation of an extensively hydrolysed casein formula (Damira 2000) in children with allergy to cow's milk proteins. *Allergol Immunopathol (Madr)*. 2010 Mar-Apr;38(2):60-8.

Iida N, Inatomi Y, Murata H, Inada A, Murata J, Lang FA, Matsuura N, Nakanishi T. A new flavone xyloside and two new flavan-3-ol glucosides from Juniperus communis var. depressa. *Chem Biodivers*. 2007 Jan;4(1):32-42.

Indrio F, Ladisa G, Mautone A, Montagna O. Effect of a fermented formula on thymus size and stool pH in healthy term infants. *Pediatr Res*. 2007 Jul;62(1):98-100.

Innis SM, Hansen JW. Plasma fatty acid responses, metabolic effects, and safety of microalgal and fungal oils rich in arachidonic and docosahexaenoic acids in adults. *Am J Clin Nutr*. 1996 Aug;64(2):159-67.

Innocenti M, Michelozzi M, Giaccherini C, Ieri F, Vincieri FF, Mulinacci N. Flavonoids and biflavonoids in Tuscan berries of Juniperus communis L.: detection and quantitation by HPLC/DAD/ESI/MS. *J Agric Food Chem*. 2007 Aug 8;55(16):6596-602.

Int J Toxicol. Final report on the safety assessment of Juniperus communis Extract, Juniperus oxycedrus Extract, Juniperus oxycedrus Tar, Juniperus phoenicea extract, and Juniperus virginiana Extract. *Int J Toxicol*. 2001;20 Suppl 2:41-56.

Ionescu JG. New insights in the pathogenesis of atopic disease. *J Med Life*. 2009 Apr-Jun;2(2):146-54.

Iribarren C, Tolstykh IV, Miller MK, Eisner MD. Asthma and the prospective risk of anaphylactic shock and other allergy diagnoses in a large integrated health care delivery system. *Ann Allergy Asthma Immunol*. 2010 May;104(5):371-7.

Ishida Y, Nakamura F, Kanzato H, Sawada D, Hirata H, Nishimura A, Kajimoto O, Fujiwara S. Clinical effects of Lactobacillus acidophilus strain L-92 on perennial allergic rhinitis: a double-blind, placebo-controlled study. *J Dairy Sci*. 2005 Feb;88(2):527-33.

Ishida Y, Nakamura F, Kanzato H, Sawada D, Yamamoto N, Kagata H, Oh-Ida M, Takeuchi H, Fujiwara S. Effect of milk fermented with Lactobacillus acidophilus strain L-92 on symptoms of Japanese cedar pollen allergy: a randomized placebo-controlled trial. *Biosci Biotechnol Biochem*. 2005 Sep;69(9):1652-60.

Ivory K, Chambers SJ, Pin C, Prieto E, Arqués JL, Nicoletti C. Oral delivery of Lactobacillus casei Shirota modifies allergen-induced immune responses in allergic rhinitis. *Clin Exp Allergy*. 2008 Aug;38(8):1282-9.

Iwańczak B, Mowszet K, Iwańczak F. Feeding disorders, ALTE syndrome, Sandifer syndrome and gastroesophageal reflux disease in the course of food hypersensitivity in 8-month old infant. *Pol Merkur Lekarski*. 2010 Jul;29(169):44-6.

Izumi K, Aihara M, Ikezawa Z. Effects of non steroidal antiinflammatory drugs (NSAIDs) on immediate-type food allergy analysis of Japanese cases from 1998 to 2009. *Arerugi*. 2009 Dec;58(12):1629-39.

Jackson PG, Lessof MH, Baker RW, Ferrett J, MacDonald DM. Intestinal permeability in patients with eczema and food allergy. *Lancet*. 1981 Jun 13;1(8233):1285-6.

Jagetia GC, Aggarwal BB. "Spicing up" of the immune system by curcumin. *J Clin Immunol*. 2007 Jan;27(1):19-35.

Jagetia GC, Nayak V, Vidyasagar MS. Evaluation of the antineoplastic activity of guduchi (Tinospora cordifolia) in cultured HeLa cells. *Cancer Lett*. 1998 May 15;127(1-2):71-82.

Jagetia GC, Rao SK. Evaluation of Cytotoxic Effects of Dichloromethane Extract of Guduchi (Tinospora cordifolia Miers ex Hook F & THOMS) on Cultured HeLa Cells. *Evid Based Complement Alternat Med*. 2006 Jun;3(2):267-72.

Janson C, Anto J, Burney P, Chinn S, de Marco R, Heinrich J, Jarvis D, Kuenzli N, Leynaert B, Luczynska C, Neukirch F, Svanes C, Sunyer J, Wjst M; European Community Respiratory Health Survey II. The European Community Respiratory Health Survey: what are the main results so far? European Community Respiratory Health Survey II. *Eur Respir J*. 2001 Sep;18(3):598-611.

Jappe U, Vieths S. Lupine, a source of new as well as hidden food allergens. *Mol Nutr Food Res*. 2010 Jan;54(1):113-26.

Jarocka-Cyrta E, Baniukiewicz A, Wasilewska J, Pawlak J, Kaczmarski M. Focal villous atrophy of the duodenum in children who have outgrown cow's milk allergy. Chromoendoscopy and magnification endoscopy evaluation. *Med Wieku Rozwoj*. 2007 Apr-Jun;11(2 Pt 1):123-7.

Järvinen KM, Amalanayagam S, Shreffler WG, Noone S, Sicherer SH, Sampson HA, Nowak-Wegrzyn A. Epinephrine treatment is infrequent and biphasic reactions are rare in food-induced reactions during oral food challenges in children. *J Allergy Clin Immunol*. 2009 Dec;124(6):1267-72.

Jazani NH, Karimzad M, Mazloomi E, Sohrabpour M, Hassan ZM, Ghasemnejad H, Roshan-Milani S, Shahabi S. Evaluation of the adjuvant activity of naloxone, an opioid receptor antagonist, in combination with heat-killed Listeria monocytogenes vaccine. *Microbes Infect*. 2010 May;12(5):382-8.

Jennings S, Prescott SL. Early dietary exposures and feeding practices: role in pathogenesis and prevention of allergic disease? *Postgrad Med J*. 2010 Feb;86(1012):94-9.

Jensen B. *Foods that Heal*. Garden City Park, NY: Avery Publ, 1988, 1993.

Jensen B. *Nature Has a Remedy*. Los Angeles: Keats, 2001.

Jeon HJ, Kang HJ, Jung HJ, Kang YS, Lim CJ, Kim YM, Park EH. Anti-inflammatory activity of Taraxacum officinale. *J Ethnopharmacol.* 2008 Jan 4;115(1):82-8.

Johansson G, Holmén A, Persson L, Högstedt B, Wassén C, Ottova L, Gustafsson JA. Long-term effects of a change from a mixed diet to a lacto-vegetarian diet on human urinary and faecal mutagenic activity. *Mutagenesis.* 1998 Mar;13(2):167-71.

Johansson G, Holmén A, Persson L, Högstedt B, Wassén C, Ottova L, Gustafsson JA. Dietary influence on some proposed risk factors for colon cancer: fecal and urinary mutagenic activity and the activity of some intestinal bacterial enzymes. *Cancer Detect Prev.* 1997;21(3):258-66.

Johansson G, Holmén A, Persson L, Högstedt R, Wassén C, Ottova L, Gustafsson JA. The effect of a shift from a mixed diet to a lacto-vegetarian diet on human urinary and fecal mutagenic activity. *Carcinogenesis.* 1992 Feb;13(2):153-7.

Johansson G, Ravald N. Comparison of some salivary variables between vegetarians and omnivores. *Eur J Oral Sci.* 1995 Apr;103(2 (Pt 1)):95-8.

Johari H. *Ayurvedic Massage: Traditional Indian Techniques for Balancing Body and Mind.* Rochester, VT: Healing Arts, 1996.

Johnson LM. Gitksan medicinal plants—cultural choice and efficacy. *J Ethnobiol Ethnomed.* 2006 Jun 21;2:29.

Jones SM, Zhong Z, Enomoto N, Schemmer P, Thurman RG. Dietary juniper berry oil minimizes hepatic reperfusion injury in the rat. *Hepatology.* 1998 Oct;28(4):1042-50.

Jones MA, Silman AJ, Whiting S, *et al.* Occurrence of rheumatoid arthritis is not increased in the first degree relatives of a population based inception cohort of inflammatory polyarthritis. *Ann Rheum Dis.* 1996;55(2): 89-93.

Julkunen-Tiitto R. A chemotaxonomic survey of phenolics in leaves of northern Salicaceae species. *Phytochemistry.* 1986;25(3):663-667.

Jung HA, Yokozawa T, Kim BW, Jung JH, Choi JS. Selective inhibition of prenylated flavonoids from Sophora flavescens against BACE1 and cholinesterases. *Am J Chin Med.* 2010;38(2):415-29.

Jurakić Toncié R, Lipozencié J. Role and significance of atopy patch test. *Acta Dermatovenerol Croat.* 2010;18(1):38-55.

Jurenka JS. Anti-inflammatory properties of curcumin, a major constituent of Curcuma longa: a review of preclinical and clinical research. *Altern Med Rev.* 2009 Feb;14(2):141-153.

Kähkönen MP, Hopia AI, Vuorela HJ, Rauha JP, Pihlaja K, Kujala TS, Heinonen M. Antioxidant activity of plant extracts containing phenolic compounds. *J Agric Food Chem.* 1999 Oct;47(10):3954-62.

Kaila M, Vanto T, Valovirta E, Koivikko A, Juntunen-Backman K. Diagnosis of food allergy in Finland: survey of pediatric practices. *Pediatr Allergy Immunol.* 2000 Nov;11(4):246-9.

Kajander K, Hatakka K, Poussa T, Färkkilä M, Korpela R. A probiotic mixture alleviates symptoms in irritable bowel syndrome patients: a controlled 6-month intervention. *Aliment Pharmacol Ther.* 2005 Sep 1;22(5):387-94.

Kajander K, Krogius-Kurikka L, Rinttilä T, Karjalainen H, Palva A, Korpela R. Effects of multispecies probiotic supplementation on intestinal microbiota in irritable bowel syndrome. *Aliment Pharmacol Ther.* 2007 Aug 1;26(3):463-73.

Kajander K, Myllyluoma E, Rajilić-Stojanović M, Kyrönpalo S, Rasmussen M, Järvenpää S, Zoetendal EG, de Vos WM, Vapaatalo H, Korpela R. Clinical trial: multispecies probiotic supplementation alleviates the symptoms of irritable bowel syndrome and stabilizes intestinal microbiota. *Aliment Pharmacol Ther.* 2008 Jan 1;27(1):48-57.

Kalach N, Benhamou PH, Campeotto F, Dupont Ch. Anemia impairs small intestinal absorption measured by intestinal permeability in children. *Eur Ann Allergy Clin Immunol.* 2007 Jan;39(1):20-2.

Kalach N, Rocchiccioli F, de Boissieu D, Benhamou PH, Dupont C. Intestinal permeability in children: variation with age and reliability in the diagnosis of cow's milk allergy. *Acta Paediatr.* 2001 May;90(5):499-504.

Kalliomäki M, Salminen S, Arvilommi H, Kero P, Koskinen P, Isolauri E. Probiotics in primary prevention of atopic disease: a randomised placebo-controlled trial. *Lancet.* 2001 Apr 7;357(9262):1076-9.

Kamdar T, Bryce PJ. Immunotherapy in food allergy. Immunotherapy. 2010 May;2(3):329-38.

Kang SK, Kim JK, Ahn SH, Oh JE, Kim JH, Lim DH, Son BK. Relationship between silent gastroesophageal reflux and food sensitization in infants and young children with recurrent wheezing. *J Korean Med Sci.* 2010 Mar;25(3):425-8.

Kanny G, Grignon G, Dauca M, Guedenet JC, Moneret-Vautrin DA. Ultrastructural changes in the duodenal mucosa induced by ingested histamine in patients with chronic urticaria. *Allergy.* 1996 Dec;51(12):935-9.

Kapil A, Sharma S. Immunopotentiating compounds from Tinospora cordifolia. *J Ethnopharmacol.* 1997 Oct;58(2):89-95.

REFERENCES AND BIBLIOGRAPHY

Kaptan K, Beyan C, Ural AU, Cetin T, Avcu F, Gülşen M, Finci R, Yalçín A. Helicobacter pylori—is it a novel causative agent in Vitamin B12 deficiency? *Arch Intern Med.* 2000 May 8;160(9):1349-53.

Karaman I, Sahin F, Güllüce M, Ogütçü H, Sengül M, Adigüzel A. Antimicrobial activity of aqueous and methanol extracts of Juniperus oxycedrus L. *J Ethnopharmacol.* 2003 Apr;85(2-3):231-5.

Karkoulias K, Patouchas D, Alahiotis S, Tsiamita M, Vrodakis K, Spiropoulos K. Specific sensitization in wheat flour and contributing factors in traditional bakers. *Eur Rev Med Pharmacol Sci.* 2007 May-Jun;11(3):141-8.

Karpińska J, Mikołuć B, Motkowski R, Piotrowska-Jastrzebska J. HPLC method for simultaneous determination of retinol, alpha-tocopherol and coenzyme Q10 in human plasma. *J Pharm Biomed Anal.* 2006 Sep 18;42(2):232-6.

Kashiwada Y, Takanaka K, Tsukada H, Miwa Y, Taga T, Tanaka S, Ikeshiro Y. Sesquiterpene glucosides from anti-leukotriene B4 release fraction of Taraxacum officinale. *J Asian Nat Prod Res.* 2001;3(3):191-7.

Kattan JD, Srivastava KD, Sampson HA, Li XM. Pharmacologic and Immunologic Effects of Individual Herbs of Food Allergy Herbal Formula 2 in a Murine Model of Peanut Allergy. *J Allergy Clin Immunol.* 2006;117(2):S34.

Kattan JD, Srivastava KD, Zou ZM, Goldfarb J, Sampson HA, Li XM. Pharmacological and immunological effects of individual herbs in the Food Allergy Herbal Formula-2 (FAHF-2) on peanut allergy. *Phytother Res.* 2008 May;22(5):651-9.

Katz Y, Rajuan N, Goldberg MR, Eisenberg E, Heyman E, Cohen A, Leshno M. Early exposure to cow's milk protein is protective against IgE-mediated cow's milk protein allergy. *J Allergy Clin Immunol.* 2010 Jul;126(1):77-82.e1.

Kazansky DB. MHC restriction and allogeneic immune responses. *J Immunotoxicol.* 2008 Oct;5(4):369-84.

Kazlowska K, Hsu T, Hou CC, Yang WC, Tsai GJ. Anti-inflammatory properties of phenolic compounds and crude extract from Porphyra dentata. *J Ethnopharmacol.* 2010 Mar 2;128(1):123-30.

Keita AV, Söderholm JD. The intestinal barrier and its regulation by neuroimmune factors. *Neurogastroenterol Motil.* 2010 Jul;22(7):718-33.

Kekkonen RA, Sysi-Aho M, Seppanen-Laakso T, Julkunen I, Vapaatalo H, Oresic M, Korpela R. Effect of probiotic Lactobacillus rhamnosus GG intervention on global serum lipidomic profiles in healthy adults. *World J Gastroenterol.* 2008 May 28;14(20):3188-94.

Kelder P. *Ancient Secret of the Fountain of Youth.* New York: Doubleday, 1998.

Keogh JB, Grieger JA, Noakes M, Clifton PM. Flow-Mediated Dilatation Is Impaired by a High-Saturated Fat Diet but Not by a High-Carbohydrate Diet. *Arterioscler Thromb Vasc Biol.* 2005 Mar 17

Kerckhoffs DA, Brouns F, Hornstra G, Mensink RP. Effects on the human serum lipoprotein profile of beta-glucan, soy protein and isoflavones, plant sterols and stanols, garlic and tocotrienols. *J Nutr.* 2002 Sep;132(9):2494-505.

Key T, Appleby P, Davey G, Allen N, Spencer E, Travis R. Mortality in British vegetarians: review and preliminary results from EPIC-Oxford. *Amer. Jour. Clin. Nutr. Suppl.* 2003;78(3): 533S-538S.

Kiefte-de Jong JC, Escher JC, Arends LR, Jaddoe VW, Hofman A, Raat H, Moll HA. Infant nutritional factors and functional constipation in childhood: the Generation R study. *Am J Gastroenterol.* 2010 Apr;105(4):940-5.

Kim DC, Choi SY, Kim SH, Yun BS, Yoo ID, Reddy NR, Yoon HS, Kim KT. Isoliquiritigenin selectively inhibits H(2) histamine receptor signaling. *Mol Pharmacol.* 2006 Aug;70(2):493-500.

Kim HM, Shin HY, Lim KH, Ryu ST, Shin TY, Chae HJ, Kim HR, Lyu YS, An NH, Lim KS. Taraxacum officinale inhibits tumor necrosis factor-alpha production from rat astrocytes. *Immunopharmacol Immunotoxicol.* 2000 Aug;22(3):519-30.

Kim JH, An S, Kim JE, Choi GS, Ye YM, Park HS. Beef-induced anaphylaxis confirmed by the basophil activation test. *Allergy Asthma Immunol Res.* 2010 Jul;2(3):206-8.

Kim JY, Kim DY, Lee YS, Lee BK, Lee KH, Ro JY. DA-9601, Artemisia asiatica herbal extract, ameliorates airway inflammation of allergic asthma in mice. *Mol Cells.* 2006;22:104–12.

Kim MN, Kim N, Lee SH, Park YS, Hwang JH, Kim JW, Jeong SH, Lee DH, Kim JS, Jung HC, Song IS. The effects of probiotics on PPI-triple therapy for Helicobacter pylori eradication. *Helicobacter.* 2008 Aug;13(4):261-8.

Kim NI, Jo Y, Ahn SB, Son BK, Kim SH, Park YS, Kim SH, Ju JE. A case of eosinophilic esophagitis with food hypersensitivity. *J Neurogastroenterol Motil.* 2010 Jul;16(3):315-8.

Kim SJ, Jung JY, Kim HW, Park T. Anti-obesity effects of Juniperus chinensis extract are associated with increased AMP-activated protein kinase expression and phosphorylation in the visceral adipose tissue of rats. *Biol Pharm Bull.* 2008 Jul;31(7):1415-21.

Kim TE, Park SW, Noh G, Lee S. Comparison of skin prick test results between crude allergen extracts from foods and commercial allergen extracts in atopic dermatitis by double-blind placebo-controlled food challenge for milk, egg, and soybean. *Yonsei Med J.* 2002 Oct;43(5):613-20.

Kim YG, Moon JT, Lee KM, Chon NR, Park H. The effects of probiotics on symptoms of irritable bowel syndrome. *Korean J Gastroenterol.* 2006 Jun;47(6):413-9.

Kim YH, Kim KS, Han CS, Yang HC, Park SH, Ko KI, Lee SH, Kim KH, Lee NH, Kim JM, Son K. Inhibitory effects of natural plants of Jeju Island on elastase and MMP-1 expression. *Int J Cosmet Sci.* 2007 Dec;29(6):487-8.

Kimata M, Inagaki N, Nagai H. Effects of luteolin and other flavonoids on IgE-mediated allergic reactions. *Planta Med.* 2000 Feb;66(1):25-9.

Kimata M, Shichijo M, Miura T, Serizawa I, Inagaki N, Nagai H. Effects of luteolin, quercetin and baicalein on immunoglobulin E-mediated mediator release from human cultured mast cells. *Clin Exp Allergy.* 2000 Apr;30(4):501-8.

Kimber I, Dearman RJ. Factors affecting the development of food allergy. *Proc Nutr Soc.* 2002 Nov;61(4):435-9.

Kimmatkar N, Thawani V, Hingorani L, Khiyani R. Efficacy and tolerability of Boswellia serrata extract in treatment of osteoarthritis of knee—a randomized double blind placebo controlled trial. *Phytomedicine.* 2003 Jan;10(1):3-7.

Kinaciyan T, Jahn-Schmid B, Radakovics A, Zwölfer B, Schreiber C, Francis JN, Ebner C, Bohle B. Successful sublingual immunotherapy with birch pollen has limited effects on concomitant food allergy to apple and the immune response to the Bet v 1 homolog Mal d 1. *J Allergy Clin Immunol.* 2007 Apr;119(4):937-43.

Kirjavainen PV, Salminen SJ, Isolauri E. Probiotic bacteria in the management of atopic disease: underscoring the importance of viability. *J Pediatr Gastroenterol Nutr.* 2003 Feb;36(2):223-7.

Kisiel W, Barszcz B. Further sesquiterpenoids and phenolics from Taraxacum officinale. *Fitoterapia.* 2000 Jun;71(3):269-73.

Kisiel W, Michalska K. Sesquiterpenoids and phenolics from Taraxacum hondoense. *Fitoterapia.* 2005 Sep;76(6):520-4.

Kjellman NI, Björkstén B, Hattevig G, Fälth-Magnusson K. Natural history of food allergy. *Ann Allergy.* 1988 Dec;61(6 Pt 2):83-7.

Klein R, Landau MG. *Healing: The Body Betrayed.* Minneapolis: DCI:Chronimed, 1992.

Klein-Galczinsky C. Pharmacological and clinical effectiveness of a fixed phytogenic combination trembling poplar (Populus tremula), true goldenrod (Solidago virgaurea) and ash (Fraxinus excelsior) in mild to moderate rheumatic complaints. *Wien Med Wochenschr.* 1999;149(8-10):248-53.

Klemola T, Vanto T, Juntunen-Backman K, Kalimo K, Korpela R, Varjonen E. Allergy to soy formula and to extensively hydrolyzed whey formula in infants with cow's milk allergy: a prospective, randomized study with a follow-up to the age of 2 years. *J Pediatr.* 2002 Feb;140(2):219-24.

Kloss J. *Back to Eden.* Twin Oaks, WI: Lotus Press, 1939-1999.

Knutson TW, Bengtsson U, Dannaeus A, Ahlstedt S, Knutson L. Effects of luminal antigen on intestinal albumin and hyaluronan permeability and ion transport in atopic patients. *J Allergy Clin Immunol.* 1996 Jun;97(6):1225-32.

Ko J, Busse PJ, Shek L, Noone SA, Sampson HA, Li XM. Effect of Chinese Herbal Formulas on T Cell Responses in Patients with Peanut Allergy or Asthma. *J Allergy Clin Immunol* .2005;115:S34.

Ko J, Lee JI, Munoz-Furlong A, Li XM, Sicherer SH. Use of complementary and alternative medicine by food-allergic patients. *Ann Allergy Asthma Immunol.* 2006;97:365–9.

Koo HN, Hong SH, Song BK, Kim CH, Yoo YH, Kim HM. Taraxacum officinale induces cytotoxicity through TNF-alpha and IL-1alpha secretion in Hep G2 cells. *Life Sci.* 2004 Jan 16;74(9):1149-57.

Kotzampassi K, Giamarellos-Bourboulis EJ, Voudouris A, Kazamias P, Eleftheriadis E. Benefits of a synbiotic formula (Synbiotic 2000Forte) in critically Ill trauma patients: early results of a randomized controlled trial. *World J Surg.* 2006 Oct;30(10):1848-55.

Kootstra HS, Vlieg-Boerstra BJ, Dubois AE. Assessment of the reduced allergenic properties of the Santana apple. *Ann Allergy Asthma Immunol.* 2007 Dec;99(6):522-5.

Kovács T, Mette H, Per B, Kun L, Schmelczer M, Barta J, Jean-Claude D, Nagy J. Relationship between intestinal permeability and antibodies against food antigens in IgA nephropathy. *Orv Hetil.* 1996 Jan 14;137(2):65-9.

Kowalchik C, Hylton W (eds). *Rodale's Illustrated Encyclopedia of Herbs.* Emmaus, PA: 1987.

Kowalczyk E, Krzesiński P, Kura M, Niedworok J, Kowalski J, Blaszczyk J. Pharmacological effects of flavonoids from Scutellaria baicalensis. *Przegl Lek.* 2006;63(2):95-6.

Kozlowski LT, Mehta NY, Sweeney CT, Schwartz SS, Vogler GP, Jarvis MJ, West RJ. Filter ventilation and nicotine content of tobacco in cigarettes from Canada, the United Kingdom, and the United States. *Tob Control.* 1998 Winter;7(4):369-75.

Kreig M. *Black Market Medicine.* New York: Bantam, 1968.

Kristjansson I, Ardal B, Jonsson JS, Sigurdsson JA, Foldevi M, Bjorksten B (1999) Adverse reactions to food and food allergy in young children in Iceland and Sweden. *Scand J Prim Health Care.* 17: 30–34.

Krogulska A, Wasowska-Królikowska K, Dynowski J. Evaluation of bronchial hyperreactivity in children with asthma undergoing food challenges. *Pol Merkur Lekarski.* 2007 Jul;23(133):30-5.

Krogulska A, Wasowska-Królikowska K, Trzeźwińska B. Food challenges in children with asthma. *Pol Merkur Lekarski.* 2007 Jul;23(133):22-9.

Krüger P, Kanzer J, Hummel J, Fricker G, Schubert-Zsilavecz M, Abdel-Tawab M. Permeation of Boswellia extract in the Caco-2 model and possible interactions of its constituents KBA and AKBA with OATP1B3 and MRP2. *Eur J Pharm Sci.* 2009 Feb 15;36(2-3):275-84.

Kuitunen M, Kukkonen K, Juntunen-Backman K, Korpela R, Poussa T, Tuure T, Haahtela T, Savilahti E. Probiotics prevent IgE-associated allergy until age 5 years in cesarean-delivered children but not in the total cohort. *J Allergy Clin Immunol.* 2009 Feb;123(2):335-41.

Kuitunen M, Savilahti E, Sarnesto A. Human alpha-lactalbumin and bovine beta-lactoglobulin absorption in infants. *Allergy.* 1994 May;49(5):354-60.

Kuitunen M, Savilahti E. Mucosal IgA, mucosal cow's milk antibodies, serum cow's milk antibodies and gastrointestinal permeability in infants. *Pediatr Allergy Immunol.* 1995 Feb;6(1):30-5.

Kukkonen K, Kuitunen M, Haahtela T, Korpela R, Poussa T, Savilahti E. High intestinal IgA associates with reduced risk of IgE-associated allergic diseases. *Pediatr Allergy Immunol.* 2010 Feb;21(1 Pt 1):67-73.

Kukkonen K, Savilahti E, Haahtela T, Juntunen-Backman K, Korpela R, Poussa T, Tuure T, Kuitunen M. Probiotics and prebiotic galacto-oligosaccharides in the prevention of allergic diseases: a randomized, double-blind, placebo-controlled trial. *J Allergy Clin Immunol.* 2007 Jan;119(1):192-8.

Kulka M. The potential of natural products as effective treatments for allergic inflammation: implications for allergic rhinitis. *Curr Top Med Chem.* 2009;9(17):1611-24.

Kull I, Bergström A, Lilja G, Pershagen G, Wickman M. Fish consumption during the first year of life and development of allergic diseases during childhood. *Allergy.* 2006 Aug;61(8):1009-15.

Kull I, Melen E, Alm J, Hallberg J, Svartengren M, van Hage M, Pershagen G, Wickman M, Bergström A. Breast-feeding in relation to asthma, lung function, and sensitization in young schoolchildren. *J Allergy Clin Immunol.* 2010 May;125(5):1013-9.

Kumar R, Singh BP, Srivastava P, Sridhara S, Arora N, Gaur SN. Relevance of serum IgE estimation in allergic bronchial asthma with special reference to food allergy. *Asian Pac J Allergy Immunol.* 2006 Dec;24(4):191-9.

Kummeling I, Mills EN, Clausen M, Dubakiene R, Pérez CF, Fernández-Rivas M, Knulst AC, Kowalski ML, Lidholm J, Le TM, Metzler C, Mustakov T, Popov T, Potts J, van Ree R, Sakellariou A, Töndury B, Tzannis K, Burney P. The EuroPrevall surveys on the prevalence of food allergies in children and adults: background and study methodology. *Allergy.* 2009 Oct;64(10):1493-7.

Kung HC, Hoyert DL, Xu J, Murphy SL. Deaths: Final Data for 2005. *National Vital Statistics Reports.* 2008;56(10). http://www.cdc.gov/nchs/data/ nvsr/nvsr56/nvsr56_10.pdf. Accessed: 2008 Jun.

Kunisawa J, Kiyono H. Aberrant interaction of the gut immune system with environmental factors in the development of food allergies. *Curr Allergy Asthma Rep.* 2010 May;10(3):215-21.

Kusano M, Zai H, Hosaka H, Shimoyama Y, Nagoshi A, Maeda M, Kawamura O, Mori M. New frontiers in gut nutrient sensor research: monosodium L-glutamate added to a high-energy, high-protein liquid diet promotes gastric emptying: a possible therapy for patients with functional dyspepsia. *J Pharmacol Sci.* 2010 Jan;112(1):33-6.

Kusunoki T, Miyanomae T, Inoue Y, Itoh M, Yoshioka T, Okafuji I, Nishikomori R, Heike T, Nakahata T. Changes in food allergen sensitization rates of Japanese allergic children during the last 15 years. *Arerugi.* 2004 Jul;53(7):683-8.

Kusunoki T, Morimoto T, Nishikomori R, Yasumi T, Heike T, Mukaida K, Fujii T, Nakahata T. Breastfeeding and the prevalence of allergic diseases in schoolchildren: Does reverse causation matter? *Pediatr Allergy Immunol.* 2010 Feb;21(1 Pt 1):60-6.

Kuvaeva IB. Permeability of the gastrointestinal tract for macromolecules in health and disease. *Hum Physiol.* 1979 Mar-Apr;4(2):272-83.

Kuznetsova TA, Shevchenko NM, Zviagintseva TN, Besednova NN. Biological activity of fucoidans from brown algae and the prospects of their use in medicine]. *Antibiot Khimioter.* 2004;49(5):24-30..

Lad V. *Ayurveda: The Science of Self-Healing.* Twin Lakes, WI: Lotus Press.

Lamaison JL, Carnat A, Petitjean-Freytet C. Tannin content and inhibiting activity of elastase in Rosaceae. *Ann Pharm Fr.* 1990;48(6):335-40.

Lappe FM. *Diet for a Small Planet.* New York: Ballantine, 1971.

Lau BH, Riesen SK, Truong KP, Lau EW, Rohdewald P, Barreta RA. Pycnogenol as an adjunct in the management of childhood asthma. *J Asthma.* 2004;41(8):825-32.

Laubereau B, Filipiak-Pittroff B, von Berg A, Grübl A, Reinhardt D, Wichmann HE, Koletzko S; GINI Study Group. Caesarean section and gastrointestinal symptoms, atopic dermatitis, and sensitisation during the first year of life. *Arch Dis Child.* 2004 Nov;89(11):993-7.

Laudat A, Arnaud P, Napoly A, Brion F. The intestinal permeability test applied to the diagnosis of food allergy in paediatrics. West Indian Med J. 1994 Sep;43(3):87-8.

Laugesen M, Elliott R. Ischaemic heart disease, Type 1 diabetes, and cow milk A1 beta-casein. N Z Med J. 2003 Jan 24;116(1168):U295.

Laurière M, Pecquet C, Bouchez-Mahiout I, Snégaroff J, Bayrou O, Raison-Peyron N, Vigan M. Hydrolysed wheat proteins present in cosmetics can induce immediate hypersensitivities. Contact Dermatitis. 2006 May;54(5):283-9.

LaValle JB. The Cox-2 Connection. Rochester, VT: Healing Arts, 2001.

Lean G. US study links more than 200 diseases to pollution. London Independent. 2004 Nov 14.

Lee BJ, Park HS. Common whelk (Buccinum undatum) allergy: identification of IgE-binding components and effects of heating and digestive enzymes. J Korean Med Sci. 2004 Dec;19(6):793-9.

Lee CK, Cheng YS. Diterpenoids from the leaves of Juniperus chinensis var. kaizuka. J Nat Prod. 2001 Apr;64(4):511-4.

Lee JH, Noh J, Noh G, Kim HS, Mun SH, Choi WS, Cho S, Lee S. Allergen-specific B cell subset responses in cow's milk allergy of late eczematous reactions in atopic dermatitis. Cell Immunol. 2010;262(1):44-51.

Lee JY, Kim CJ. Determination of allergenic egg proteins in food by protein-, mass spectrometry-, and DNA-based methods. J AOAC Int. 2010 Mar-Apr;93(2):462-77.

Lee YS, Kim SH, Jung SH, Kim JK, Pan CH, Lim SS. Aldose reductase inhibitory compounds from Glycyrrhiza uralensis. Biol Pharm Bull. 2010;33(5):917-21.

Leffler DA, Schuppan D. Update on serologic testing in celiac disease. Am J Gastroenterol. 2010 Dec;105(12):2520-4.

Lehmann B. The vitamin D3 pathway in human skin and its role for regulation of biological processes. Photochem Photobiol. 2005 Nov-Dec;81(6):1246-51.

Lehto M, Airaksinen L, Puustinen A, Tillander S, Hannula S, Nyman T, Toskala E, Alenius H, Lauerma A. Thaumatin-like protein and baker's respiratory allergy. Ann Allergy Asthma Immunol. 2010 Feb;104(2):139-46.

Lehto M, Airaksinen L, Puustinen A, Tillander S, Hannula S, Nyman T, Toskala E, Alenius H, Lauerma A. Thaumatin-like protein and baker's respiratory allergy. Ann Allergy Asthma Immunol. 2010 Feb;104(2):139-46.

Leitzmann C. Vegetarian diets: what are the advantages? Forum Nutr. 2005;(57):147-56.

Leu YL, Shi LS, Damu AG. Chemical constituents of Taraxacum formosanum. Chem Pharm Bull. 2003 May;51(5):599-601.

Leu YL, Wang YL, Huang SC, Shi LS. Chemical constituents from roots of Taraxacum formosanum. Chem Pharm Bull. 2005 Jul;53(7):853-5.

Leung DY, Sampson HA, Yunginger JW, Burks AW Jr, Schneider LC, Wortel CH, Davis FM, Hyun JD, Shanahan WR Jr; Avon Longitudinal Study of Parents and Children Study Team. Effect of anti-IgE therapy in patients with peanut allergy. N Engl J Med. 2003 Mar 13;348(11):986-93.

Leung DY, Shanahan WR Jr, Li XM, Sampson HA. New approaches for the treatment of anaphylaxis. Novartis Found Symp. 2004;257:248-60; discussion 260-4, 276-85.

Lewerin C, Jacobsson S, Lindstedt G, Nilsson-Ehle H. Serum biomarkers for atrophic gastritis and antibodies against Helicobacter pylori in the elderly: Implications for vitamin B12, folic acid and iron status and response to oral vitamin therapy. Scand J Gastroenterol. 2008;43(9):1050-6.

Lewis SA, Grimshaw KE, Warner JO, Hourihane JO. The promiscuity of immunoglobulin E binding to peanut allergens, as determined by Western blotting, correlates with the severity of clinical symptoms. Clin Exp Allergy. 2005 Jun;35(6):767-73.

Lewis WH, Elvin-Lewis MPF. Medical Botany: Plants Affecting Man's Health. New York: Wiley, 1977.

Lewontin R. The Genetic Basis of Evolutionary Change. New York: Columbia Univ Press, 1974.

Leyel CF. Culpeper's English Physician & Complete Herbal. Hollywood, CA: Wilshire, 1971.

Leynadier F. Mast cells and basophils in asthma. Ann Biol Clin (Paris). 1989;47(6):351-6.

Li H, Tan G, Jiang X, Qiao H, Pan S, Jiang H, Kanwar JR, Sun X. Therapeutic effects of matrine on primary and metastatic breast cancer. Am J Chin Med. 2010;38(6):1115-30.

Li S, Li W, Wang Y, Asada Y, Koike K. Prenylflavonoids from Glycyrrhiza uralensis and their protein tyrosine phosphatase-1B inhibitory activities. Bioorg Med Chem Lett. 2010 Sep 15;20(18):5398-401.

Li XM, Huang CK, Zhang TF, Teper AA, Srivastava K, Schofield BH, Sampson HA. The chinese herbal medicine formula MSSM-002 suppresses allergic airway hyperreactivity and modulates TH1/TH2 responses in a murine model of allergic asthma. J Allergy Clin Immunol. 2000;106:660-8.

Li XM, Schofield BH, Huang CK, Kleiner GA, Sampson HA. A Murine Model of IgE Mediated Cow Milk Hypersensitivity. J Allergy Clin Immunol. 1999;103:206-14.

Li XM, Serebrisky D, Lee SY, Huang CK, Bardina L, Schofield BH, Stanley JS, Burks AW, Bannon GA, Sampson HA. A murine model of peanut anaphylaxis: T- and B-cell responses to a major peanut allergen mimic human responses. J Allergy Clin Immunol. 2000;106:150-8.

Li XM, Zhang TF, Huang CK, Srivastava K, Teper AA, Zhang L, Schofield BH, Sampson HA. Food Allergy Herbal Formula-1 (FAHF-1) blocks peanut-induced anaphylaxis in a murine model. *J Allergy Clin Immunol.* 2001;108:639–46.

Li XM, Zhang TF, Sampson H, Zou ZM, Beyer K, Wen MC, Schofield B. The potential use of Chinese herbal medicines in treating allergic asthma. *Ann Allergy Asthma Immunol.* 2004;93:S35–S44.

Li XM. Beyond allergen avoidance: update on developing therapies for peanut allergy. *Curr Opin Allergy Clin Immunol.* 2005;5:287–92.

Lidén M, Kristjánsson G, Valtysdottir S, Venge P, Hällgren R. Cow's milk protein sensitivity assessed by the mucosal patch technique is related to irritable bowel syndrome in patients with primary Sjögren's syndrome. *Clin Exp Allergy.* 2008 Jun;38(6):929-35.

Lidén M, Kristjánsson G, Valtysdottir S, Venge P, Hällgren R. Self-reported food intolerance and mucosal reactivity after rectal food protein challenge in patients with rheumatoid arthritis. *Scand J Rheumatol.* 2010 Aug;39(4):292-8.

Lied GA, Lillestol K, Valeur J, Berstad A. Intestinal B cell-activating factor: an indicator of non-IgE-mediated hypersensitivity reactions to food? *Aliment Pharmacol Ther.* 2010 Jul;32(1):66-73.

Lillestol K, Berstad A, Lind R, Florvaag E, Arslan Lied G, Tangen T. Anxiety and depression in patients with self-reported food hypersensitivity. *Gen Hosp Psychiatry.* 2010 Jan-Feb;32(1):42-8.

Lillestol K, Helgeland L, Arslan Lied G, Florvaag E, Valeur J, Lind R, Berstad A. Indications of 'atopic bowel' in patients with self-reported food hypersensitivity. *Aliment Pharmacol Ther.* 2010 May;31(10):1112-22.

Lim JP, Song YC, Kim JW, Ku CH, Eun JS, Leem KH, Kim DK. Free radical scavengers from the heartwood of Juniperus chinensis. *Arch Pharm Res.* 2002 Aug;25(4):449-52.

Ling WH, Hänninen O. Shifting from a conventional diet to an uncooked vegan diet reversibly alters fecal hydrolytic activities in humans. *J Nutr.* 1992 Apr;122(4):924-30.

Lininger S, Gaby A, Austin S, Brown D, Wright J, Duncan A. *The Natural Pharmacy.* New York: Three Rivers, 1999.

Linsalata M, Russo F, Berloco P, Caruso ML, Matteo GD, Cifone MG, Simone CD, Ierardi E, Di Leo A. The influence of Lactobacillus brevis on ornithine decarboxylase activity and polyamine profiles in Helicobacter pylori-infected gastric mucosa. Helicobacter. 2004 Apr;9(2):165-72. Madden JA, Plummer SF, Tang J, Garaiova I, Plummer NT, Herbison M, Hunter JO, Shimada T, Cheng L, Shirakawa T. Effect of probiotics on preventing disruption of the intestinal microflora following antibiotic therapy: a double-blind, placebo-controlled pilot study. *Int Immunopharmacol.* 2005 Jun;5(6):1091-7.

Lipozencić J, Wolf R. The diagnostic value of atopy patch testing and prick testing in atopic dermatitis: facts and controversies. *Clin Dermatol.* 2010 Jan-Feb;28(1):38-44.

Lipski E. *Digestive Wellness.* Los Angeles, CA: Keats, 2000.

Liu GM, Cao MJ, Huang YY, Cai QF, Weng WY, Su WJ. Comparative study of in vitro digestibility of major allergen tropomyosin and other food proteins of Chinese mitten crab (Eriocheir sinensis). *J Sci Food Agric.* 2010 Aug 15;90(10):1614-20.

Liu HY, Giday Z, Moore BF. Possible pathogenetic mechanisms producing bovine milk protein inducible malabsorption: a hypothesis. *Ann Allergy.* 1977 Jul;39(1):1-7.

Liu JY, Hu JH, Zhu QG, Li FQ, Wang J, Sun HJ. Effect of matrine on the expression of substance P receptor and inflammatory cytokines production in human skin keratinocytes and fibroblasts. *Int Immunopharmacol.* 2007 Jun;7(6):816-23.

Liu X, Beaty TH, Deindl P, Huang SK, Lau S, Sommerfeld C, Fallin MD, Kao WH, Wahn U, Nickel R. Associations between specific serum IgE response and 6 variants within the genes IL4, IL13, and IL4RA in German children: the German Multicenter Atopy Study. *J Allergy Clin Immunol.* 2004 Mar;113(3):489-95.

Liu XJ, Cao MA, Li WH, Shen CS, Yan SQ, Yuan CS. Alkaloids from Sophora flavescens Aition. *Fitoterapia.* 2010 Sep;81(6):524-7.

Lloyd JU. *American Materia Medica, Therapeutics and Pharmacognosy.* Portland, OR: Eclectic Medical Publications, 1989-1983.

Lloyd-Still JD, Powers CA, Hoffman DR, Boyd-Trull K, Lester LA, Benisek DC, Arterburn LM. Bioavailability and safety of a high dose of docosahexaenoic acid triacylglycerol of algal origin in cystic fibrosis patients: a randomized, controlled study. *Nutrition.* 2006 Jan;22(1):36-46.

Loizzo MR, Saab AM, Tundis R, Statti GA, Menichini F, Lampronti I, Gambari R, Cinatl J, Doerr HW. Phytochemical analysis and in vitro antiviral activities of the essential oils of seven Lebanon species. *Chem Biodivers.* 2008 Mar;5(3):461-70.

Lomax AR, Calder PC. Probiotics, immune function, infection and inflammation: a review of the evidence from studies conducted in humans. *Curr Pharm Des.* 2009;15(13):1428-518.

Longo G, Barbi E, Berti I, Meneghetti R, Pittalis A, Ronfani L, Ventura A. Specific oral tolerance induction in children with very severe cow's milk-induced reactions. *J Allergy Clin Immunol.* 2008 Feb;121(2):343-7.

López N, de Barros-Mazón S, Vilela MM, Silva CM, Ribeiro JD. Genetic and environmental influences on atopic immune response in early life. *J Investig Allergol Clin Immunol.* 1999 Nov-Dec;9(6):392-8.

Lopez-Garcia E, Schulze MB, Meigs JB, Manson JE, Rifai N, Stampfer MJ, Willett WC, Hu FB. Consumption of trans fatty acids is related to plasma biomarkers of inflammation and endothelial dysfunction. *J Nutr.* 2005 Mar;135(3):562-6.

Lorca Baroja M, Kirjavainen PV, Hekmat S, Reid G. Anti-inflammatory effects of probiotic yogurt in inflammatory bowel disease patients. *Clin Exp Immunol.* 2007 Sep;149(3):470-9.

Lovchik MA, Fráter G, Goeke A, Hug W. Total synthesis of junionone, a natural monoterpenoid from Juniperus communis L., and determination of the absolute configuration of the naturally occurring enantiomer by ROA spectroscopy. *Chem Biodivers.* 2008 Jan;5(1):126-39.

Lu MK, Shih YW, Chang Chien TT, Fang LH, Huang HC, Chen PS. α-Solanine inhibits human melanoma cell migration and invasion by reducing matrix metalloproteinase-2/9 activities. Biol Pharm Bull. 2010;33(10):1685-91.

Lykken DT, Tellegen A, DeRubeis R: Volunteer bias in twin research: the rule of two-thirds. *Soc Biol* 1978, 25(1): 1-9. Phillips DI: Twin studies in medical research: can they tell us whether diseases are genetically determined? *Lancet* 1993;341(8851): 1008-1009.

Mabey R, ed. *The New Age Herbalist.* New York: Simon & Schuster, 1941.

Macdonald TT, Monteleone G. Immunity, inflammation, and allergy in the gut. *Science.* 2005 Mar 25;307(5717):1920-5. Review. PubMed PMID: 15790845.

Maciorkowska E, Kaczmarski M, Andrzej K. Endoscopic evaluation of upper gastrointestinal tract mucosa in children with food hypersensitivity. *Med Wieku Rozwoj.* 2000 Jan-Mar;4(1):37-48.

Maeda N, Inomata N, Morita A, Kirino M, Ikezawa Z. Correlation of oral allergy syndrome due to plant-derived foods with pollen sensitization in Japan. *Ann Allergy Asthma Immunol.* 2010 Mar;104(3):205-10.

Maes HH, Silberg JL, Neale MC, Eaves LJ. Genetic and cultural transmission of antisocial behavior: an extended twin parent model. *Twin Res Hum Genet.* 2007 Feb;10(1):136-50.

Mahady GB, Pendland SL, Stoia A, Hamill FA, Fabricant D, Dietz BM, Chadwick LR. In vitro susceptibility of Helicobacter pylori to botanical extracts used traditionally for the treatment of gastrointestinal disorders. *Phytother Res.* 2005 Nov;19(11):988-91.

Mai XM, Kull I, Wickman M, Bergström A. Antibiotic use in early life and development of allergic diseases: respiratory infection as the explanation. *Clin Exp Allergy.* 2010 Aug;40(8):1230-7.

Majamaa H, Isolauri E. Probiotics: a novel approach in the management of food allergy. *J Allergy Clin Immunol.* 1997 Feb;99(2):179-85.

Makrides M, Neumann M, Gibson R. Effect of maternal docosahexaenoic acid (DHA) supplementation on breast milk composition. *Europ Jrnl of Clin Nutr.* 1996;50:352-357.

Maliakal PP, Wanwimolruk S. Effect of herbal teas on hepatic drug metabolizing enzymes in rats. *J Pharm Pharmacol.* 2001 Oct;53(10):1323-9.

Mälkönen T, Alanko K, Jolanki R, Luukkonen R, Aalto-Korte K, Lauerma A, Susitaival P. Long-term follow-up study of occupational hand eczema. Br J Dermatol. 2010 Aug 13.

Månsson HL. Fatty acids in bovine milk fat. *Food Nutr Res.* 2008;52. doi: 10.3402/fnr.v52i0.1821.

Manz F. Hydration and disease. *J Am Coll Nutr.* 2007 Oct;26(5 Suppl):535S-541S.

Marcucci F, Duse M, Frati F, Incorvaia C, Marseglia GL, La Rosa M. The future of sublingual immunotherapy. *Int J Immunopathol Pharmacol.* 2009 Oct-Dec;22(4 Suppl):31-3.

Margioris AN. Fatty acids and postprandial inflammation. *Curr Opin Clin Nutr Metab Care.* 2009 Mar;12(2):129-37.

Martinez M. Docosahexaenoic acid therapy in docosahexaenoic acid-deficient patients with disorders of peroxisomal biogenesis. *Versicherungsmedizin.* 1996;31 Suppl:145-152

Martin-Venegas R, Roig-Perez S, Ferrer R, Moreno JJ. Arachidonic acid cascade and epithelial barrier function during Caco-2 cell differentiation. J Lipid Res. 2006 Apr;3.

Martínez-Augustin O, Boza JJ, Del Pino JI, Lucena J, Martínez-Valverde A, Gil A. Dietary nucleotides might influence the humoral immune response against cow's milk proteins in preterm neonates. *Biol Neonate.* 1997;71(4):215-23.

Massey DG, Chien YK, Fournier-Massey G. Mamane: scientific therapy for asthma? *Hawaii Med J.* 1994;53:350-1. 363.

Massicot JG, Cohen SG. Epidemiologic and socioeconomic aspects of allergic diseases. *J Allergy Clin Immunol.* 1986 Nov;78(5 Pt 2):954-8.

Matheson MC, Haydn Walters E, Burgess JA, Jenkins MA, Giles GG, Hopper JL, Abramson MJ, Dharmage SC. Childhood immunization and atopic disease into middle-age—a prospective cohort study. *Pediatr Allergy Immunol.* 2010 Mar;21(2 Pt 1):301-6.

Matricardi PM, Bockelbrink A, Beyer K, Keil T, Niggemann B, Grüber C, Wahn U, Lau S. Primary versus secondary immunoglobulin E sensitization to soy and wheat in the Multi-Centre Allergy Study cohort. *Clin Exp Allergy*. 2008 Mar;38(3):493-500.

Matsuda T, Maruyama T, Iizuka H, Kondo A, Tamai T, Kurohane K, Imai Y. Phthalate esters reveal skin-sensitizing activity of phenethyl isothiocyanate in mice. *Food Chem Toxicol*. 2010 Jun;48(6):1704-8.

Mayes MD. Epidemiologic studies of environmental agents and systemic autoimmune diseases. *Environ Health Perspect*. 1999 Oct;107 Suppl 5:743-8.

McAlindon TE. Nutraceuticals: do they work and when should we use them? *Best Pract Res Clin Rheumatol*. 2006 Feb;20(1):99-115.

McBride C, McBride-Henry K, Wissen K. Parenting a child with medically diagnosed severe food allergies in New Zealand: The experience of being unsupported in keeping their children healthy and safe. *Contemp Nurse*. 2010 Apr;35(1):77-87.

McConnaughey E. *Sea Vegetables*. Happy Camp, CA: Naturegraph, 1985.

McCune LM, Johns T. Antioxidant activity in medicinal plants associated with the symptoms of diabetes mellitus used by the indigenous peoples of the North American boreal forest. *J Ethnopharmacol*. 2002 Oct;82(2-3):197-205.

McDougall J, McDougall M. *The McDougal Plan*. Clinton, NJ: New Win, 1983.

McKenzie H, Main J, Pennington CR, Parratt D. Antibody to selected strains of Saccharomyces cerevisiae (baker's and brewer's yeast) and Candida albicans in Crohn's disease. *Gut*. 1990 May;31(5):536-8.

McLachlan CN. beta-casein A1, ischaemic heart disease mortality, and other illnesses. *Med Hypotheses*. 2001 Feb;56(2):262-72.

McLean S, Sheikh A. Does avoidance of peanuts in early life reduce the risk of peanut allergy? *BMJ*. 2010 Mar 11;340:c424. doi: 10.1136/bmj.c424.

McNally ME, Atkinson SA, Cole DE. Contribution of sulfate and sulfoesters to total sulfur intake in infants fed human milk. *J Nutr*. 1991 Aug;121(8):1250-4.

Meglio P, Bartone E, Plantamura M, Arabito E, Giampietro PG. A protocol for oral desensitization in children with IgE-mediated cow's milk allergy. *Allergy*. 2004 Sep;59(9):980-7.

Mehra PN, Puri HS. Studies on Gaduchi satwa. *Indian J Pharm*. 1969;31:180-2.

Meier B, Shao Y, Julkunen-Tiitto R, Bettschart A, Sticher O. A chemotaxonomic survey of phenolic compounds in Swiss willow species. *Planta Med*. 1992;58:A698.

Meier B, Sticher O, Julkunen-Tiitto R. Pharmaceutical aspects of the use of willows in herbal remedies. *Planta Med*. 1988;54(6):559-560.

Melcion C, Verroust P, Baud L, Ardaillou N, Morel-Maroger L, Ardaillou R. Protective effect of procyanidolic oligomers on the heterologous phase of glomerulonephritis induced by anti-glomerular basement membrane antibodies. *C R Seances Acad Sci III*. 1982 Dec 6;295(12):721-6.

Melzig MF. Goldenrod—a classical exponent in the urological phytotherapy. *Wien Med Wochenschr*. 2004 Nov;154(21-22):523-7.

Merchant RE and Andre CA. 2001. A review of recent clinical trials of the nutritional supplement Chlorella pyrenoidosa in the treatment of fibromyalgia, hypertension, and ulcerative colitis. *Altern Ther Health Med*. May-Jun;7(3):79-91.

Metsälä J, Lundqvist A, Kaila M, Gissler M, Klaukka T, Virtanen SM. Maternal and perinatal characteristics and the risk of cow's milk allergy in infants up to 2 years of age: a case-control study nested in the Finnish population. *Am J Epidemiol*. 2010 Jun 15;171(12):1310-6.

Meyer A, Kirsch H, Domergue F, Abbadi A, Sperling P, Bauer J, Cirpus P, Zank TK, Moreau H, Roscoe TJ, Zahringer U, Heinz E. Novel fatty acid elongases and their use for the reconstitution of docosahexaenoic acid biosynthesis. *J Lipid Res*. 2004 Oct;45(10):1899-909.

Miceli N, Trovato A, Dugo P, Cacciola F, Donato P, Marino A, Bellinghieri V, La Barbera TM, Güvenç A, Taviano MF. Comparative Analysis of Flavonoid Profile, Antioxidant and Antimicrobial Activity of the Berries of Juniperus communis L. var. communis and Juniperus communis L. var. saxatilis Pall. *J Agric Food Chem*. 2009 Jul 6.

Michaelsen KF. Probiotics, breastfeeding and atopic eczema. *Acta Derm Venereol Suppl (Stockh)*. 2005 Nov;(215):21-4.

Michalska K, Kisiel W. Sesquiterpene lactones from Taraxacum obovatum. *Planta Med*. 2003 Feb;69(2):181-3.

Michetti P, Dorta G, Wiesel PH, Brassart D, Verdu E, Herranz M, Felley C, Porta N, Rouvet M, Blum AL, Corthésy-Theulaz I. Effect of whey-based culture supernatant of Lactobacillus acidophilus (johnsonii) La1 on Helicobacter pylori infection in humans. *Digestion*. 1999;60(3):203-9.

Mikoluc B, Motkowski R, Karpinska J, Piotrowska-Jastrzebska J. Plasma levels of vitamins A and E, coenzyme Q10, and anti-ox-LDL antibody titer in children treated with an elimination diet due to food hypersensitivity. *Int J Vitam Nutr Res*. 2009 Sep;79(5-6):328-36.

Miller GT. *Living in the Environment*. Belmont, CA: Wadsworth, 1996.

Miller K. Cholesterol and In-Hospital Mortality in Elderly Patients. *Am Family Phys*. 2004 May.

Mindell E, Hopkins V. *Prescription Alternatives*. New Canaan, CT: Keats, 1998.

Miranda H, Outeiro TF. The sour side of neurodegenerative disorders: the effects of protein glycation. J Pathol. 2010 May;221(1):13-25.

Mitchell AE, Hong YJ, Koh E, Barrett DM, Bryant DE, Denison RF, Kaffka S. Ten-year comparison of the influence of organic and conventional crop management practices on the content of flavonoids in tomatoes. *J Agric Food Chem.* 2007 Jul 25;55(15):6154-9.

Mittag D, Akkerdaas J, Ballmer-Weber BK, Vogel L, Wensing M, Becker WM, Koppelman SJ, Knulst AC, Helbling A, Hefle SL, Van Ree R, Vieths S. Ara h 8, a Bet v 1-homologous allergen from peanut, is a major allergen in patients with combined birch pollen and peanut allergy. *J Allergy Clin Immunol.* 2004 Dec;114(6):1410-7.

Mittag D, Vieths S, Vogel L, Becker WM, Rihs HP, Helbling A, Wüthrich B, Ballmer-Weber BK. Soybean allergy in patients allergic to birch pollen: clinical investigation and molecular characterization of allergens. *J Allergy Clin Immunol.* 2004 Jan;113(1):148-54.

Miyazawa T, Itahashi K, Imai T. Management of neonatal cow's milk allergy in high-risk neonates. *Pediatr Int.* 2009 Aug;51(4):544-7.

Molkhou P, Dupont C. Ketotifen in prevention and therapy of food allergy. *Ann Allergy.* 1987 Nov;59(5 Pt 2):187-93.

Monarca S. Zerbini I, Simonati C, Gelatti U. Drinking water hardness and chronic degenerative diseases. Part II. Cardiovascular diseases. *Ann. Ig.* 2003;15:41-56.

Moneret-Vautrin DA, Kanny G, Thévenin F. Asthma caused by food allergy. *Rev Med Interne.* 1996;17(7):551-7.

Moneret-Vautrin DA, Morisset M. Adult food allergy. *Curr Allergy Asthma Rep.* 2005 Jan;5(1):80-5.

Monks H, Gowland MH, Mackenzie H, Erlewyn-Lajeunesse M, King R, Lucas JS, Roberts G. How do teenagers manage their food allergies? *Clin Exp Allergy.* 2010 Aug 2.

Moorhead KJ, Morgan HC. *Spirulina: Nature's Superfood*. Kailua-Kona, HI: Nutrex, 1995.

Morel AF, Dias GO, Porto C, Simionatto E, Stuker CZ, Dalcol II. Antimicrobial activity of extractives of Solidago microglossa. *Fitoterapia.* 2006 Sep;77(6):453-5.

Morgan JE, Daul CB, Hughes J, McCants M, Lehrer SB. Food specific skin-test reactivity in atopic subjects. *Clin Exp Allergy.* 1989 Jul;19(4):431-5.

Mori F, Bianchi L, Pucci N, Azzari C, De Martino M, Novembre E. CD4+CD25+Foxp3+ T regulatory cells are not involved in oral desensitization. *Int J Immunopathol Pharmacol.* 2010 Jan-Mar;23(1):359-61.

Morisset M, Moneret-Vautrin DA, Guenard L, Cuny JM, Frentz P, Hatahet R, Hanss Ch, Beaudouin E, Petit N, Kanny G. Oral desensitization in children with milk and egg allergies obtains recovery in a significant proportion of cases. A randomized study in 60 children with cow's milk allergy and 90 children with egg allergy. *Eur Ann Allergy Clin Immunol.* 2007 Jan;39(1):12-9.

Morisset M, Moneret-Vautrin DA, Kanny G, Guénard L, Beaudouin E, Flabbée J, Hatahet R. Thresholds of clinical reactivity to milk, egg, peanut and sesame in immunoglobulin E-dependent allergies: evaluation by double-blind or single-blind placebo-controlled oral challenges. *Clin Exp Allergy.* 2003 Aug;33(8):1046-51.

Morisset M, Moneret-Vautrin DA, Kanny G; Allergo-Vigilance Network. Prevalence of peanut sensitization in a population of 4,737 subjects—an Allergo-Vigilance Network enquiry carried out in 2002. *Eur Ann Allergy Clin Immunol.* 2005 Feb;37(2):54-7.

Morisset M, Moneret-Vautrin DA, Maadi F, Frémont S, Guénard L, Croizier A, Kanny G. Prospective study of mustard allergy: first study with double-blind placebo-controlled food challenge trials (24 cases). *Allergy.* 2003 Apr;58(4):295-9.

Moujir L, Seca AM, Silva AM, Barreto MC. Cytotoxic activity of diterpenes and extracts of Juniperus brevifolia. *Planta Med.* 2008 Jun;74(7):751-3.

Moussaieff A, Shein NA, Tsenter J, Grigoriadis S, Simeonidou C, Alexandrovich AG, Trembovler V, Ben-Neriah Y, Schmitz ML, Fiebich BL, Munoz E, Mechoulam R, Shohami E. Incensole acetate: a novel neuroprotective agent isolated from Boswellia carterii. *J Cereb Blood Flow Metab.* 2008 Jul;28(7):1341-52.

Mozaffarian D, Aro A, Willett WC. Health effects of trans-fatty acids: experimental and observational evidence. *Eur J Clin Nutr.* 2009 May;63 Suppl 2:S5-21.

Mrowietz-Ruckstuhl B. Bacteriological stool examinations. *Dtsch Arztebl Int.* 2010 Jan;107(3):40; author reply 40-1.

Mullin GE, Swift KM, Lipski L, Turnbull LK, Rampertab SD. Testing for food reactions: the good, the bad, and the ugly. *Nutr Clin Pract.* 2010 Apr;25(2):192-8.

Murray M, Pizzorno J. *Encyclopedia of Natural Medicine*. 2nd Edition. Roseville, CA: Prima Publishing, 1998.

Na HJ, Koo HN, Lee GG, Yoo SJ, Park JH, Lyu YS, Kim HM. Juniper oil inhibits the heat shock-induced apoptosis via preventing the caspase-3 activation in human astrocytes CCF-STTG1 cells. *Clin Chim Acta.* 2001 Dec;314(1-2):215-20.

Nadkarni AK, Nadkarni KM. *Indian Materia Medica.* (Vols 1 and 2). Bombay, India: Popular Pradashan, 1908, 1976.

Nagel G, Weinmayr G, Kleiner A, Garcia-Marcos L, Strachan DP; ISAAC Phase Two Study Group. Effect of diet on asthma and allergic sensitisation in the International Study on Allergies and Asthma in Childhood (ISAAC) Phase Two. *Thorax.* 2010 Jun;65(6):516-22.

Naghii MR, Samman S. The role of boron in nutrition and metabolism. *Prog Food Nutr Sci.* 1993 Oct-Dec;17(4):331-49.

Nair PK, Rodriguez S, Ramachandran R, Alamo A, Melnick SJ, Escalon E, Garcia PI Jr, Wnuk SF, Ramachandran C. Immune stimulating properties of a novel polysaccharide from the medicinal plant Tinospora cordifolia. *Int Immunopharmacol.* 2004 Dec 15;4(13):1645-59.

Nakano T, Shimojo N, Morita Y, Arima T, Tomiita M, Kohno Y. Sensitization to casein and beta-lactoglobulin (BLG) in children with cow's milk allergy (CMA). *Arerugi.* 2010 Feb;59(2):117-22.

Napoli, J.E., Brand-Miller, J.C., Conway, P. (2003) Bifidogenic effects of feeding infant formula containing galactooligosaccharides in healthy formula-fed infants. *Asia Pac J Clin Nutr.* 12(Suppl): S60

Nariya M, Shukla V, Jain S, Ravishankar B. Comparison of enteroprotective efficacy of triphala formulations (Indian Herbal Drug) on methotrexate-induced small intestinal damage in rats. *Phytother Res.* 2009 Aug;23(8):1092-8.

Naruszewicz M, Johansson ML, Zapolska-Downar D, Bukowska H. Effect of Lactobacillus plantarum 299v on cardiovascular disease risk factors in smokers. *Am J Clin Nutr.* 2002 Dec;76(6):1249-55.

NDL, BHNRC, ARS, USDA. *Oxygen Radical Absorbance Capacity (ORAC) of Selected Foods - 2007.* Beltsville, MD: USDA-ARS. 2007.

Nehra V. New clinical issues in celiac disease. *Gastroenterol Clin North Am.* 1998 Jun;27(2):453-65.

Neilan NA, Dowling PJ, Taylor DL, Ryan P, Schurman JV, Friesen CA. Useful biomarkers in pediatric eosinophilic duodenitis and their existence: a case-control, single-blind, observational pilot study. *J Pediatr Gastroenterol Nutr.* 2010 Apr;50(4):377-84.

Nentwich I, Michková E, Nevoral J, Urbanek R, Szépfalusi Z. Cow's milk-specific cellular and humoral immune responses and atopy skin symptoms in infants from atopic families fed a partially (pHF) or extensively (eHF) hydrolyzed infant formula. *Allergy.* 2001 Dec;56(12):1144-56.

Nermes M, Karvonen H, Sarkkinen E, Isolauri E. Safety of barley starch syrup in patients with allergy to cereals. *Br J Nutr.* 2009 Jan;101(2):165-8.

Newall CA, Anderson LA, Philpson JD. *Herbal Medicine: A Guide for Healthcare Professionals.* London: Pharmaceutical Press, 1996.

Newmark T, Schulick P. *Beyond Aspirin.* Prescott, AZ: Holm, 2000.

Neyestani TR, Shariatzadeh N, Gharavi A, Kalayi A, Khalaji N. Physiological dose of lycopene suppressed oxidative stress and enhanced serum levels of immunoglobulin M in patients with Type 2 diabetes mellitus: a possible role in the prevention of long-term complications. *J Endocrinol Invest.* 2007 Nov;30(10):833-8.

Nicholls SJ, Lundman P, Harmer JA, Cutri B, Griffiths KA, Rye KA, Barter PJ, Celermajer DS. Consumption of saturated fat impairs the anti-inflammatory properties of high-density lipoproteins and endothelial function. *J Am Coll Cardiol.* 2006 Aug 15;48(4):715-20.

Nicolaou N, Poorafshar M, Murray C, Simpson A, Winell H, Kerry G, Härlin A, Woodcock A, Ahlstedt S, Custovic A. Allergy or tolerance in children sensitized to peanut: prevalence and differentiation using component-resolved diagnostics. *J Allergy Clin Immunol.* 2010 Jan;125(1):191-7.e1-13.

Niederau C, Göpfert E. The effect of chelidonium- and turmeric root extract on upper abdominal pain due to functional disorders of the biliary system. Results from a placebo-controlled double-blind study. *Med Klin.* 1999 Aug 15;94(8):425-30.

Niederberger V, Horak F, Vrtala S, Spitzauer S, Krauth MT, Valent P, Reisinger J, Pelzmann M, Hayek B, Kronqvist M, Gafvelin G, Grönlund H, Purohit A, Suck R, Fiebig H, Cromwell O, Pauli G, van Hage-Hamsten M, Valenta R. Vaccination with genetically engineered allergens prevents progression of allergic disease. *Proc Natl Acad Sci U S A.* 2004 Oct 5;101 Suppl 2:14677-82.

Niedzielin K, Kordecki H, Birkenfeld B. A controlled, double-blind, randomized study on the efficacy of Lactobacillus plantarum 299V in patients with irritable bowel syndrome. *Eur J Gastroenterol Hepatol.* 2001 Oct;13(10):1143-7.

Nielsen RG, Bindslev-Jensen C, Kruse-Andersen S, Husby S. Severe gastroesophageal reflux disease and cow milk hypersensitivity in infants and children: disease association and evaluation of a new challenge procedure. *J Pediatr Gastroenterol Nutr.* 2004 Oct;39(4):383-91.

Nielsen WW, Lindsey K. When there is no school nurse—are teachers prepared for students with peanut allergies? *School Nurse News.* 2010 Jan;27(1):12-5.

Niggemann B, Binder C, Dupont C, Hadji S, Arvola T, Isolauri E. Prospective, controlled, multi-center study on the effect of an amino-acid-based formula in infants with cow's milk allergy/intolerance and atopic dermatitis. *Pediatr Allergy Immunol.* 2001 Apr;12(2):78-82.

307

Niggemann B, Celik-Bilgili S, Ziegert M, Reibel S, Sommerfeld C, Wahn U. Specific IgE levels do not indicate persistence or transience of food allergy in children with atopic dermatitis. *J Investig Allergol Clin Immunol.* 2004;14(2):98-103.

Niggemann B, von Berg A, Bollrath C, Berdel D, Schauer U, Rieger C, Haschke-Becher E, Wahn U. Safety and efficacy of a new extensively hydrolyzed formula for infants with cow's milk protein allergy. *Pediatr Allergy Immunol.* 2008 Jun;19(4):348-54.

Nobaek S, Johansson ML, Molin G, Ahrné S, Jeppsson B. Alteration of intestinal microflora is associated with reduction in abdominal bloating and pain in patients with irritable bowel syndrome. *Am J Gastroenterol.* 2000 May;95(5):1231-8.

Nodake Y, Fukumoto S, Fukasawa M, Sakakibara R, Yamasaki N. Reduction of the immunogenicity of beta-lactoglobulin from cow's milk by conjugation with a dextran derivative. *Biosci Biotechnol Biochem.* 2010;74(4):721-6.

Noh J, Lee JH, Noh G, Bang SY, Kim HS, Choi WS, Cho S, Lee SS. Characterisation of allergen-specific responses of IL-10-producing regulatory B cells (Br1) in Cow Milk Allergy. *Cell Immunol.* 2010;264(2):143-9.

Noorbakhsh R, Mortazavi SA, Sankian M, Shahidi F, Assarehzadegan MA, Varasteh A. Cloning, expression, characterization, and computational approach for cross-reactivity prediction of manganese superoxide dismutase allergen from pistachio nut. *Allergol Int.* 2010 Sep;59(3):295-304.

Nowak-Wegrzyn A, Fiocchi A. Is oral immunotherapy the cure for food allergies? *Curr Opin Allergy Clin Immunol.* 2010 Jun;10(3):214-9.

Nowak-Wegrzyn A, Muraro A. Food protein-induced enterocolitis syndrome. *Curr Opin Allergy Clin Immunol.* 2009 Aug;9(4):371-7.

Nowak-Wegrzyn A, Sampson HA, Wood RA, Sicherer SH. Food protein-induced enterocolitis syndrome caused by solid food proteins. *Pediatrics.* 2003 Apr;111(4 Pt 1):829-35.

Nuñez YO, Salabarria IS, Collado IG, Hernández-Galán R. Sesquiterpenes from the wood of Juniperus lucayana. *Phytochemistry.* 2007 Oct;68(19):2409-14.

O'Connor J., Bensky D. (ed). *Shanghai College of Traditional Chinese Medicine: Acupuncture: A Comprehensive Text.* Seattle: Eastland Press, 1981.

O'Connor MI. Warming strengthens an herbivore-plant interaction. *Ecology.* 2009 Feb;90(2):388-98.

O'Neil C, Helbling AA, Lehrer SB. Allergic reactions to fish. *Clin Rev Allergy.* 1993 Summer;11(2):183-200.

Odamaki T, Xiao JZ, Iwabuchi N, Sakamoto M, Takahashi N, Kondo S, Miyaji K, Iwatsuki K, Togashi H, Enomoto T, Benno Y. Influence of Bifidobacterium longum BB536 intake on faecal microbiota in individuals with Japanese cedar pollinosis during the pollen season. *J Med Microbiol.* 2007 Oct;56(Pt 10):1301-8.

Oehme FW (ed.). *Toxicity of heavy metals in the environment. Part 1.* New York: M.Dekker, 1979.

Oh CK, Lücker PW, Wetzelsberger N, Kuhlmann F. The determination of magnesium, calcium, sodium and potassium in assorted foods with special attention to the loss of electrolytes after various forms of food preparations. *Mag.-Bull.* 1986;8:297-302.

Oh JW, Pyun BY, Choung JT, Ahn KM, Kim CH, Song SW, Son JA, Lee SY, Lee SI. Epidemiological change of atopic dermatitis and food allergy in school-aged children in Korea between 1995 and 2000. *J Korean Med Sci.* 2004 Oct;19(5):716-23.

Oh SY, Chung J, Kim MK, Kwon SO, Cho BH. Antioxidant nutrient intakes and corresponding biomarkers associated with the risk of atopic dermatitis in young children. *Eur J Clin Nutr.* 2010 Mar;64(3):245-52.

Okasaka M, Takaishi Y, Kashiwada Y, Kodzhimatov OK, Ashurmetov O, Lin AJ, Consentino LM, Lee KH.Terpenoids from Juniperus polycarpus var. seravschanica. *Phytochemistry.* 2006 Dec;67(24):2635-40.

Oldak E, Kurzatkowska B, Stasiak-Barmuta A. Natural course of sensitization in children: follow-up study from birth to 6 years of age, I. Evaluation of total serum IgE and specific IgE antibodies with regard to atopic family history. *Rocz Akad Med Bialymst.* 2000;45:87-95.

O'Mahony L, McCarthy J, Kelly P, Hurley G, Luo F, Chen K, O'Sullivan GC, Kiely B, Collins JK, Shanahan F, Quigley EM. Lactobacillus and bifidobacterium in irritable bowel syndrome: symptom responses and relationship to cytokine profiles. *Gastroenterology.* 2005 Mar;128(3):541-51.

O'Neil C, Helbling AA, Lehrer SB. Allergic reactions to fish. *Clin Rev Allergy.* 1993;11(2):183-200.

Orhan F, Karakas T, Cakir M, Aksoy A, Baki A, Gedik Y. Prevalence of immunoglobulin E-mediated food allergy in 6-9-year-old urban schoolchildren in the eastern Black Sea region of Turkey. *Clin Exp Allergy.* 2009 Jul;39(7):1027-35.

Ortiz-Andrellucchi A, Sánchez-Villegas A, Rodríguez-Gallego C, Lemes A, Molero T, Soria A, Peña-Quintana L, Santana M, Ramírez O, García J, Cabrera F, Cobo J, Serra-Majem L. Immunomodulatory effects of the intake of fermented milk with Lactobacillus casei DN114001 in lactating mothers and their children. *Br J Nutr.* 2008 Oct;100(4):834-45.

Osguthorpe JD. Immunotherapy. *Curr Opin Otolaryngol Head Neck Surg.* 2010 Jun;18(3):206-12.

Otto SJ, van Houwelingen AC, Hornstra G. The effect of supplementation with docosahexaenoic and arachidonic acid derived from single cell oils on plasma and erythrocyte fatty acids of pregnant women in the second trimester. *Prostaglandins Leukot Essent Fatty Acids.* 2000 Nov;63(5):323-8.

Ou CC, Tsao SM, Lin MC, Yin MC. Protective action on human LDL against oxidation and glycation by four organosulfur compounds derived from garlic. *Lipids.* 2003 Mar;38(3):219-24.

Ouwehand AC, Nermes M, Collado MC, Rautonen N, Salminen S, Isolauri E. Specific probiotics alleviate allergic rhinitis during the birch pollen season. *World J Gastroenterol.* 2009 Jul 14;15(26):3261-8.

Ouwehand AC, Tiihonen K, Saarinen M, Putaala H, Rautonen N. Influence of a combination of Lactobacillus acidophilus NCFM and lactitol on healthy elderly: intestinal and immune parameters. *Br J Nutr.* 2009 Feb;101(3):367-75.

Ozdemir O. Any benefits of probiotics in allergic disorders? *Allergy Asthma Proc.* 2010 Mar;31(2):103-11.

Paajanen L, Tuure T, Poussa T, Korpela R. No difference in symptoms during challenges with homogenized and unhomogenized cow's milk in subjects with subjective hypersensitivity to homogenized milk. *J Dairy Res.* 2003 May;70(2):175-9.

Paganelli R, Pallone F, Montano S, Le Moli S, Matricardi PM, Fais S, Paoluzi P, D'Amelio R, Aiuti F. Isotypic analysis of antibody response to a food antigen in inflammatory bowel disease. *Int Arch Allergy Appl Immunol.* 1985;78(1):81-5.

Pahud JJ, Schwarz K. Research and development of infant formulae with reduced allergenic properties. *Ann Allergy.* 1984 Dec;53(6 Pt 2):609-14.

Pak CH, Oleneva VA, Agadzhanov SA. Dietetic aspects of preventing urolithiasis in patients with gout and uric acid diathesis. *Vopr Pitan.* 1985 Jan-Feb;(1):21-4.

Palacin A, Bartra J, Muñoz R, Diaz-Perales A, Valero A, Salcedo G. Anaphylaxis to wheat flour-derived foodstuffs and the lipid transfer protein syndrome: a potential role of wheat lipid transfer protein Tri a 14. *Int Arch Allergy Immunol.* 2010;152(2):178-83.

Paller AS, Nimmagadda S, Schachner L, Mallory SB, Kahn T, Willis I, Eichenfield LF. Fluocinolone acetonide 0.01% in peanut oil: therapy for childhood atopic dermatitis, even in patients who are peanut sensitive. *J Am Acad Dermatol.* 2003 Apr;48(4):569-77.

Palmer DJ, Gold MS, Makrides M. Effect of cooked and raw egg consumption on ovalbumin content of human milk: a randomized, double-blind, cross-over trial. *Clin Exp Allergy.* 2005 Feb;35(2):173-8.

Panzani R, Ariano R, Mistrello G. Cypress pollen does not cross-react to plant-derived foods. *Eur Ann Allergy Clin Immunol.* 2010 Jun;42(3):125-6.

Parcell S. Sulfur in human nutrition and applications in medicine. *Altern Med Rev.* 2002 Feb;7(1):22-44.

Pastorello EA, Farioli L, Conti A, Pravettoni V, Bonomi S, Iametti S, Fortunato D, Scibilia J, Bindslev-Jensen C, Ballmer-Weber B, Robino AM, Ortolani C. Wheat IgE-mediated food allergy in European patients: alpha-amylase inhibitors, lipid transfer proteins and low-molecular-weight glutenins. Allergenic molecules recognized by double-blind, placebo-controlled food challenge. Int Arch Allergy Immunol. 2007;144(1):10-22.

Pastorello EA, Farioli L, Pravettoni V, Robino AM, Scibilia J, Fortunato D, Conti A, Borgonovo L, Bengtsson A, Ortolani C. Lipid transfer protein and vicilin are important walnut allergens in patients not allergic to pollen. *J Allergy Clin Immunol.* 2004 Oct;114(4):908-14.

Pastorello EA, Farioli L, Pravettoni V, Scibilia J, Conti A, Fortunato D, Borgonovo L, Bonomi S, Primavesi L, Ballmer-Weber B. Maize food allergy: lipid-transfer proteins, endochitinases, and alpha-zein precursor are relevant maize allergens in double-blind placebo-controlled maize-challenge-positive patients. *Anal Bioanal Chem.* 2009 Sep;395(1):93-102.

Pastorello EA, Pompei C, Pravettoni V, Farioli L, Calamari AM, Scibilia J, Robino AM, Conti A, Iametti S, Fortunato D, Bonomi S, Ortolani C. Lipid-transfer protein is the major maize allergen maintaining IgE-binding activity after cooking at 100 degrees C, as demonstrated in anaphylactic patients and patients with positive double-blind, placebo-controlled food challenge results. *J Allergy Clin Immunol.* 2003 Oct;112(4):775-83.

Pastorello EA, Vieths S, Pravettoni V, Farioli L, Trambaioli C, Fortunato D, Lüttkopf D, Calamari M, Ansaloni R, Scibilia J, Ballmer-Weber BK, Poulsen LK, Wütrich B, Hansen KS, Robino AM, Ortolani C, Conti A. Identification of hazelnut major allergens in sensitive patients with positive double-blind, placebo-controlled food challenge results. *J Allergy Clin Immunol.* 2002 Mar;109(3):563-70.

Patriarca G, Nucera E, Pollastrini E, Roncallo C, De Pasquale T, Lombardo C, Pedone C, Gasbarrini G, Buonomo A, Schiavino D. Oral specific desensitization in food-allergic children. *Dig Dis Sci.* 2007 Jul;52(7):1662-72.

Patriarca G, Nucera E, Roncallo C, Pollastrini E, Bartolozzi F, De Pasquale T, Buonomo A, Gasbarrini G, Di Campli C, Schiavino D. Oral desensitizing treatment in food allergy: clinical and immunological results. *Aliment Pharmacol Ther.* 2003 Feb;17(3):459-65.

Patwardhan B, Gautam M. Botanical immunodrugs: scope and opportunities. *Drug Discov Today.* 2005 Apr 1;10(7):495-502.

Payment P, Franco E, Richardson L, Siemiatyck, J. Gastrointestinal health effects associated with the consumption of drinking water produced by point-of-use domestic reverse-osmosis filtration units. *Appl. Environ. Microbiol.* 1991;57:945-948.

Peeters KA, Koppelman SJ, van Hoffen E, van der Tas CW, den Hartog Jager CF, Penninks AH, Hefle SL, Bruijnzeel-Koomen CA, Knol EF, Knulst AC. Does skin prick test reactivity to purified allergens correlate with clinical severity of peanut allergy? *Clin Exp Allergy.* 2007 Jan;37(1):108-15.

Pehowich DJ, Gomes AV, Barnes JA. Fatty acid composition and possible health effects of coconut constituents. *West Indian Med J.* 2000 Jun;49(2):128-33.

Peña AS, Crusius JB. Food allergy, coeliac disease and chronic inflammatory bowel disease in man. *Vet Q.* 1998;20 Suppl 3:S49-52.

Pepeljnjak S, Kosalec I, Kalodera Z, Blazević N. Antimicrobial activity of juniper berry essential oil (Juniperus communis L., Cupressaceae). *Acta Pharm.* 2005 Dec;55(4):417-22.

Pereira B, Venter C, Grundy J, Clayton CB, Arshad SH, Dean T (2005) Prevalence of sensitization to food allergens, reported adverse reaction to foods, food avoidance, and food hypersensitivity among teenagers. *J Allergy Clin Immunol.* 116: 884–892.

Perez-Galvez A, Martin HD, Sies H, Stahl W. Incorporation of carotenoids from paprika oleoresin into human chylomicrons. *Br J Nutr.* 2003 Jun;89(6):787-93.

Perez-Pena R. Secrets of the Mummy's Medicine Chest. *NY Times.* 2005 Sept 10.

Permaul P, Stutius LM, Sheehan WJ, Rangsithienchai P, Walter JE, Twarog FJ, Young MC, Scott JE, Schneider LC, Phipatanakul W. Sesame allergy: role of specific IgE and skin-prick testing in predicting food challenge results. *Allergy Asthma Proc.* 2009 Nov-Dec;30(6):643-8.

Perrier C, Thierry AC, Mercenier A, Corthésy B. Allergen-specific antibody and cytokine responses, mast cell reactivity and intestinal permeability upon oral challenge of sensitized and tolerized mice. *Clin Exp Allergy.* 2010 Jan;40(1):153-62.

Pessi T, Sütas Y, Hurme M, Isolauri E. Interleukin-10 generation in atopic children following oral Lactobacillus rhamnosus GG. *Clin Exp Allergy.* 2000 Dec;30(12):1804-8.

Peterson CG, Hansson T, Skott A, Bengtsson U, Ahlstedt S, Magnussons J. Detection of local mast-cell activity in patients with food hypersensitivity. *J Investig Allergol Clin Immunol.* 2007;17(5):314-20.

Petlevski R, Hadzija M, Slijepcević M, Juretić D, Petrik J. Glutathione S-transferases and malondialdehyde in the liver of NOD mice on short-term treatment with plant mixture extract P-9801091. *Phytother Res.* 2003 Apr;17(4):311-4.

Petlevski R, Hadzija M, Slijepcević M, Juretić D. Toxicological assessment of P-9801091 plant mixture extract after chronic administration in CBA/HZg mice—a biochemical and histological study. *Coll Antropol.* 2008 Jun;32(2):577-81.

Pfefferle PI, Sel S, Ege MJ, Büchele G, Blümer N, Krauss-Etschmann S, Herzum I, Albers CE, Lauener RP, Roponen M, Hirvonen MR, Vuitton DA, Riedler J, Brunekreef B, Dalphin JC, Braun-Fahrländer C, Pekkanen J, von Mutius E, Renz H; PASTURE Study Group. Cord blood allergen-specific IgE is associated with reduced IFN-gamma production by cord blood cells: the Protection against Allergy-Study in Rural Environments (PASTURE) Study. *J Allergy Clin Immunol.* 2008 Oct;122(4):711-6.

Pfundstein B, El Desouky SK, Hull WE, Haubner R, Erben G, Owen RW. Polyphenolic compounds in the fruits of Egyptian medicinal plants (Terminalia bellerica, Terminalia chebula and Terminalia horrida): characterization, quantitation and determination of antioxidant capacities. *Phytochemistry.* 2010 Jul;71(10):1132-48.

Pharmacopoeia of the People's Republic of China. English. Beijing: Chemical Industry Press; 2005. The State Pharmacopoeia Commission of The People's Republic of China.Nusem D, Panasoff J. Beer anaphylaxis. *Isr Med Assoc J.* 2009 Jun;11(6):380-1.

Physicians' Desk Reference. Montvale, NJ: Thomson, 2003-2008

Phytochemical investigation of juniper rufescens Juniperus oxycedrus L. leaves and fruits. *Georgian Med News.* 2009 Mar;(168):107-11.

Piboonpocanun S, Boonchoo S, Pariyaprasert W, Visitsunthorn N, Jirapongsananuruk O. Determination of storage conditions for shrimp extracts: analysis of specific IgE-allergen profiles. *Asian Pac J Allergy Immunol.* 2010 Mar;28(1):47-52.

Pierce SK, Klinman NR. Antibody-specific immunoregulation. *J Exp Med.* 1977 Aug 1;146(2):509-19.

Piirainen L, Haahtela S, Helin T, Korpela R, Haahtela T, Vaarala O. Effect of Lactobacillus rhamnosus GG on rBet v1 and rMal d1 specific IgA in the saliva of patients with birch pollen allergy. *Ann Allergy Asthma Immunol.* 2008 Apr;100(4):338-42.

Pike MG, Heddle RJ, Boulton P, Turner MW, Atherton DJ. Increased intestinal permeability in atopic eczema. *J Invest Dermatol.* 1986 Feb;86(2):101-4.

Pitt-Rivers R, Trotter WR. *The Thyroid Gland.* London: Butterworth Publ, 1954.

Plein K, Hotz J. Therapeutic effects of Saccharomyces boulardii on mild residual symptoms in a stable phase of Crohn's disease with special respect to chronic diarrhea—a pilot study. *Z Gastroenterol.* 1993 Feb;31(2):129-34.

Plohmann B, Bader G, Hiller K, Franz G. Immunomodulatory and antitumoral effects of triterpenoid saponins. *Pharmazie.* 1997 Dec;52(12):953-7.

Poblocka-Olech L, Krauze-Baranowska M. SPE-HPTLC of procyanidins from the barks of different species and clones of Salix. *J Pharm Biomed Anal.* 2008 Nov 4;48(3):965-8.

Pochard P, Vickery B, Berin MC, Grishin A, Sampson HA, Caplan M, Bottomly K. Targeting Toll-like receptors on dendritic cells modifies the T(H)2 response to peanut allergens in vitro. *J Allergy Clin Immunol.* 2010 Jul;126(1):92-7.e5.

Pohjavuori E, Viljanen M, Korpela R, Kuitunen M, Tiittanen M, Vaarala O, Savilahti E. Lactobacillus GG effect in increasing IFN-gamma production in infants with cow's milk allergy. *J Allergy Clin Immunol.* 2004 Jul;114(1):131-6.

Pollini F, Capristo C, Boner AL. Upper respiratory tract infections and atopy. *Int J Immunopathol Pharmacol.* 2010 Jan-Mar;23(1 Suppl):32-7.

Ponsonby AL, McMichael A, van der Mei I. Ultraviolet radiation and autoimmune disease: insights from epidemiological research. *Toxicology.* 2002 Dec 27;181-182:71-8.

Potterton D. (Ed.) *Culpeper's Color Herbal.* New York: Sterling, 1983.

Poulos LM, Waters AM, Correll PK, Loblay RH, Marks GB. Trends in hospitalizations for anaphylaxis, angioedema, and urticaria in Australia, 1993-1994 to 2004-2005. *J Allergy Clin Immunol.* 2007 Oct;120(4):878-84.

Prescott SL, Wickens K, Westcott L, Jung W, Currie H, Black PN, Stanley TV, Mitchell EA, Fitzharris P, Siebers R, Wu L, Crane J; Probiotic Study Group. Supplementation with Lactobacillus rhamnosus or Bifidobacterium lactis probiotics in pregnancy increases cord blood interferon-gamma and breast milk transforming growth factor-beta and immunoglobin A detection. *Clin Exp Allergy.* 2008 Oct;38(10):1606-14.

Prieto A, Razzak E, Lindo DP, Alvarez-Perea A, Rueda M, Baeza ML. Recurrent anaphylaxis due to lupin flour: primary sensitization through inhalation. *J Investig Allergol Clin Immunol.* 2010;20(1):76-9.

Prioult G, Fliss I, Pecquet S. Effect of probiotic bacteria on induction and maintenance of oral tolerance to beta-lactoglobulin in gnotobiotic mice. *Clin Diagn Lab Immunol.* 2003 Sep;10(5):787-92.

Proujansky R, Winter HS, Walker WA. Gastrointestinal syndromes associated with food sensitivity. *Adv Pediatr.* 1988;35:219-37.

Prucksunand C, Indrasukhsri B, Leethochawalit M, Hungspreugs K. Phase II clinical trial on effect of the long turmeric (Curcuma longa Linn) on healing of peptic ulcer. *Southeast Asian J Trop Med Public Health.* 2001 Mar;32(1):208-15.

Prussin C, Lee J, Foster B. Eosinophilic gastrointestinal disease and peanut allergy are alternatively associated with IL-5+ and IL-5(-) T(H)2 responses. *J Allergy Clin Immunol.* 2009 Dec;124(6):1326-32.e6.

Pruthi S, Thapa MM. Infectious and inflammatory disorders. *Magn Reson Imaging Clin N Am.* 2009 Aug;17(3):423-38, v.

Pulcini JM, Sease KK, Marshall GD. Disparity between the presence and absence of food allergy action plans in one school district. *Allergy Asthma Proc.* 2010 Mar;31(2):141-6.

Pustisek N, Jaklin-Kekez A, Frkanec R, Sikanić-Dugić N, Misak Z, Jadresin O, Kolacek S. Our experiences with the use of atopy patch test in the diagnosis of cow's milk hypersensitivity. Acta Dermatovenerol Croat. 2010;18(1):14-20. Kim JH, Kim JE, Choi GS, Hwang EK, An S, Ye YM, Park HS. A case of occupational rhinitis caused by rice powder in the grain industry. *Allergy Asthma Immunol Res.* 2010 Apr;2(2):141-3.

Qin HL, Zheng JJ, Tong DN, Chen WX, Fan XB, Hang XM, Jiang YQ. Effect of Lactobacillus plantarum enteral feeding on the gut permeability and septic complications in the patients with acute pancreatitis. *Eur J Clin Nutr.* 2008 Jul;62(7):923-30.

Qu C, Srivastava K, Ko J, Zhang TF, Sampson HA, Li XM. Induction of tolerance after establishment of peanut allergy by the food allergy herbal formula-2 is associated with up-regulation of interferon-gamma. *Clin Exp Allergy.* 2007 Jun;37(6):846-55.

Rafter J, Bennett M, Caderni G, Clune Y, Hughes R, Karlsson PC, Klinder A, O'Riordan M, O'Sullivan GC, Pool-Zobel B, Rechkemmer G, Roller M, Rowland I, Salvadori M, Thijs H, Van Loo J, Watzl B, Collins JK. Dietary synbiotics reduce cancer risk factors in polypectomized and colon cancer patients. *Am J Clin Nutr.* 2007 Feb;85(2):488-96.

Raherison C, Pénard-Morand C, Moreau D, Caillaud D, Charpin D, Kopferschmitt C, Lavaud F, Taytard A, Maesano IA. Smoking exposure and allergic sensitization in children according to maternal allergies. *Ann Allergy Asthma Immunol.* 2008 Apr;100(4):351-7.

Rahman MM, Bhattacharya A, Fernandes G. Docosahexaenoic acid is more potent inhibitor of osteoclast differentiation in RAW 264.7 cells than eicosapentaenoic acid. *J Cell Physiol.* 2008 Jan;214(1):201-9.

Railey MD, Burks AW. Therapeutic approaches for the treatment of food allergy. *Expert Opin Pharmacother.* 2010 May;11(7):1045-8.

Raimondi F, Indrio F, Crivaro V, Araimo G, Capasso L, Paludetto R. Neonatal hyperbilirubinemia increases intestinal protein permeability and the prevalence of cow's milk protein intolerance. *Acta Paediatr.* 2008 Jun;97(6):751-3.

Raithel M, Weidenhiller M, Abel R, Baenkler HW, Hahn EG. Colorectal mucosal histamine release by mucosa oxygenation in comparison with other established clinical tests in patients with gastrointestinally mediated allergy. *World J Gastroenterol.* 2006 Aug 7;12(29):4699-705.

Ramagopalan SV, Dyment DA, Guimond C, Orton SM, Yee IM, Ebers GC, Sadovnick AD. Childhood cow's milk allergy and the risk of multiple sclerosis: a population based study. *J Neurol Sci.* 2010 Apr 15;291(1-2):86-8.

Rampton DS, Murdoch RD, Sladen GE. Rectal mucosal histamine release in ulcerative colitis. *Clin Sci (Lond).* 1980 Nov;59(5):389-91.

Rancé F, Abbal M, Lauwers-Cancès V. Improved screening for peanut allergy by the combined use of skin prick tests and specific IgE assays. *J Allergy Clin Immunol.* 2002 Jun;109(6):1027-33.

Rancé F, Bidat E, Bourrier T, Sabouraud D. Cashew allergy: observations of 42 children without associated peanut allergy. *Allergy.* 2003 Dec;58(12):1311-4.

Rance F, Kanny G, Dutau G, Moneret-Vautrin DA. Food allergens in children. *Arch Pediatr.* 1999;6(Suppl 1):61S-66S.

Randal Bollinger R, Barbas AS, Bush EL, Lin SS, Parker W. Biofilms in the large bowel suggest an apparent function of the human vermiform appendix. *J Theor Biol.* 2007 Dec 21;249(4):826-31.

Rao SK, Rao PS, Rao BN. Preliminary investigation of the radiosensitizing activity of guduchi (Tinospora cordifolia) in tumor-bearing mice. *Phytother Res.* 2008 Nov;22(11):1482-9.

Rapin JR, Wiernsperger N. Possible links between intestinal permeablity and food processing: A potential therapeutic niche for glutamine. *Clinics (Sao Paulo).* 2010 Jun;65(6):635-43.

Rappoport J. Both sides of the pharmaceutical death coin. *Townsend Letter for Doctors and Patients.* 2006 Oct.

Rauha JP, Remes S, Heinonen M, Hopia A, Kähkönen M, Kujala T, Pihlaja K, Vuorela H, Vuorela P. Antimicrobial effects of Finnish plant extracts containing flavonoids and other phenolic compounds. *Int J Food Microbiol.* 2000 May 25;56(1):3-12.

Rauma A. Antioxidant status in vegetarians versus omnivores. *Nutrition.* 2003;16(2): 111-119.

Rautava S, Isolauri E. Cow's milk allergy in infants with atopic eczema is associated with aberrant production of interleukin-4 during oral cow's milk challenge. *J Pediatr Gastroenterol Nutr.* 2004 Nov;39(5):529-35.

Reger D, Goode S, Mercer E. *Chemistry: Principles & Practice.* Fort Worth, TX: Harcourt Brace, 1993.

Reha CM, Ebru A. Specific immunotherapy is effective in the prevention of new sensitivities. *Allergol Immunopathol (Madr).* 2007 Mar-Apr;35(2):44-51.

Reichling J, Schmökel H, Fitzi J, Bucher S, Saller R. Dietary support with Boswellia resin in canine inflammatory joint and spinal disease. *Schweiz Arch Tierheilkd.* 2004 Feb;146(2):71-9.

Reuter A, Lidholm J, Andersson K, Ostling J, Lundberg M, Scheurer S, Enrique E, Cistero-Bahima A, San Miguel-Moncin M, Ballmer-Weber BK, Vieths S. A critical assessment of allergen component-based in vitro diagnosis in cherry allergy across Europe. *Clin Exp Allergy.* 2006 Jun;36(6):815-23.

Rimbaud L, Heraud F, La Vieille S, Leblanc JC, Crepet A. Quantitative risk assessment relating to adventitious presence of allergens in food: a probabilistic model applied to peanut in chocolate. *Risk Anal.* 2010 Jan;30(1):7-19.

Rinne M, Kalliomaki M, Arvilommi H, Salminen S, Isolauri E. Effect of probiotics and breastfeeding on the bifidobacterium and lactobacillus/enterococcus microbiota and humoral immune responses. *J Pediatr.* 2005 Aug;147(2):186-91.

Río ME, Zago Beatriz L, Garcia H, Winter L. The nutritional status change the effectiveness of a dietary supplement of lactic bacteria on the emerging of respiratory tract diseases in children. *Arch Latinoam Nutr.* 2002 Mar;52(1):29-34.

Robert AM, Groult N, Six C, Robert L. The effect of procyanidolic oligomers on mesenchymal cells in culture II—Attachment of elastic fibers to the cells. *Pathol Biol.* 1990 Jun;38(6):601-7.

Robert AM, Groult N, Six C, Robert L. The effect of procyanidolic oligomers on mesenchymal cells in culture II—Attachment of elastic fibers to the cells. *Pathol Biol.* 1990 Jun;38(6):601-7.

Roberts G, Lack G. Diagnosing peanut allergy with skin prick and specific IgE testing. *J Allergy Clin Immunol.* 2005 Jun;115(6):1291-6.

Rodriguez J, Crespo JF, Burks W, Rivas-Plata C, Fernandez-Anaya S, Vives R, Daroca P. Randomized, double-blind, crossover challenge study in 53 subjects reporting adverse reactions to melon (Cucumis melo). *J Allergy Clin Immunol.* 2000 Nov;106(5):968-72.

Rodriguez-Fragoso L, Reyes-Esparza J, Burchiel SW, Herrera-Ruiz D, Torres E. Risks and benefits of commonly used herbal medicines in Mexico. *Toxicol Appl Pharmacol.* 2008 Feb 15;227(1):125-35.

REFERENCES AND BIBLIOGRAPHY

Rodríguez-Ortiz PG, Muñoz-Mendoza D, Arias-Cruz A, González-Díaz SN, Herrera-Castro D, Vidaurri-Ojeda AC. Epidemiological characteristics of patients with food allergy assisted at Regional Center of Allergies and Clinical Immunology of Monterrey. *Rev Alerg Mex.* 2009 Nov-Dec;56(6):185-91.

Roduit C, Scholtens S, de Jongste JC, Wijga AH, Gerritsen J, Postma DS, Brunekreef B, Hoekstra MO, Aalberse R, Smit HA. Asthma at 8 years of age in children born by caesarean section. *Thorax.* 2009 Feb;64(2):107-13.

Roessler A, Friedrich U, Vogelsang H, Bauer A, Kaatz M, Hipler UC, Schmidt I, Jahreis G. The immune system in healthy adults and patients with atopic dermatitis seems to be affected differently by a probiotic intervention. *Clin Exp Allergy.* 2008 Jan;38(1):93-102.

Romeo J, Wärnberg J, Nova E, Díaz LE, González-Gross M, Marcos A. Changes in the immune system after moderate beer consumption. *Ann Nutr Metab.* 2007;51(4):359-66.

Rona RJ, Keil T, Summers C, Gislason D, Zuidmeer L, Sodergren E, Sigurdardottir ST, Lindner T, Goldhahn K, Dahlstrom J, McBride D, Madsen C. The prevalence of food allergy: a meta-analysis. *J Allergy Clin Immunol.* 2007 Sep;120(3):638-46.

Ronteltap A, van Schaik J, Wensing M, Rynja FJ, Knulst AC, de Vries JH. Sensory testing of recipes masking peanut or hazelnut for double-blind placebo-controlled food challenges. Allergy. 2004 Apr;59(4):457-60. Clark S, Bock SA, Gaeta TJ, Brenner BE, Cydulka RK, Camargo CA; Multicenter Airway Research Collaboration-8 Investigators. Multicenter study of emergency department visits for food allergies. *J Allergy Clin Immunol.* 2004 Feb;113(2):347-52.

Ros E, Mataix J. Fatty acid composition of nuts—implications for cardiovascular health. *Br J Nutr.* 2006 Nov;96 Suppl 2:S29-35.

Rosenfeldt V, Benfeldt E, Valerius NH, Paerregaard A, Michaelsen KF. Effect of probiotics on gastrointestinal symptoms and small intestinal permeability in children with atopic dermatitis. *J Pediatr.* 2004 Nov;145(5):612-6.

Rozycki VR, Baigorria CM, Freyre MR, Bernard CM, Zannier MS, Charpentier M. Nutrient content in vegetable species from the Argentine Chaco. *Arch Latinoam Nutr.* 1997 Sep;47(3):265-70.

Rubin E., Farber JL. *Pathology.* 3rd Ed. Philadelphia: Lippincott-Raven, 1999.

Rudders SA, Espinola JA, Camargo CA Jr. North-south differences in US emergency department visits for acute allergic reactions. *Ann Allergy Asthma Immunol.* 2010 May;104(5):413-6.

Saarinen KM, Juntunen-Backman K, Järvenpää AL, Klemetti P, Kuitunen P, Lope L, Renlund M, Siivola M, Vaarala O, Savilahti E. Breast-feeding and the development of cows' milk protein allergy. *Adv Exp Med Biol.* 2000;478:121-30.

Saggioro A. Probiotics in the treatment of irritable bowel syndrome. *J Clin Gastroenterol.* 2004 Jul;38(6 Suppl):S104-6.

Sahagún-Flores JE, López-Peña LS, de la Cruz-Ramírez Jaimes J, García-Bravo MS, Peregrina-Gómez R, de Alba-García JE. Eradication of Helicobacter pylori: triple treatment scheme plus Lactobacillus vs. triple treatment alone. *Cir Cir.* 2007 Sep-Oct;75(5):333-6.

Sahin-Yilmaz A, Nocon CC, Corey JP. Immunoglobulin E-mediated food allergies among adults with allergic rhinitis. *Otolaryngol Head Neck Surg.* 2010 Sep;143(3):379-85.

Salem N, Wegher B, Mena P, Uauy R. Arachidonic and docosahexaenoic acids are biosynthesized from their 18-carbon precursors in human infants. *Proc Natl Acad Sci.* 1996;93:49-54.

Salido S, Altarejos J, Nogueras M, Sánchez A, Pannecouque C, Witvrouw M, De Clercq E. Chemical studies of essential oils of Juniperus oxycedrus ssp. badia. *J Ethnopharmacol.* 2002 Jun;81(1):129-34.

Salim AS. Sulfhydryl-containing agents in the treatment of gastric bleeding induced by nonsteroidal antiinflammatory drugs. *Can J Surg.* 1993 Feb;36(1):53-8.

Salim, A.S., Role of oxygen-derived free radical scavengers in the management of recurrent attacks of ulcerative colitis: A new approach. *J. Lab Clin Med.* 1992;119:740-747.

Salmi H, Kuitunen M, Viljanen M, Lapatto R. Cow's milk allergy is associated with changes in urinary organic acid concentrations. *Pediatr Allergy Immunol.* 2010 Mar;21(2 Pt 2):e401-6.

Salminen S, Isolauri E, Salminen E. Clinical uses of probiotics for stabilizing the gut mucosal barrier: successful strains and future challenges. *Antonie Van Leeuwenhoek.* 1996 Oct;70(2-4):347-58.

Salom IL, Silvis SE, Doscherholmen A. Effect of cimetidine on the absorption of vitamin B12. *Scand J Gastroenterol.* 1982;17:129-31.

Salpietro CD, Gangemi S, Briuglia S, Meo A, Merlino MV, Muscolino G, Bisignano G, Trombetta D, Saija A. The almond milk: a new approach to the management of cow-milk allergy/intolerance in infants. *Minerva Pediatr.* 2005 Aug;57(4):173-80.

Samoylenko V, Dunbar DC, Gafur MA, Khan SI, Ross SA, Mossa JS, El-Feraly FS, Tekwani BL, Bosselaers J, Muhammad I. Antiparasitic, nematicidal and antifouling constituents from Juniperus berries. *Phytother Res.* 2008 Dec;22(12):1570-6.

Sancho AI, Hoffmann-Sommergruber K, Alessandri S, Conti A, Giuffrida MG, Shewry P, Jensen BM, Skov P, Vieths S. Authentication of food allergen quality by physicochemical and immunological methods. *Clin Exp Allergy.* 2010 Jul;40(7):973-86.

Sandin A, Annus T, Björkstén B, Nilsson L, Riikjärv MA, van Hage-Hamsten M, Bråbäck L. Prevalence of self-reported food allergy and IgE antibodies to food allergens in Swedish and Estonian schoolchildren. *Eur J Clin Nutr.* 2005 Mar;59(3):399-403.

Santos A, Dias A, Pinheiro JA. Predictive factors for the persistence of cow's milk allergy. *Pediatr Allergy Immunol.* 2010 Apr 27.

Sanz Ortega J, Martorell Aragonés A, Michavila Gómez A, Nieto García A; Grupo de Trabajo para el Estudio de la Alergia Alimentaria. Incidence of IgE-mediated allergy to cow's milk proteins in the first year of life. *An Esp Pediatr.* 2001 Jun;54(6):536-9.

Sato S, Tachimoto H, Shukuya A, Kurosaka N, Yanagida N, Utsunomiya T, Iguchi M, Komata T, Imai T, Tomikawa M, Ebisawa M. Basophil activation marker CD203c is useful in the diagnosis of hen's egg and cow's milk allergies in children. *Int Arch Allergy Immunol.* 2010;152 Suppl 1:54-61.

Sato Y, Akiyama H, Matsuoka H, Sakata K, Nakamura R, Ishikawa S, Inakuma T, Totsuka M, Sugita-Konishi Y, Ebisawa M, Teshima R. Dietary carotenoids inhibit oral sensitization and the development of food allergy. *J Agric Food Chem.* 2010 Jun 23;58(12):7180-6.

Satyanarayana S, Sushruta K, Sarma GS, Srinivas N, Subba Raju GV. Antioxidant activity of the aqueous extracts of spicy food additives—evaluation and comparison with ascorbic acid in in-vitro systems. *J Herb Pharmacother.* 2004;4(2):1-10.

Savage JH, Kaeding AJ, Matsui EC, Wood RA. The natural history of soy allergy. *J Allergy Clin Immunol.* 2010 Mar;125(3):683-6.

Savilahti EM, Karinen S, Salo HM, Klemetti P, Saarinen KM, Klemola T, Kuitunen M, Hautaniemi S, Savilahti E, Vaarala O. Combined T regulatory cell and Th2 expression profile identifies children with cow's milk allergy. *Clin Immunol.* 2010 Jul;136(1):16-20.

Savilahti EM, Rantanen V, Lin JS, Karinen S, Saarinen KM, Goldis M, Mäkelä MJ, Hautaniemi S, Savilahti E, Sampson HA. Early recovery from cow's milk allergy is associated with decreasing IgE and increasing IgG4 binding to cow's milk epitopes. *J Allergy Clin Immunol.* 2010 Jun;125(6):1315-1321.e9.

Savilahti EM, Rantanen V, Lin JS, Karinen S, Saarinen KM, Goldis M, Mäkelä MJ, Hautaniemi S, Savilahti E, Sampson HA. Early recovery from cow's milk allergy is associated with decreasing IgE and increasing IgG4 binding to cow's milk epitopes. *J Allergy Clin Immunol.* 2010 Jun;125(6):1315-1321.e9.

Sazanova NE, Varnacheva LN, Novikova AV, Pletneva NB. Immunological aspects of food intolerance in children during first years of life. *Pediatriia.* 1992;(3):14-8. Russian.

Scadding G, Bjarnason I, Brostoff J, Levi AJ, Peters TJ. Intestinal permeability to 51Cr-labelled ethylenediaminetetraacetate in food-intolerant subjects. *Digestion.* 1989;42(2):104-9.

Scalabrin DM, Johnston WH, Hoffman DR, P'Pool VL, Harris CL, Mitmesser SH. Growth and tolerance of healthy term infants receiving hydrolyzed infant formulas supplemented with Lactobacillus rhamnosus GG: randomized, double-blind, controlled trial. *Clin Pediatr (Phila).* 2009 Sep;48(7):734-44.

Schabelman E, Witting M. The Relationship of Radiocontrast, Iodine, and Seafood Allergies: A Medical Myth Exposed. *J Emerg Med.* 2009 Dec 31.

Schade RP, Meijer Y, Pasmans SG, Knulst AC, Kimpen JL, Bruijnzeel-Koomen CA. Double blind placebo controlled cow's milk provocation for the diagnosis of cow's milk allergy in infants and children. *Ned Tijdschr Geneeskd.* 2002 Sep 14;146(37):1739-42.

Schauenberg P, Paris F. *Guide to Medicinal Plants.* New Canaan, CT: Keats Publ, 1977.

Schauss AG, Wu X, Prior RL, Ou B, Huang D, Owens J, Agarwal A, Jensen GS, Hart AN, Shanbrom E. Antioxidant capacity and other bioactivities of the freeze-dried Amazonian palm berry, Euterpe oleracea mart. (acai). *J Agric Food Chem.* 2006 Nov 1;54(22):8604-10.

Schempp H, Weiser D, Elstner EF. Biochemical model reactions indicative of inflammatory processes. Activities of extracts from Fraxinus excelsior and Populus tremula. *Arzneimittelforschung.* 2000 Apr;50(4):362-72.

Schepetkin IA, Faulkner CL, Nelson-Overton LK, Wiley JA, Quinn MT. Macrophage immunomodulatory activity of polysaccharides isolated from Juniperus scopolorum. *Int Immunopharmacol.* 2005 Dec;5(13-14):1783-99.

Schilcher H, Leuschner F. The potential nephrotoxic effects of essential juniper oil. *Arzneimittelforschung.* 1997 Jul;47(7):855-8.

Schillaci D, Arizza V, Dayton T, Camarda L, Di Stefano V. In vitro anti-biofilm activity of Boswellia spp. oleogum resin essential oils. *Lett Appl Microbiol.* 2008 Nov;47(5):433-8.

Schmid B, Kötter I, Heide L. Pharmacokinetics of salicin after oral administration of a standardised willow bark extract. *Eur J Clin Pharmacol.* 2001 Aug;57(5):387-91.

Schmitt DA, Maleki SJ (2004) Comparing the effects of boiling, frying and roasting on the allergenicity of peanuts. *J Allergy Clin Immunol.* 113: S155.

REFERENCES AND BIBLIOGRAPHY

Schnappinger M, Sausenthaler S, Linseisen J, Hauner H, Heinrich J. Fish consumption, allergic sensitisation and allergic diseases in adults. *Ann Nutr Metab.* 2009;54(1):67-74.

Schneider I, Gibbons S, Bucar F. Inhibitory activity of Juniperus communis on 12(S)-HETE production in human platelets. *Planta Med.* 2004 May;70(5):471-4.

Schönfeld P. Phytanic Acid toxicity: implications for the permeability of the inner mitochondrial membrane to ions. *Toxicol Mech Methods.* 2004;14(1-2):47-52.

Schottner M, Gansser D, Spiteller G. Lignans from the roots of Urtica dioica and their metabolites bind to human sex hormone binding globulin (SHBG). *Planta Med.* 1997;63:529–532.

Schouten B, van Esch BC, Hofman GA, Boon L, Knippels LM, Willemsen LE, Garssen J. Oligosaccharide-induced whey-specific CD25(+) regulatory T-cells are involved in the suppression of cow milk allergy in mice. *J Nutr.* 2010 Apr;140(4):835-41.

Schouten B, van Esch BC, van Thuijl AO, Blokhuis BR, Groot Kormelink T, Hofman GA, Moro GE, Boehm G, Arslanoglu S, Sprikkelman AB, Willemsen LE, Knippels LM, Redegeld FA, Garssen J. Contribution of IgE and immunoglobulin free light chain in the allergic reaction to cow's milk proteins. *J Allergy Clin Immunol.* 2010 Jun;125(6):1308-14.

Schroecksnadel S, Jenny M, Fuchs D. Sensitivity to sulphite additives. *Clin Exp Allergy.* 2010 Apr;40(4):688-9.

Schulick P. *Ginger: Common Spice & Wonder Drug.* Brattleboro, VT: Herbal Free Perss, 1996.

Schumacher P. *Biophysical Therapy Of Allergies.* Stuttgart: Thieme, 2005.

Schütz K, Carle R, Schieber A. Taraxacum—a review on its phytochemical and pharmacological profile. *J Ethnopharmacol.* 2006 Oct 11;107(3):313-23.

Schwab D, Hahn EG, Raithel M. Enhanced histamine metabolism: a comparative analysis of collagenous colitis and food allergy with respect to the role of diet and NSAID use. *Inflamm Res.* 2003 Apr;52(4):142-7.

Schwab D, Müller S, Aigner T, Neureiter D, Kirchner T, Hahn EG, Raithel M. Functional and morphologic characterization of eosinophils in the lower intestinal mucosa of patients with food allergy. *Am J Gastroenterol.* 2003 Jul;98(7):1525-34.

Schwelberger HG. Histamine intolerance: a metabolic disease? *Inflamm Res.* 2010 Mar;59 Suppl 2:S219-21.

Scibilia J, Pastorello EA, Zisa G, Ottolenghi A, Ballmer-Weber B, Pravettoni V, Scovena E, Robino A, Ortolani C. Maize food allergy: a double-blind placebo-controlled study. *Clin Exp Allergy.* 2008 Dec;38(12):1943-9.

Scott-Taylor TH, O'B Hourihane J, Strobel S. Correlation of allergen-specific IgG subclass antibodies and T lymphocyte cytokine responses in children with multiple food allergies. *Pediatr Allergy Immunol.* 2010 Sep;21(6):935-44.

Scurlock AM, Jones SM. An update on immunotherapy for food allergy. *Curr Opin Allergy Clin Immunol.* 2010 Dec;10(6):587-93.

Sealey-Voyksner JA, Khosla C, Voyksner RD, Jorgenson JW. Novel aspects of quantitation of immunogenic wheat gluten peptides by liquid chromatography-mass spectrometry/mass spectrometry. *J Chromatogr A.* 2010 Jun 18;1217(25):4167-183.

Seca AM, Silva AM, Bazzocchi IL, Jimenez IA. Diterpene constituents of leaves from Juniperus brevifolia. *Phytochemistry.* 2008 Jan;69(2):498-505.

Seca AM, Silva AM. The chemical composition of hexane extract from bark of Juniperus brevifolia. *Nat Prod Res.* 2008;22(11):975-83.

Senna G, Gani F, Leo G, Schiappoli M. Alternative tests in the diagnosis of food allergies. *Recenti Prog Med.* 2002 May;93(5):327-34.

Seo K, Jung S, Park M, Song Y, Choung S. Effects of leucocyanidines on activities of metabolizing enzymes and antioxidant enzymes. *Biol Pharm Bull.* 2001 May;24(5):592-3.

Seo SW, Koo HN, An HJ, Kwon KB, Lim BC, Seo EA, Ryu DG, Moon G, Kim HY, Kim HM, Hong SH. Taraxacum officinale protects against cholecystokinin-induced acute pancreatitis in rats. *World J Gastroenterol.* 2005 Jan 28;11(4):597-9.

Seppo L, Korpela R, Lönnerdal B, Metsäniitty L, Juntunen-Backman K, Klemola T, Paganus A, Vanto T. A follow-up study of nutrient intake, nutritional status, and growth in infants with cow milk allergy fed either a soy formula or an extensively hydrolyzed whey formula. *Am J Clin Nutr.* 2005 Jul;82(1):140-5.

Settipane RA, Siri D, Bellanti JA. Egg allergy and influenza vaccination. *Allergy Asthma Proc.* 2009 Nov-Dec;30(6):660-5.

Shahani KM, Meshbesher BF, Mangalampalli V. *Cultivate Health From Within.* Danbury, CT: Vital Health Publ, 2005.

Shakib F, Brown HM, Phelps A, Redhead R. Study of IgG sub-class antibodies in patients with milk intolerance. *Clin Allergy.* 1986 Sep;16(5):451-8.

Shao J, Sheng J, Dong W, Li YZ, Yu SC. Effects of feeding intervention on development of eczema in atopy high-risk infants: an 18-month follow-up study. *Zhonghua Er Ke Za Zhi.* 2006 Sep;44(9):684-7. Chinese.

Sharma P, Sharma BC, Puri V, Sarin SK. An open-label randomized controlled trial of lactulose and probiotics in the treatment of minimal hepatic encephalopathy. *Eur J Gastroent Hepatol.* 2008 Jun;20(6):506-11.

Sharma SC, Sharma S, Gulati OP. Pycnogenol inhibits the release of histamine from mast cells. *Phytother Res.* 2003 Jan;17(1):66-9.

Sharnan J, Kumar L, Singh S. Comparison of results of skin prick tests, enzyme-linked immunosorbent assays and food challenges in children with respiratory allergy. *J Trop Pediatr.* 2001 Dec;47(6):367-8.

Shaw J, Roberts G, Grimshaw K, White S, Hourihane J. Lupin allergy in peanut-allergic children and teenagers. *Allergy.* 2008 Mar;63(3):370-3.

Shawcross DL, Wright G, Olde Damink SW, Jalan R. Role of ammonia and inflammation in minimal hepatic encephalopathy. *Metab Brain Dis.* 2007 Mar;22(1):125-38.

Shea-Donohue T, Stiltz J, Zhao A, Notari L. Mast Cells. *Curr Gastroenterol Rep.* 2010 Aug 14.

Sheth SS, Waserman S, Kagan R, Alizadchfar R, Primeau MN, Elliot S, St Pierre Y, Wickett R, Joseph L, Harada L, Dufresne C, Allen M, Allen M, Godefroy SB, Clarke AE. Role of food labels in accidental exposures in food-allergic individuals in Canada. *Ann Allergy Asthma Immunol.* 2010 Jan;104(1):60-5.

Shi S, Zhao Y, Zhou H, Zhang Y, Jiang X, Huang K. Identification of antioxidants from Taraxacum mongolicum by high-performance liquid chromatography-diode array detection-radical-scavenging detection-electrospray ionization mass spectrometry and nuclear magnetic resonance experiments. *J Chromatogr A.* 2008 Oct 31;1209(1-2):145-52

Shi S, Zhou H, Zhang Y, Huang K, Liu S. Chemical constituents from Neo-Taraxacum siphonathum. *Zhongguo Zhong Yao Za Zhi.* 2009 Apr;34(8):1002-4.

Shi SY, Zhou CX, Xu Y, Tao QF, Bai H, Lu FS, Lin WY, Chen HY, Zheng W, Wang LW, Wu YH, Zeng S, Huang KX, Zhao Y, Li XK, Qu J. Studies on chemical constituents from herbs of Taraxacum mongolicum. *Zhongguo Zhong Yao Za Zhi.* 2008 May;33(10):1147-57.

Shibata H, Nabe T, Yamamura H, Kohno S. l-Ephedrine is a major constituent of Mao-Bushi-Saishin-To, one of the formulas of Chinese medicine, which shows immediate inhibition after oral administration of passive cutaneous anaphylaxis in rats. *Inflamm Res.* 2000 Aug;49(8):398-403.

Shimoi T, Ushiyama H, Kan K, Saito K, Kamata K, Hirokado M. Survey of glycoalkaloids content in the various potatoes. Shokuhin Eiseigaku Zasshi. 2007 Jun;48(3):77-82.

Shishehbor F, Behroo L, Ghafouriyan Broujerdnia M, Namjoyan F, Latifi SM. Quercetin effectively quells peanut-induced anaphylactic reactions in the peanut sensitized rats. *Iran J Allergy Asthma Immunol.* 2010 Mar;9(1):27-34.

Shoaf, K., Muvey, G.L., Armstrong, G.D., Hutkins, R.W. (2006) Prebiotic galactooligosaccharides reduce adherence of enteropathogenic Escherichia coli to tissue culture cells. *Infect Immun.* Dec;74(12):6920-8.

Sicherer SH, Muñoz-Furlong A, Godbold JH, Sampson HA. US prevalence of self-reported peanut, tree nut, and sesame allergy: 11-year follow-up. *J Allergy Clin Immunol.* 2010 Jun;125(6):1322-6.

Sicherer SH, Munoz-Furlong A, Sampson HA (2003) Prevalence of peanut and tree nut allergy in the United States determined by means of a random digit dial telephone survey: a 5-year follow-up study. *J Allergy Clin Immunol.* 112: 1203–1207.

Sicherer SH, Noone SA, Koerner CB, Christie L, Burks AW, Sampson HA. Hypoallergenicity and efficacy of an amino acid-based formula in children with cow's milk and multiple food hypersensitivities. *J Pediatr.* 2001 May;138(5):688-93.

Sicherer SH, Sampson HA. Food allergy. *J Allergy Clin Immunol.* 2010 Feb;125(2 Suppl 2):S116-25.

Sicherer SH, Wood RA, Stablein D, Burks AW, Liu AH, Jones SM, Fleischer DM, Leung DY, Grishin A, Mayer L, Shreffler W, Lindblad R, Sampson HA. Immunologic features of infants with milk or egg allergy enrolled in an observational study (Consortium of Food Allergy Research) of food allergy. *J Allergy Clin Immunol.* 2010 May;125(5):1077-1083.e8.

Sigstedt SC, Hooten CJ, Callewaert MC, Jenkins AR, Romero AE, Pullin MJ, Kornienko A, Lowrey TK, Slambrouck SV, Steelant WF. Evaluation of aqueous extracts of Taraxacum officinale on growth and invasion of breast and prostate cancer cells. *Int J Oncol.* 2008 May;32(5):1085-90.

Silman AJ, MacGregor AJ, Thomson W, Holligan S, Carthy D, Farhan A, Ollier WE. Twin concordance rates for rheumatoid arthritis: results from a nationwide study. *Br J Rheumatol.* 1993 Oct;32(10):903-7.

Silva MF, Kamphorst AO, Hayashi EA, Bellio M, Carvalho CR, Faria AM, Sabino KC, Coelho MG, Nobrega A, Tavares D, Silva AC. Innate profiles of cytokines implicated in oral tolerance correlate with low- or high-suppression of humoral response. *Immunology.* 2010 Jul;130(3):447-57.

Simeone D, Miele E, Boccia G, Marino A, Troncone R, Staiano A. Prevalence of atopy in children with chronic constipation. *Arch Dis Child.* 2008 Dec;93(12):1044-7.

Simonte SJ, Ma S, Mofidi S, Sicherer SH. Relevance of casual contact with peanut butter in children with peanut allergy. *J Allergy Clin Immunol.* 2003 Jul;112(1):180-2.

Simopoulos AP. Essential fatty acids in health and chronic disease. *Am J Clin Nutr.* 1999 Sep;70(3 Suppl):560S-569S.

Simpson AB, Yousef E, Hossain J. Association between peanut allergy and asthma morbidity. *J Pediatr.* 2010 May;156(5):777-81, 781.e1.

Singer P, Shapiro H, Theilla M, Anbar R, Singer J, Cohen J. Anti-inflammatory properties of omega-3 fatty acids in critical illness: novel mechanisms and an integrative perspective. *Intensive Care Med.* 2008 Sep;34(9):1580-92.

Singh S, Khajuria A, Taneja SC, Johri RK, Singh J, Qazi GN. Boswellic acids: A leukotriene inhibitor also effective through topical application in inflammatory disorders. *Phytomedicine.* 2008 Jun;15(6-7):400-7.

Sirvent S, Palomares O, Vereda A, Villalba M, Cuesta-Herranz J, Rodríguez R. nsLTP and profilin are allergens in mustard seeds: cloning, sequencing and recombinant production of Sin a 3 and Sin a 4. *Clin Exp Allergy.* 2009 Dec;39(12):1929-36.

Skamstrup Hansen K, Vieths S, Vestergaard H, Skov PS, Bindslev-Jensen C, Poulsen LK. Seasonal variation in food allergy to apple. *J Chromatogr B Biomed Sci Appl.* 2001 May 25;756(1-2):19-32.

Skripak JM, Nash SD, Rowley H, Brereton NH, Oh S, Hamilton RG, Matsui EC, Burks AW, Wood RA. A randomized, double-blind, placebo-controlled study of milk oral immunotherapy for cow's milk allergy. *J Allergy Clin Immunol.* 2008 Dec;122(6):1154-60.

Sletten GB, Halvorsen R, Egaas E, Halstensen TS. Changes in humoral responses to beta-lactoglobulin in tolerant patients suggest a particular role for IgG4 in delayed, non-IgE-mediated cow's milk allergy. *Pediatr Allergy Immunol.* 2006 Sep;17(6):435-43.

Smith J. *Genetic Roulette: The Documented Health Risks of Genetically Engineered Foods.* White River Jct, Vermont: Chelsea Green, 2007.

Smith K, Warholak T, Armstrong E, Leib M, Rehfeld R, Malone D. Evaluation of risk factors and health outcomes among persons with asthma. *J Asthma.* 2009 Apr;46(3):234-7.

Smith S, Sullivan K. Examining the influence of biological and psychological factors on cognitive performance in chronic fatigue syndrome: a randomized, double-blind, placebo-controlled, crossover study. *Int J Behav Med.* 2003;10(2):162-73.

Sofic E, Denisova N, Youdim K, Vatrenjak-Velagic V, De Filippo C, Mehmedagic A, Causevic A, Cao G, Joseph JA, Prior RL. Antioxidant and pro-oxidant capacity of catecholamines and related compounds. Effects of hydrogen peroxide on glutathione and sphingomyelinase activity in pheochromocytoma PC12 cells: potential relevance to age-related diseases. *J Neural Transm.* 2001;108(5):541-57.

Soleo L, Colosio C, Alinovi R, Guarneri D, Russo A, Lovreglio P, Vimercati L, Birindelli S, Cortesi I, Flore C, Carta P, Colombi A, Parrinello G, Ambrosi L. Immunologic effects of exposure to low levels of inorganic mercury. *Med Lav.* 2002 May-Jun;93(3):225-32. Italian.

Sompamit K, Kukongviriyapan U, Nakmareong S, Pannangpetch P, Kukongviriyapan V. Curcumin improves vascular function and alleviates oxidative stress in non-lethal lipopolysaccharide-induced endotoxaemia in mice. *Eur J Pharmacol.* 2009 Aug 15;616(1-3):192-9.

Soyland Wasenius AK, Halvorsen R. Oral provocation tests for adverse reactions to food. *Tidsskr Nor Laegeforen.* 2003 Jun 26;123(13-14):1829-30.

Spence A. *Basic Human Anatomy.* Menlo Park, CA: Benjamin/Commings, 1986.

Spiller G. *The Super Pyramid.* New York: HRS Press, 1993.

Srivastava K, Zou ZM, Sampson HA, Dansky H, Li XM. Direct Modulation of Airway Reactivity by the Chinese Anti-Asthma Herbal Formula ASHMI. *J Allergy Clin Immunol.* 2005;115:S7.

Srivastava KD, Kattan JD, Zou ZM, Li JH, Zhang L, Wallenstein S, Goldfarb J, Sampson HA, Li XM. The Chinese herbal medicine formula FAHF-2 completely blocks anaphylactic reactions in a murine model of peanut allergy. *J Allergy Clin Immunol.* 2005;115:171-8.

Srivastava KD, Qu C, Zhang T, Goldfarb J, Sampson HA, Li XM. Food Allergy Herbal Formula-2 silences peanut-induced anaphylaxis for a prolonged posttreatment period via IFN-gamma-producing CD8+ T cells. *J Allergy Clin Immunol.* 2009 Feb;123(2):443-51.

Srivastava KD, Zhang TF, Qu C, Sampson HA, Li XM. Silencing Peanut Allergy: A Chinese Herbal Formula, FAHF-2, Completely Blocks Peanut-induced Anaphylaxis for up to 6 Months Following Therapy in a Murine Model Of Peanut Allergy. *J Allergy Clin Immunol.* 2006;117:S328.

Staden U, Rolinck-Werninghaus C, Brewe F, Wahn U, Niggemann B, Beyer K. Specific oral tolerance induction in food allergy in children: efficacy and clinical patterns of reaction. *Allergy.* 2007 Nov;62(11):1261-9.

Stahl SM. Selective histamine H1 antagonism: novel hypnotic and pharmacologic actions challenge classical notions of antihistamines. *CNS Spectr.* 2008 Dec;13(12):1027-38.

Stenberg JA, Hambäck PA, Ericson L. Herbivore-induced "rent rise" in the host plant may drive a diet breadth enlargement in the tenant. *Ecology.* 2008 Jan;89(1):126-33.

Stengler M. *The Natural Physician's Healing Therapies.* Stamford, CT: Bottom Line Books, 2008.

Stratiki Z, Costalos C, Sevastiadou S, Kastanidou O, Skouroliakou M, Giakoumatou A, Petrohilou V. The effect of a bifidobacter supplemented bovine milk on intestinal permeability of preterm infants. *Early Hum Dev.* 2007 Sep;83(9):575-9.

Stirapongsasuti P, Tanglertsampan C, Aunhachoke K, Sangasapaviliya A. Anaphylactic reaction to phuk-waan-ban in a patient with latex allergy. *J Med Assoc Thai.* 2010 May;93(5):616-9.

Strinnholm A, Brulin C, Lindh V. Experiences of double-blind, placebo-controlled food challenges (DBPCFC): a qualitative analysis of mothers' experiences. *J Child Health Care.* 2010 Jun;14(2):179-88.

Stutius LM, Sheehan WJ, Rangsithienchai P, Bharmanee A, Scott JE, Young MC, Dioun AF, Schneider LC, Phipatanakul W. Characterizing the relationship between sesame, coconut, and nut allergy in children. *Pediatr Allergy Immunol.* 2010 Dec;21(8):1114-8.

Sugawara G, Nagino M, Nishio H, Ebata T, Takagi K, Asahara T, Nomoto K, Nimura Y. Perioperative synbiotic treatment to prevent postoperative infectious complications in biliary cancer surgery: a ran-domized controlled trial. *Ann Surg.* 2006 Nov;244(5):706-14.

Suh KY. Food allergy and atopic dermatitis: separating fact from fiction. *Semin Cutan Med Surg.* 2010 Jun;29(2):72-8.

Sumantran VN, Kulkarni AA, Harsulkar A, Wele A, Koppikar SJ, Chandwaskar R, Gaire V, Dalvi M, Wagh UV. Hyaluronidase and collagenase inhibitory activities of the herbal formulation Triphala guggulu. *J Biosci.* 2007 Jun;32(4):755-61.

Sumiyoshi M, Sakanaka M, Kimura Y. Effects of Red Ginseng extract on allergic reactions to food in Balb/c mice. *J Ethnopharmacol.* 2010 Aug 14.

Sung JH, Lee JO, Son JK, Park NS, Kim MR, Kim JG, Moon DC. Cytotoxic constituents from Solidago virga-aurea var. gigantea MIQ. *Arch Pharm Res.* 1999 Dec;22(6):633-7.

Suomalainen H, Isolauri E. New concepts of allergy to cow's milk. *Ann Med.* 1994 Aug;26(4):289-96.

Sütas Y, Kekki OM, Isolauri E. Late onset reactions to oral food challenge are linked to low serum inter-leukin-10 concentrations in patients with atopic dermatitis and food allergy. *Clin Exp Allergy.* 2000 Aug;30(8):1121-8.

Sweeney B, Vora M, Ulbricht C, Basch E. Evidence-based systematic review of dandelion (Taraxacum officinale) by natural standard research collaboration. *J Herb Pharmacother.* 2005;5(1):79-93.

Svendsen AJ, Holm NV, Kyvik K, *et al.* Relative importance of genetic effects in rheumatoid arthritis: historical cohort study of Danish nationwide twin population. *BMJ* 2002;324(7332): 264-266.

Swiderska-Kielbik S, Krakowiak A, Wiszniewska M, Dudek W, Walusiak-Skorupa J, Krawczyk-Szulc P, Michowicz A, Pałczyński C. Health hazards associated with occupational exposure to birds. *Med Pr.* 2010;61(2):213-22.

Szyf M, McGowan P, Meaney MJ. The social environment and the epigenome. *Environ Mol Mutagen.* 2008 Jan;49(1):46-60.

Takada Y, Ichikawa H, Badmaev V, Aggarwal BB. Acetyl-11-keto-beta-boswellic acid potentiates apoptosis, inhibits invasion, and abolishes osteoclastogenesis by suppressing NF-kappa B and NF-kappa B-regulated gene expression. *J Immunol.* 2006 Mar 1;176(5):3127-40.

Takahashi N, Eisenhuth G, Lee I, Schachtele C, Laible N, Binion S. Nonspecific antibacterial factors in milk from cows immunized with human oral bacterial pathogens. *J Dairy Sci.* 1992 Jul;75(7):1810-20.

Takasaki M, Konoshima T, Tokuda H, Masuda K, Arai Y, Shiojima K, Ageta H. Anti-carcinogenic activity of Taraxacum plant. I. *Biol Pharm Bull.* 1999 Jun;22(6):602-5.

Tamura M, Shikina T, Morihana T, Hayama M, Kajimoto O, Sakamoto A, Kajimoto Y, Watanabe O, Nonaka C, Shida K, Nanno M. Effects of probiotics on allergic rhinitis induced by Japanese cedar pol-len: randomized double-blind, placebo-controlled clinical trial. *Int Arch Allergy Imml.* 2007;143(1):75-82.

Tapiero H, Ba GN, Couvreur P, Tew KD. Polyunsaturated fatty acids (PUFA) and eicosanoids in human health and pathologies. *Biomed Pharmacother.* 2002 Jul;56(5):215-22.

Tapsell LC, Hemphill I, Cobiac L, Patch CS, Sullivan DR, Fenech M, Roodenrys S, Keogh JB, Clifton PM, Williams PG, Fazio VA, Inge KE. Health benefits of herbs and spices: the past, the present, the fu-ture. *Med J Aust.* 2006 Aug 21;185(4 Suppl):S4-24.

Tasli L, Mat C, De Simone C, Yazici H. Lactobacilli lozenges in the management of oral ulcers of Behçet's syndrome. *Clin Exp Rheumatol.* 2006 Sep-Oct;24(5 Suppl 42):S83-6.

Taussig SJ, Batkin S. Bromelain, the enzyme complex of pineapple (Ananas comosus) and its clinical applica-tion. An update. *J Ethnopharmacol.* 1988 Feb-Mar;22(2):191-203.

Taylor AL, Dunstan JA, Prescott SL. Probiotic supplementation for the first 6 months of life fails to reduce the risk of atopic dermatitis and increases the risk of allergen sensitization in high-risk children: a ran-domized controlled trial. *J Allergy Clin Immunol.* 2007 Jan;119(1):184-91.

Taylor AL, Hale J, Wiltschut J, Lehmann H, Dunstan JA, Prescott SL. Effects of probiotic supplementation for the first 6 months of life on allergen- and vaccine-specific immune responses. *Clin Exp Allergy.* 2006 Oct;36(10):1227-35.

Taylor RB, Lindquist N, Kubanek J, Hay ME. Intraspecific variation in palatability and defensive chemistry of brown seaweeds: effects on herbivore fitness. *Oecologia.* 2003 Aug;136(3):412-23.

REFERENCES AND BIBLIOGRAPHY

Taylor SL, Moneret-Vautrin DA, Crevel RW, Sheffield D, Morisset M, Dumont P, Remington BC, Baumert JL. Threshold dose for peanut: Risk characterization based upon diagnostic oral challenge of a series of 286 peanut-allergic individuals. *Food Chem Toxicol.* 2010 Mar;48(3):814-9.

Teitelbaum J. *From Fatigue to Fantastic.* New York: Avery, 2001.

Terheggen-Lagro SW, Khouw IM, Schaafsma A, Wauters EA. Safety of a new extensively hydrolysed formula in children with cow's milk protein allergy: a double blind crossover study. *BMC Pediatr.* 2002 Oct 14;2:10.

Terracciano L, Bouygue GR, Sarratud T, Veglia F, Martelli A, Fiocchi A. Impact of dietary regimen on the duration of cow's milk allergy: a random allocation study. *Clin Exp Allergy.* 2010 Apr;40(4):637-42.

Tham KW, Zuraimi MS, Koh D, Chew FT, Ooi PL. Associations between home dampness and presence of molds with asthma and allergic symptoms among young children in the tropics. *Pediatr Allergy Immunol.* 2007 Aug;18(5):418-24.

Thampithak A, Jaisin Y, Meesarapee B, Chongthammakun S, Piyachaturawat P, Govitrapong P, Supavilai P, Sanvarinda Y. Transcriptional regulation of iNOS and COX-2 by a novel compound from Curcuma comosa in lipopolysaccharide-induced microglial activation. *Neurosci Lett.* 2009 Sep 22;462(2):171-5.

Theler B, Brockow K, Ballmer-Weber BK. Clinical presentation and diagnosis of meat allergy in Switzerland and Southern Germany. *Swiss Med Wkly.* 2009 May 2;139(17-18):264-70.

Theofilopoulos AN, Kono DH: The genes of systemic autoimmunity. *Proc Assoc Am Physicians.* 1999;111(3): 228-240.

Thomas, R.G., Gebhardt, S.E. 2008. Nutritive value of pomegranate fruit and juice. *Maryland Dietetic Association Annual Meeting, USDA-ARS.* 2008 April 11.

Thompson RL, Miles LM, Lunn J, Devereux G, Dearman RJ, Strid J, Buttriss JL. Peanut sensitisation and allergy: influence of early life exposure to peanuts. *Br J Nutr.* 2010 May;103(9):1278-86.

Thompson T, Lee AR, Grace T. Gluten contamination of grains, seeds, and flours in the United States: a pilot study. *J Am Diet Assoc.* 2010 Jun;110(6):937-40.

Tierra L. *The Herbs of Life.* Freedom, CA: Crossing Press, 1992.

Tierra M. *The Way of Herbs.* New York: Pocket Books, 1990.

Tisserand R. *The Art of Aromatherapy.* New York: Inner Traditions, 1979.

Tiwari M. *Ayurveda: A Life of Balance.* Rochester, VT: Healing Arts, 1995.

Tlaskalová-Hogenová H, Stepánková R, Hudcovic T, Tucková L, Cukrowska B, Lodinová-Zádníková R, Kozáková H, Rossmann P, Bártová J, Sokol D, Funda DP, Borovská D, Reháková Z, Sinkora J, Hofman J, Drastich P, Kokesová A. Commensal bacteria (normal microflora), mucosal immunity and chronic inflammatory and autoimmune diseases. *Immunol Lett.* 2004 May 15;93(2-3):97-108.

Todd GR, Acerini CL, Ross-Russell R, Zahra S, Warner JT, McCance D. Survey of adrenal crisis associated with inhaled corticosteroids in the United Kingdom. *Arch Dis Child.* 2002 Dec;87(6):457-61.

Tomicić S, Norrman G, Fälth-Magnusson K, Jenmalm MC, Devenney I, Böttcher MF. High levels of IgG4 antibodies to foods during infancy are associated with tolerance to corresponding foods later in life. *Pediatr Allergy Immunol.* 2009 Feb;20(1):35-41.

Tonkal AM, Morsy TA. An update review on Commiphora molmol and related species. *J Egypt Soc Parasitol.* 2008 Dec;38(3):763-96.

Topçu G, Erenler R, Cakmak O, Johansson CB, Celik C, Chai HB, Pezzuto JM. Diterpenes from the berries of Juniperus excelsa. *Phytochemistry.* 1999 Apr;50(7):1195-9.

Tordesillas L, Pacios LF, Palacín A, Cuesta-Herranz J, Madero M, Díaz-Perales A. Characterization of IgE epitopes of Cuc m 2, the major melon allergen, and their role in cross-reactivity with pollen profilins. *Clin Exp Allergy.* 2010 Jan;40(1):174-81.

Towers GH. FAHF-1 purporting to block peanut-induced anaphylaxis. *J Allergy Clin Immunol.* 2003 May;111(5):1140; author reply 1140-1.

Towle A. *Modern Biology.* Austin: Harcourt Brace, 1993.

Trojanová I, Rada V, Kokoska L, Vlková E. The bifidogenic effect of Taraxacum officinale root. *Fitoterapia.* 2004 Dec;75(7-8):760-3.

Troncone R, Caputo N, Florio G, Finelli E. Increased intestinal sugar permeability after challenge in children with cow's milk allergy or intolerance. *Allergy.* 1994 Mar;49(3):142-6.

Truswell AS. The A2 milk case: a critical review. *Euro J Clin Nutr.* 2005:59;623–631.

Tsai JC, Tsai S, Chang WC. Comparison of two Chinese medical herbs, Huangbai and Qianniuzi, on influence of short circuit current across the rat intestinal epithelia. *J Ethnopharmacol.* 2004 Jul;93(1):21-5.

Tsong T. Deciphering the language of cells. *Trends in Biochem Sci.* 1989;14:89-92.

Tsuchiya J, Barreto R, Okura R, Kawakita S, Fesce E, Marotta F. Single-blind follow-up study on the effectiveness of a symbiotic preparation in irritable bowel syndrome. *Chin J Dig Dis.* 2004;5(4):169-74.

Tulk HM, Robinson LE. Modifying the n-6/n-3 polyunsaturated fatty acid ratio of a high-saturated fat challenge does not acutely attenuate postprandial changes in inflammatory markers in men with metabolic syndrome. *Metabolism.* 2009 Jul 20.

Tursi A, Brandimarte G, Giorgetti GM, Elisei W. Mesalazine and/or Lactobacillus casei in maintaining long-term remission of symptomatic uncomplicated diverticular disease of the colon. *Hepatogastroenterology.* 2008 May-Jun;55(84):916-20.

U.S. Food and Drug Administration CfDEaR. *Guidance for Industry Botanical Drug Products.* 2000

Ueno H, Yoshioka K, Matsumoto T. Usefulness of the skin index in predicting the outcome of oral challenges in children. *J Investig Allergol Clin Immunol.* 2007;17(4):207-10.

Ueno M, Adachi A, Fukumoto T, Nishitani N, Fujiwara N, Matsuo H, Kohno K, Morita E. Analysis of causative allergen of the patient with baker's asthma and wheat-dependent exercise-induced anaphylaxis (WDEIA). *Arerugi.* 2010 May;59(5):552-7.

Ukabam SO, Mann RJ, Cooper BT. Small intestinal permeability to sugars in patients with atopic eczema. *Br J Dermatol.* 1984 Jun;110(6):649-52.

Unsel M, Ardeniz O, Mete N, Ersoy R, Sin AZ, Gulbahar O, Kokuludag A. Food allergy due to olive. J Investig Allergol Clin Immunol. 2009;19(6):497-9. García BE, Gamboa PM, Asturias JA, López-Hoyos M, Sanz ML, Caballero MT, García JM, Labrador M, Lahoz C, Longo Areso N, Martínez Quesada J, Mayorga L, Monteseirín FJ; Clinical Immunology Committee; Spanish Society of Allergology and Clinical Immunology. Guidelines on the clinical usefulness of determination of specific immunoglobulin E to foods. *J Investig Allergol Clin Immunol.* 2009;19(6):423-32.

Unsel M, Sin AZ, Ardeniz O, Erdem N, Ersoy R, Gulbahar O, Mete N, Kokuludağ A. New onset egg allergy in an adult. *J Investig Allergol Clin Immunol.* 2007;17(1):55-8.

Untersmayr E, Vestergaard H, Malling HJ, Jensen LB, Platzer MH, Boltz-Nitulescu G, Scheiner O, Skov PS, Jensen-Jarolim E, Poulsen LK. Incomplete digestion of codfish represents a risk factor for anaphylaxis in patients with allergy. *J Allergy Clin Immunol.* 2007 Mar;119(3):711-7.

Upadhyay AK, Kumar K, Kumar A, Mishra HS. Tinospora cordifolia (Willd.) Hook. f. and Thoms. (Guduchi) - validation of the Ayurvedic pharmacology through experimental and clinical studies. *Int J Ayurveda Res.* 2010 Apr;1(2):112-21.

Vally H, Thompson PJ, Misso NL. Changes in bronchial hyperresponsiveness following high- and low-sulphite wine challenges in wine-sensitive asthmatic patients. *Clin Exp Allergy.* 2007 Jul;37(7):1062-6.

van Beelen VA, Roeleveld J, Mooibroek H, Sijtsma L, Bino RJ, Bosch D, Rietjens IM, Alink GM. A comparative study on the effect of algal and fish oil on viability and cell proliferation of Caco-2 cells. *Food Chem Toxicol.* 2007 May;45(5):716-24.

van Elburg RM, Uil JJ, de Monchy JG, Heymans HS. Intestinal permeability in pediatric gastroenterology. *Scand J Gastroenterol Suppl.* 1992;194:19-24.

van Kampen V, Merget R, Rabstein S, Sander I, Bruening T, Broding HC, Keller C, Muesken H, Overlack A, Schultze-Werninghaus G, Walusiak J, Raulf-Heimsoth M. Comparison of wheat and rye flour solutions for skin prick testing: a multi-centre study (Stad 1). *Clin Exp Allergy.* 2009 Dec;39(12):1896-902.

van Odijk J, Peterson CG, Ahlstedt S, Bengtsson U, Borres MP, Hulthén L, Magnusson J, Hansson T. Measurements of eosinophil activation before and after food challenges in adults with food hypersensitivity. *Int Arch Allergy Immunol.* 2006;140(4):334-41.

Vanderhoof JA. Probiotics in allergy management. *J Pediatr Gastroenterol Nutr.* 2008 Nov;47 Suppl 2:S38-40.

Vanto T, Helppilä S, Juntunen-Backman K, Kalimo K, Klemola T, Korpela R, Koskinen P. Prediction of the development of tolerance to milk in children with cow's milk hypersensitivity. *J Pediatr.* 2004 Feb;144(2):218-22.

Vassallo MF, Banerji A, Rudders SA, Clark S, Mullins RJ, Camargo CA Jr. Season of birth and food allergy in children. *Ann Allergy Asthma Immunol.* 2010 Apr;104(4):307-13.

Vendt N, Grünberg H, Tuure T, Malminiemi O, Wuolijoki E, Tillmann V, Sepp E, Korpela R. Growth during the first 6 months of life in infants using formula enriched with Lactobacillus rhamnosus GG: double-blind, randomized trial. *J Hum Nutr Diet.* 2006 Feb;19(1):51-8.

Venkatachalam KV. Human 3'-phosphoadenosine 5'-phosphosulfate (PAPS) synthase: biochemistry, molecular biology and genetic deficiency. *IUBMB Life.* 2003 Jan;55(1):1-11.

Venter C, Hasan Arshad S, Grundy J, Pereira B, Bernie Clayton C, Voigt K, Higgins B, Dean T. Time trends in the prevalence of peanut allergy: three cohorts of children from the same geographical location in the UK. *Allergy.* 2010 Jan;65(1):103-8.

Venter C, Meyer R. Session 1: Allergic disease: The challenges of managing food hypersensitivity. *Proc Nutr Soc.* 2010 Feb;69(1):11-24.

Venter C, Pereira B, Grundy J, Clayton CB, Arshad SH, Dean T (2006a) Prevalence of sensitization reported and objectively assessed food hypersensitivity amongst six-year-old children: A population-based study. *Pediatr Allergy Immunol.* 17: 356–363.

Venter C, Pereira B, Grundy J, Clayton CB, Roberts G, Higgins B, Dean T (2006b) Incidence of parentally reported and clinically diagnosed food hypersensitivity in the first year of life. *J Allergy Clin Immunol.* 117: 1118–1124.

Ventura MT, Polimeno L, Amoruso AC, Gatti F, Annoscia E, Marinaro M, Di Leo E, Matino MG, Buquicchio R, Bonini S, Tursi A, Francavilla A. Intestinal permeability in patients with adverse reactions to food. *Dig Liver Dis.* 2006 Oct;38(10):732-6.

Venturi A, Gionchetti P, Rizzello F, Johansson R, Zucconi E, Brigidi P, Matteuzzi D, Campieri M. Impact on the composition of the faecal flora by a new probiotic preparation: preliminary data on maintenance treatment of patients with ulcerative colitis. *Aliment Pharmacol Ther.* 1999 Aug;13(8):1103-8.

Verhasselt V. Oral tolerance in neonates: from basics to potential prevention of allergic disease. *Mucosal Immunol.* 2010 Jul;3(4):326-33.

Verstege A, Mehl A, Rolinck-Werninghaus C, Staden U, Nocon M, Beyer K, Niggemann B. The predictive value of the skin prick test weal size for the outcome of oral food challenges. Clin Exp Allergy. 2005 Sep;35(9):1220-6. Rolinck-Werninghaus C, Staden U, Mehl A, Hamelmann E, Beyer K, Niggemann B. Specific oral tolerance induction with food in children: transient or persistent effect on food allergy? *Allergy.* 2005 Oct;60(10):1320-2.

Vidgren HM, Agren JJ, Schwab U, Rissanen T, Hanninen O, Uusitupa MI. Incorporation of n-3 fatty acids into plasma lipid fractions, and erythrocyte membranes and platelets during dietary supplementation with fish, fish oil, and docosahexaenoic acid-rich oil among healthy young men. *Lipids.* 1997 Jul;32(7):697-705.

Vila R, Mundina M, Tomi F, Furlán R, Zacchino S, Casanova J, Cañigueral S. Composition and antifungal activity of the essential oil of Solidago chilensis. *Planta Med.* 2002 Feb;68(2):164-7.

Viljanen M, Kuitunen M, Haahtela T, Juntunen-Backman K, Korpela R, Savilahti E. Probiotic effects on faecal inflammatory markers and on faecal IgA in food allergic atopic eczema/dermatitis syndrome infants. *Pediatr Allergy Immunol.* 2005 Feb;16(1):65-71.

Viljanen M, Savilahti E, Haahtela T, Juntunen-Backman K, Korpela R, Poussa T, Tuure T, Kuitunen M. Probiotics in the treatment of atopic eczema/dermatitis syndrome in infants: a double-blind placebo-controlled trial. *Allergy.* 2005 Apr;60(4):494-500.

Vinson JA, Proch J, Bose P. MegaNatural((R)) Gold Grapeseed Extract: In Vitro Antioxidant and In Vivo Human Supplementation Studies. *J Med Food.* 2001 Spring;4(1):17-26.

Visness CM, London SJ, Daniels JL, Kaufman JS, Yeatts KB, Siega-Riz AM, Liu AH, Calatroni A, Zeldin DC. Association of obesity with IgE levels and allergy symptoms in children and adolescents: results from the National Health and Nutrition Examination Survey 2005-2006. *J Allergy Clin Immunol.* 2009 May;123(5):1163-9, 1169.e1-4.

Vlieg-Boerstra BJ, Dubois AE, van der Heide S, Bijleveld CM, Wolt-Plompen SA, Oude Elberink JN, Kukler J, Jansen DF, Venter C, Duiverman EJ. Ready-to-use introduction schedules for first exposure to allergenic foods in children at home. Allergy. 2008 Jul;63(7):903-9.

Vlieg-Boerstra BJ, van der Heide S, Bijleveld CM, Kukler J, Duiverman EJ, Dubois AE. Placebo reactions in double-blind, placebo-controlled food challenges in children. *Allergy.* 2007 Aug;62(8):905-12.

Vlieg-Boerstra BJ, van der Heide S, Bijleveld CM, Kukler J, Duiverman EJ, Wolt-Plompen SA, Dubois AE. Dietary assessment in children adhering to a food allergen avoidance diet for allergy prevention. *Eur J Clin Nutr.* 2006 Dec;60(12):1384-90.

Vojdani A. Antibodies as predictors of complex autoimmune diseases. *Int J Immunopathol Pharmacol.* 2008 Apr-Jun;21(2):267-78.

von Berg A, Filipiak-Pittroff B, Krämer U, Link E, Bollrath C, Brockow I, Koletzko S, Grübl A, Heinrich J, Wichmann HE, Bauer CP, Reinhardt D, Berdel D; GINIplus study group. Preventive effect of hydrolyzed infant formulas persists until age 6 years: long-term results from the German Infant Nutritional Intervention Study (GINI). *J Allergy Clin Immunol.* 2008 Jun;121(6):1442-7.

von Berg A, Koletzko S, Grübl A, Filipiak-Pittroff B, Wichmann HE, Bauer CP, Reinhardt D, Berdel D; German Infant Nutritional Intervention Study Group. The effect of hydrolyzed cow's milk formula for allergy prevention in the first year of life: the German Infant Nutritional Intervention Study, a randomized double-blind trial. J Allergy Clin Immunol. 2003 Mar;111(3):533-40.

von Kruedener S, Schneider W, Elstner EF. A combination of Populus tremula, Solidago virgaurea and Fraxinus excelsior as an anti-inflammatory and antirheumatic drug. A short review. *Arzneimittelforschung.* 1995 Feb;45(2):169-71.

Vulevic J, Drakoularakou A, Yaqoob P, Tzortzis G and Gibson GR; Modulation of the fecal microflora profile and immune function by a novel trans-galactooligosaccharide mixture (B-GOS) in healthy elderly volunteers. *Am J Clin Nutr.* 1988 88;1438-1446.

Waddell L. Food allergies in children: the difference between cow's milk protein allergy and food intolerance. *J Fam Health Care.* 2010;20(3):104.

Wahler D, Gronover CS, Richter C, Foucu F, Twyman RM, Moerschbacher BM, Fischer R, Muth J, Prufer D. Polyphenoloxidase silencing affects latex coagulation in Taraxacum spp. *Plant Physiol.* 2009 Jul 15.

Wahn U, Warner J, Simons FE, de Benedictis FM, Diepgen TL, Naspitz CK, de Longueville M, Bauchau V; EPAAC Study Group. IgE antibody responses in young children with atopic dermatitis. *Pediatr Allergy Immunol.* 2008 Jun;19(4):332-6.

Wainstein BK, Yee A, Jelley D, Ziegler M, Ziegler JB. Combining skin prick, immediate skin application and specific-IgE testing in the diagnosis of peanut allergy in children. Pediatr Allergy Immunol. 2007 May;18(3):231-9. Nolan RC, Richmond P, Prescott SL, Mallon DF, Gong G, Franzmann AM, Naidoo R, Loh RK. Skin prick testing predicts peanut challenge outcome in previously allergic or sensitized children with low serum peanut-specific IgE antibody concentration. *Pediatr Allergy Immunol.* 2007 May;18(3):224-30.

Walker S, Wing A. Allergies in children. *J Fam Health Care.* 2010;20(1):24-6.

Walker WA. Antigen absorption from the small intestine and gastrointestinal disease. *Pediatr Clin North Am.* 1975 Nov;22(4):731-46.

Walker WA. Antigen handling by the small intestine. *Clin Gastroenterol.* 1986 Jan;15(1):1-20.

Walle UK, Walle T. Transport of the cooked-food mutagen 2-amino-1-methyl-6-phenylimidazo- 4,5-b pyridine (PhIP) across the human intestinal Caco-2 cell monolayer: role of efflux pumps. *Carcinogenesis.* 1999 Nov;20(11):2153-7.

Walsh SJ, Rau LM. Autoimmune diseases: a leading cause of death among young and middle-aged women in the United States. *Am J Public Health* 2000, 90(9): 1463-1466.

Wan KS, Yang W, Wu WF. A survey of serum specific-IgE to common allergens in primary school children of Taipei City. *Asian Pac J Allergy Immunol.* 2010 Mar;28(1):1-6.

Wang J, Lin J, Bardina L, Goldis M, Nowak-Wegrzyn A, Shreffler WG, Sampson HA. Correlation of IgE/IgG4 milk epitopes and affinity of milk-specific IgE antibodies with different phenotypes of clinical milk allergy. *J Allergy Clin Immunol.* 2010 Mar;125(3):695-702, 702.e1-702.e6.

Wang J, Patil SP, Yang N, Ko J, Lee J, Noone S, Sampson HA, Li XM. Safety, tolerability, and immunologic effects of a food allergy herbal formula in food allergic individuals: a randomized, double-blinded, pla- cebo-controlled, dose escalation, phase 1 study. *Ann Allergy Asthma Immunol.* 2010 Jul;105(1):75-84.

Wang J. Management of the patient with multiple food allergies. *Curr Allergy Asthma Rep.* 2010 Jul;10(4):271-7.

Wang KY, Li SN, Liu CS, Perng DS, Su YC, Wu DC, Jan CM, Lai CH, Wang TN, Wang WM. Effects of ingesting Lactobacillus- and Bifidobacterium-containing yogurt in subjects with colonized Helicobacter pylori. *Am J Clin Nutr.* 2004 Sep;80(3):737-41.

Wang WS, Li EW, Jia ZJ. Terpenes from Juniperus przewalskii and their antitumor activities. *Pharmazie.* 2002 May;57(5):343-5.

Wang YM, Huan GX. *Utilization of Classical Formulas.* Beijing, China: Chinese Medicine and Pharmacology Publishing Co, 1998.

Waring G, Levy D. Challenging adverse reactions in children with food allergies. *Paediatr Nurs.* 2010 Jul;22(6):16-22.

Waser M, Michels KB, Bieli C, Flöistrup H, Pershagen G, von Mutius E, Ege M, Riedler J, Schram-Bijkerk D, Brunekreef B, van Hage M, Lauener R, Braun-Fahrländer C; PARSIFAL Study team. Inverse asso- ciation of farm milk consumption with asthma and allergy in rural and suburban populations across Europe. *Clin Exp Allergy.* 2007 May;37(5):661-70.

Watkins BA, Hannon K, Ferruzzi M, Li Y. Dietary PUFA and flavonoids as deterrents for environmental pollutants. *J Nutr Biochem.* 2007 Mar;18(3):196-205.

Watzl B, Bub A, Blockhaus M, Herbert BM, Lührmann PM, Neuhäuser-Berthold M, Rechkemmer G. Prolonged tomato juice consumption has no effect on cell-mediated immunity of well-nourished eld- erly men and women. *J Nutr.* 2000 Jul;130(7):1719-23.

Webber CM, England RW. Oral allergy syndrome: a clinical, diagnostic, and therapeutic challenge. *Ann Allergy Asthma Immunol.* 2010 Feb;104(2):101-8; quiz 109-10, 117.

Webster D, Taschereau P, Belland RJ, Sand C, Rennie RP. Antifungal activity of medicinal plant extracts; preliminary screening studies. *J Ethnopharmacol.* 2008 Jan 4;115(1):140-6.

Wedge DE, Tabanca N, Sampson BJ, Werle C, Demirci B, Baser KH, Nan P, Duan J, Liu Z. Antifungal and insecticidal activity of two Juniperus essential oils. *Nat Prod Commun.* 2009 Jan;4(1):123-7.

Wei A, Shibamoto T. Antioxidant activities and volatile constituents of various essential oils. *J Agric Food Chem.* 2007 Mar 7;55(5):1737-42.

Weiner MA. *Secrets of Fijian Medicine.* Berkeley, CA: Univ. of Calif., 1969.

Weiss RF. *Herbal Medicine.* Gothenburg, Sweden: Beaconsfield, 1988.

Wen MC, Huang CK, Srivastava KD, Zhang TF, Schofield B, Sampson HA, Li XM. Ku–Shen (Sophora flavescens Ait), a single Chinese herb, abrogates airway hyperreactivity in a murine model of asthma. *J Allergy Clin Immunol.* 2004;113:218.

Wen MC, Taper A, Srivastava KD, Huang CK, Schofield B, Li XM. Immunology of T cells by the Chinese Herbal Medicine Ling Zhi (Ganoderma lucidum) *J Allergy Clin Immunol.* 2003;111:S320.

Wen MC, Wei CH, Hu ZQ, Srivastava K, Ko J, Xi ST, Mu DZ, Du JB, Li GH, Wallenstein S, Sampson H, Kattan M, Li XM. Efficacy and tolerability of anti-asthma herbal medicine intervention in adult patients with moderate-severe allergic asthma. *J Allergy Clin Immunol.* 2005;116:517–24.

Wensing M, Penninks AH, Hefle SL, Akkerdaas JH, van Ree R, Koppelman SJ, Bruijnzeel-Koomen CA, Knulst AC. The range of minimum provoking doses in hazelnut-allergic patients as determined by double-blind, placebo-controlled food challenges. *Clin Exp Allergy.* 2002 Dec;32(12):1757-62.

Werbach M. *Nutritional Influences on Illness.* Tarzana, CA: Third Line Press, 1996.

West CE, Hammarström ML, Hernell O. Probiotics during weaning reduce the incidence of eczema. *Pediatr Allergy Immunol.* 2009 Aug;20(5):430-7.

West R. Risk of death in meat and non-meat eaters. *BMJ.* 1994 Oct 8;309(6959):955.

Westerholm-Ormio M, Vaarala O, Tiittanen M, Savilahti E. Infiltration of Foxp3- and Toll-like receptor-4-positive cells in the intestines of children with food allergy. *J Pediatr Gastroenterol Nutr.* 2010 Apr;50(4):367-76.

Wheeler JG, Shema SJ, Bogle ML, Shirrell MA, Burks AW, Pittler A, Helm RM. Immune and clinical impact of Lactobacillus acidophilus on asthma. *Ann Allergy Asthma Immunol.* 1997 Sep;79(3):229-33.

Whitfield KE, Wiggins SA, Belue R, Brandon DT. Genetic and environmental influences on forced expiratory volume in African Americans: the Carolina African-American Twin Study of Aging. *Ethn Dis.* 2004 Spring;14(2):206-11.

WHO. *Guidelines for Drinking-water Quality.* 2nd ed, vol. 2. Geneva: World Health Organization, 1996.

WHO. Health effects of the removal of substances occurring naturally in drinking water, with special reference to demineralized and desalinated water. Report on a working group (Brussels, 20-23 March 1978). *EURO Reports and Studies.* 1979;16.

WHO. How trace elements in water contribute to health. *WHO Chronicle.* 1978;32:382-385.

WHO. *INFOSAN Food Allergies. Information Note No. 3.* Geneva, Switzerland: World Health Organization, 2006.

Whorwell PJ, Altringer L, Morel J, Bond Y, Charbonneau D, O'Mahony L, Kiely B, Shanahan F, Quigley EM. Efficacy of an encapsulated probiotic Bifidobacterium infantis 35624 in women with irritable bowel syndrome. *Am J Gastroenterol.* 2006 Jul;101(7):1581-90.

Wildt S, Munck LK, Vinter-Jensen L, Hanse BF, Nordgaard-Lassen I, Christensen S, Avnstroem S, Rasmussen SN, Rumessen JJ. Probiotic treatment of collagenous colitis: a randomized, double-blind, placebo-controlled trial with Lactobacillus acidophilus and Bifidobacterium animalis subsp. *Lactis. Inflamm Bowel Dis.* 2006 May;12(5):395-401.

Willard T, Jones K. *Reishi Mushroom: Herb of Spiritual Potency and Medical Wonder.* Issaquah, Washington: Sylvan Press, 1990.

Willard T. *Edible and Medicinal Plants of the Rocky Mountains and Neighbouring Territories.* Calgary: 1992.

Willemsen LE, Koetsier MA, Balvers M, Beermann C, Stahl B, van Tol EA. Polyunsaturated fatty acids support epithelial barrier integrity and reduce IL-4 mediated permeability in vitro. *Eur J Nutr.* 2008 Jun;47(4):183-91.

Wilson D, Evans M, Guthrie N, Sharma P, Baisley J, Schonlau F, Burki C. A randomized, double-blind, placebo-controlled exploratory study to evaluate the potential of pycnogenol for improving allergic rhinitis symptoms. *Phytother Res.* 2010 Aug;24(8):1115-9.

Wilson K, McDowall L, Hodge D, Chetcuti P, Cartledge P. Cow's milk protein allergy. *Community Pract.* 2010 May;83(5):40-1.

Wilson L. *Nutritional Balancing and Hair Mineral Analysis.* Prescott, AZ: LD Wilson, 1998.

Winchester AM. *Biology and its Relation to Mankind.* New York: Van Nostrand Reinhold, 1969.

Wittenberg JS. *The Rebellious Body.* New York: Insight, 1996.

Wöhrl S, Hemmer W, Focke M, Rappersberger K, Jarisch R. Histamine intolerance-like symptoms in healthy volunteers after oral provocation with liquid histamine. *Allergy Asthma Proc.* 2004 Sep-Oct;25(5):305-11.

Wolvers DA, van Herpen-Broekmans WM, Logman MH, van der Wielen RP, Albers R. Effect of a mixture of micronutrients, but not of bovine colostrum concentrate, on immune function parameters in healthy volunteers: a randomized placebo-controlled study. *Nutr J.* 2006 Nov 21;5:28.

Wood M. *The Book of Herbal Wisdom.* Berkeley, CA: North Atlantic, 1997.

Wood RA, Kraynak J. *Food Allergies for Dummies.* Hoboken, NJ: Wiley Publ, 2007.

Woods RK, Abramson M, Bailey M, Walters EH (2001) International prevalences of reported food allergies and intolerances. Comparisons arising from the European Community Respiratory Health Survey (ECRHS) 1991–1994. *Eur J Clin Nutr* 55: 298–304.

Woods RK, Abramson M, Bailey M, Walters EH. International prevalences of reported food allergies and intolerances. Comparisons arising from the European Community Respiratory Health Survey (ECRHS) 1991-1994. *Eur J Clin Nutr.* 2001 Apr;55(4):298-304.

Woods RK, Abramson M, Raven JM, Bailey M, Weiner JM, Walters EH (1998) Reported food intolerance and respiratory symptoms in young adults. *Eur Respir J.* 11: 151–155.

Worm M, Hompes S, Fiedler EM, Illner AK, Zuberbier T, Vieths S. Impact of native, heat-processed and encapsulated hazelnuts on the allergic response in hazelnut-allergic patients. *Clin Exp Allergy.* 2009 Jan;39(1):159-66.

Xiao P, Kubo H, Ohsawa M, Higashiyama K, Nagase H, Yan YN, Li JS, Kamei J, Ohmiya S. kappa-Opioid receptor-mediated antinociceptive effects of stereoisomers and derivatives of (+)-matrine in mice. *Planta Med.* 1999 Apr;65(3):230-3.

Xu X, Zhang D, Zhang H, Wolters PJ, Killeen NP, Sullivan BM, Locksley RM, Lowell CA, Caughey GH. Neutrophil histamine contributes to inflammation in mycoplasma pneumonia. *J Exp Med.* 2006 Dec 25;203(13):2907-17.

Yadav VS, Mishra KP, Singh DP, Mehrotra S, Singh VK. Immunomodulatory effects of curcumin. *Immunopharmacol Immunotoxicol.* 2005;27(3):485-97.

Yadzir ZH, Misnan R, Abdullah N, Bakhtiar F, Arip M, Murad S. Identification of Ige-binding proteins of raw and cooked extracts of Loligo edulis (white squid). *Southeast Asian J Trop Med Public Health.* 2010 May;41(3):653-9.

Yang Z. Are peanut allergies a concern for using peanut-based formulated foods in developing countries? *Food Nutr Bull.* 2010 Jun;31(2 Suppl):S147-53.

Yarnell E. Botanical medicines for the urinary tract. *World J Urol.* 2002 Nov;20(5):285-93.

Yeager S. *The Doctor's Book of Food Remedies.* Emmaus, PA: Rodale Press, 1998.

Yu LC. The epithelial gatekeeper against food allergy. *Pediatr Neonatol.* 2009 Dec;50(6):247-54.

Yusoff NA, Hampton SM, Dickerson JW, Morgan JB. The effects of exclusion of dietary egg and milk in the management of asthmatic children: a pilot study. *J R Soc Promot Health.* 2004 Mar;124(2):74-80.

Zanjanian MH. The intestine in allergic diseases. *Ann Allergy.* 1976 Sep;37(3):208-18.

Zarkadas M, Scott FW, Salminen J, Ham Pong A. Common Allergenic Foods and Their Labelling in Canada. *Can J Allerg Clin Immun.* 1999; 4:118-141.

Zeiger RS, Heller S. The development and prediction of atopy in high-risk children: follow-up at age seven years in a prospective randomized study of combined maternal and infant food allergen avoidance. *J Allergy Clin Immunol.* 1995 Jun;95(6):1179-90.

Zhang J, Zhang X, Lei G, Li B, Chen J, Zhou T. A new phenolic glycoside from the aerial parts of Solidago canadensis. *Fitoterapia.* 2007 Jan;78(1):69-71.

Zheng M. Experimental study of 472 herbs with antiviral action against the herpes simplex virus. *Zhong Xi Yi Jie He Za Zhi.* 1990 Jan;10(1):39-41, 6.

Zhou Q, Zhang B, Verne GN. Intestinal membrane permeability and hypersensitivity in the irritable bowel syndrome. *Pain.* 2009 Nov;146(1-2):41-6.

Ziemniak W. Efficacy of Helicobacter pylori eradication taking into account its resistance to antibiotics. *J Physiol Pharmacol.* 2006 Sep;57 Suppl 3:123-41.

Zizza, C. The nutrient content of the Italian food supply 1961-1992. *Euro J Clin Nutr.* 1997;51: 259-265.

Zoccatelli G, Pokoj S, Foetisch K, Bartra J, Valero A, Del Mar San Miguel-Moncin M, Vieths S, Scheurer S. Identification and characterization of the major allergen of green bean (Phaseolus vulgaris) as a non-specific lipid transfer protein (Pha v 3). *Mol Immunol.* 2010 Apr;47(7-8):1561-8.

Zuidmeer L, Goldhahn K, Rona RJ, Gislason D, Madsen C, Summers C, Sodergren E, Dahlstrom J, Lindner T, Sigurdardottir ST, McBride D, Keil T. The prevalence of plant food allergies: a systematic review. *J Allergy Clin Immunol.* 2008 May;121(5):1210-1218.e4.

Zwolińska-Wcisło M, Brzozowski T, Mach T, Budak A, Trojanowska D, Konturek PC, Pajdo R, Drozdowicz D, Kwiecień S. Are probiotics effective in the treatment of fungal colonization of the gastrointestinal tract? Experimental and clinical studies. *J Physiol Pharmacol.* 2006 Nov;57 Suppl 9:35-49.

Index

(foods and herbs too numerous to index)

Made in the USA
Las Vegas, NV
17 March 2023

69227346R00198